Heart Valve Surgery

Jan Dominik • Pavel Zacek

Heart Valve Surgery

An Illustrated Guide

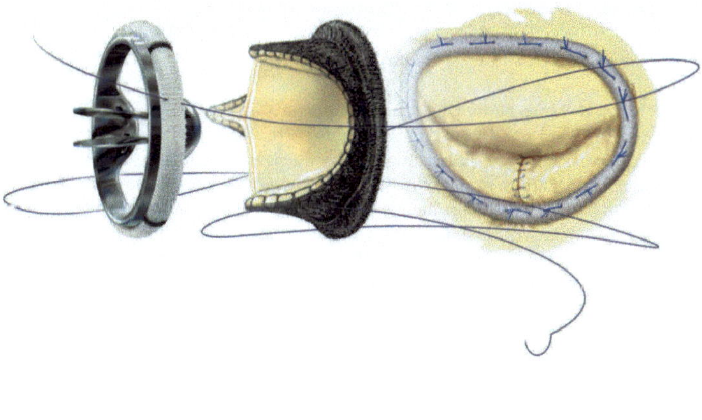

Springer

Dr. Jan Dominik
Dr. Pavel Zacek
Department of Cardiac Surgery
Charles University in Prague
Faculty of Medicine in Hradec Kralove
University Hospital Hradec Kralove
500 05 Hradec Kralove
Czech Republic
zacek@fnhk.cz

Originally published in 2008 by Grada Publishing, a.s. Czech Republic with the following title: "Chirurgie srdečních chlopní (...nejen pro kardiochirurgy)".

ISBN 978-3-642-12205-7 ISBN 978-3-642-12206-4 (eBook)
DOI 10.1007/978-3-642-12206-4
Springer Heidelberg Dordrecht London New York

Library of Congress Control Number: 2010928389

Cover design: eStudio Calamar, Figures/Berlin

Printed on acid-free paper

Springer is part of Springer Science+Business Media (www.springer.com)

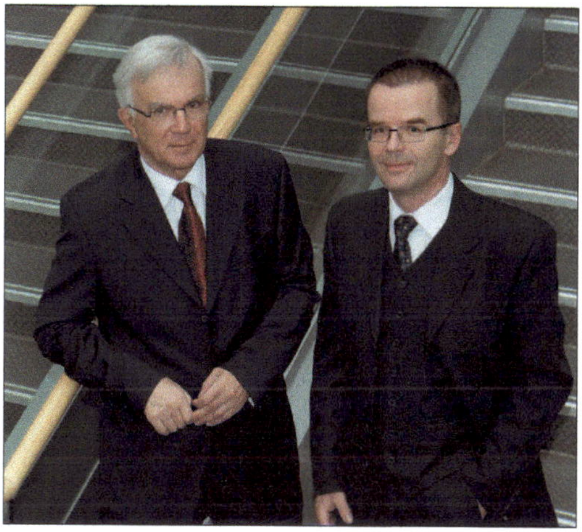

Preface

The four heart valves reside in the center of the heart. This indicates their crucial role in cardiac performance. Faultless function of the valves is a prerequisite for unidirectional forward movement of the blood, and such function is necessary to support the efforts of the cardiac atria and ventricles. Healthy heart valves function gracefully and offer mechanical durability. Bioengineers have to marvel at the biomechanical evolution of these perfectly placed valves.

Heart valves can be involved in pathological processes, however, and only then do we realize just how indispensable they really are. At one time, serious valve disorders used to be a matter of life and death for patients. Only in recent decades have surgeons been able to reverse the ominous course of heart valve disease and offer patients a quality of life and life span comparable to that of healthy persons. The story of this effort began approximately 100 years ago, and today heart valve surgery is a substantial subspecialty of cardiac surgery, with accumulated experience in indications, procedures, risks, and outcomes.

The aim of this book is to present a richly illustrated compendium of the present knowledge related to heart valve surgery, based on the clinical expertise of the authors as well as the newest treatment modalities.

The authors thank Dr. Alireeza Matloobi from the Mayo Clinic for his help in preparating the book.

March 2010

Jan Dominik
Pavel Zacek

Prof. Jan Dominik, MD, Ph.D., was born in 1944 and graduated from Masaryk University, Brno, in 1967. He practiced at the 1st Department of Surgery, University Hospital, Brno, from 1967 to 1977. From 1977 to 1990 he worked at the Center of Cardiovascular and Transplant Surgery in Brno. He was the Head of the Department of Cardiac Surgery, Charles University Hospital, Hradec Kralove, Czech Republic from 1991–2005 and the vice-dean of the Faculty of Medicine in Hradec Králové from 1997 to 2003.

Prof. Dominik has published more than 300 scientific papers. His specific field of interest is heart valve surgery. He is the author of the textbook "Kardiochirurgie" (Karolinum, Prague, 1997) and the monograph "Kardiochirurgie" (Grada Publishing, Prague, 1998), and a co-author of "Interactive Cardiac Surgery" (Springer, 2005). He is an Honorary Member of the Czech Society of Cardiology and a fellow of several international scientific societies.

Assoc. Prof. Pavel Zacek, MD, Ph.D., was born in 1959 and graduated from Charles University, Prague, in 1984. After a brief period of practice at a district surgery department he began his cardiosurgical career at the Department of Cardiac Surgery, Charles University Hospital, Hradec Kralove, Czech Republic, where he is presently a consultant cardiac surgeon for adult cardiac surgery. He also teaches medical students at the Faculty of Medicine in Hradec Kralove. He is the author and co-author of 107 papers and the main author of the multimedia electronic textbook "Interactive Cardiac Surgery" (Grada Prague 2003, Springer Heidelberg 2005).

Besides his medical profession, Pavel Zacek is also a devoted painter and he has illustrated several medical monographs. His artwork has been presented at many solo exhibitions (www.pavelzacek.cz).

Contents

History of Heart Valve Surgery

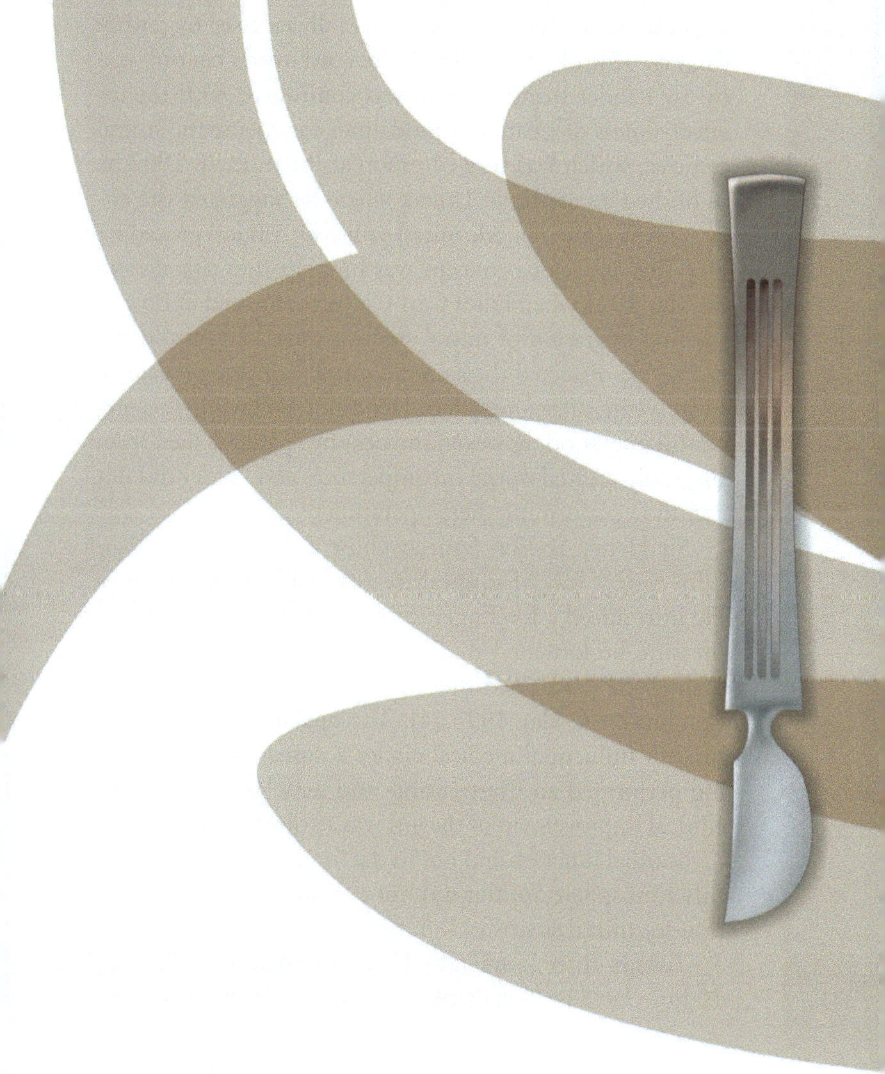

1 History of Heart Valve Surgery

Unfavorable prognosis of patients with severe and worsening heart valve disease can be successfully reversed by cardiac surgery. This idea was first put forward over a century ago by Sir Lauder Brunton, who was confronted with the ineffectiveness of treatment modalities for rheumatic mitral stenosis, which was very common at the time. In 1902 he published an article in Lancet where he suggested the enlargement of the stenotic mitral orifice by surgical procedure [1]. This audacious concept was brought into practice on 20 May 1923 when Elliot Carr Cutler performed in Boston the first operation of mitral stenosis on a 12-year-old girl [2, 3]. He dissected the stenotic mitral orifice by means of a transventriculary-introduced tenotom. Following this successful operation, however, the next five patients died from surgically created mitral incompetence, and Cutler did not continue performing these operations.

Sir Henry Session Souttar chose a different and logically correct way of surgical treatment for mitral stenosis. He introduced a forefinger into the left atrium, and by its pressure he loosened the fused commissures and in this manner he performed the first digital commissurolysis in London on 6 May 1925 [4]. The operation was successful, but influential medical circles accused Souttar of having performed an irresponsible and senseless surgery. The clinical improvement of the girl was attributed to improved myocardial function and not to the surgical intervention. In this atmosphere Souttar did not perform any other operation for mitral stenosis [3, 5, 6].

Twenty-three years later, Charles Philamore Bailey, on 10 June 1948 in Philadelphia, and Dwight Emary Harken,

J. Dominik and P. Zacek, *Heart Valve Surgery: An Illustrated Guide*,
DOI 10.1007/978-3-642-12206-4_1,

on 16 June 1948 in Boston, performed independently the first successful mitral commissurolyses (preceded by several unsuccessful attempts since 1945) [5–9]. In Europe Russell Claude Baron Brock of Wimbledon performed his first successful mitral commissurolysis on 16 September 1948 in London [10, 11].

The first successful pulmonary valvulotomy for pulmonary valve stenosis was performed by Thomas Holmes Sellors on 4 December 1947 in London by means of a tenotom introduced through the right ventricle [12].

A landmark procedure, not only in heart valve surgery but in cardiac surgery in general, occurred in Philadelphia on 6 May 1953 when John Heysham Gibbon successfully performed cardiopulmonary bypass for open-heart closure of the atrial septal defect [13].

The possibility to operate using cardiopulmonary bypass inside the heart chambers enabled performance, under direct visual control, of not only open mitral commissurotomies but also valve repairs and later valve replacement.

The 1960 is the year of the first artificial valves implantations. Nina Braunwald and Andrew Morrow in Bethesda implanted a polyurethane heart valve of their own design into the mitral orifice on 10 March and the other one on 11 March 1960 [3]. In regards to only short survival of their patients literature attributes the priority to Albert Starr from Portland who implanted a ball cage valve into the mitral position on 21 September 1960 followed by a long-term survival of the patient [3, 14].

The first aortic valve replacement into the subcoronary position was performed by Dwight Harken in Boston on 10 March 1960 [15]. Almost eight years before that, Charles Hufnagel (Washington) had treated the patients with aortic regurgitation by implantation of a ball valve into the descending aorta (first performed on 11 September 1952) [3, 16].

Robert Cartwright (Pittsburg) carried out the first combined aortic and mitral valve replacement on 1 November 1961 and Albert Starr the first simultaneous aortic, mitral, and tricuspid valve replacement on 21 February 1963 [3].

Soon after the first mechanical heart valve implantations, the era of biological valves in human cardiac surgery was launched. Donald Nixon Ross (London) performed the first subcoronary implantation of the aortic allograft on 24 July 1962 [17]. Two months later, he was followed by the second pioneer of allograft surgery, Sir Brian Gerald Barratt-Boyes (Auckland, New Zealand) [18].

The pioneering work of Alain Frederick Carpentier on the research and development of the porcine aortic valve xenograft resulted in the first human implantation into the aortic position in Paris in 1965 (together with Jean-Paul Binet) [3, 19, 20]. In 1967 Carpentier (together with Charles Dubost) implanted a stented xenograft into the mitral position. Also in 1967 Donald Ross used for the first time the patient's pulmonary valve as an autograft for aortic valve replacement and reconstructed the pulmonary outflow tract with an allograft [21, 22].

In 1968 Hugh Bentall and Anthony DeBono reported the surgical treatment of the annulo-aortic ectasia. They replaced the aortic valve with a mechanical Starr–Edwards valve mounted on a Teflon (DuPont, Wilmington, Del.) vascular graft. The coronary ostia were anastomosed to the graft, which then replaced the ascending aorta (inclusion technique) [23].

The expansion of reconstructive mitral valve surgery owes much to Alain Carpentier (Paris) who, since the 1980s, has been the leading promoter of valve-sparing procedures on the mitral valve [24]. Aortic valve-sparing surgery in patients with aortic incompetence has, contrary to this, attracted the growing interest of cardiac surgeons only in the past decade. The contributions of Sir Magdi Yacoub (London) and Tirone David (Toronto) in this field are fundamental. Techniques of aortic valve reconstruction surgery have been adopted at the majority of cardiac surgery units, and current progress has been influenced primarily by Hans Joachim Schäfers (Homburg) and Gebrine El Khoury (Brussels).

At the present authors' institution (Charles University Hospital in Hradec Králové) heart valve surgery has a long tradition: Jan Bedrna performed the first mitral and pulmonary commissurotomies there in 1951. At the same institution, Jaroslav Procházka in 1958 performed the first cardiac surgery with use of cardiopulmonary bypass and in 1966 the first aortic and mitral valve replacements.

References

1. Brunton L (1902) Treating mitral stenosis by surgical methods. Lancet 1:352
2. Cutler EC, Levine SA (1923) Cardiotomy and valvulotomy for mitral stenosis. Boston Med Surg J 188:1023
3. Westaby S (1997) Development of surgery for valvular heart disease. In: Westaby S (ed) Landmarks in cardiac surgery. ISIS Medical Media, Oxford
4. Souttar HS (1925) Surgical treatment of mitral stenosis. Br Med J 2:603–606
5. Gonzalez-Lavin L (1992) Charles P. Bailey and Dwight E. Harken: the dawn of the modern era of mitral valve surgery. Ann Thorac Surg 53:916–919

6. Litwak RS (1971) The growth of cardiac surgery: historical notes. Cardiovasc Clin 3:5–50
7. Bailey CP (1949) The surgical treatment of mitral stenosis (mitral commissurotomy). Dis Chest 15:377–397
8. Davila JC (1998) The birth of intracardiac surgery: a semicentennial tribute (June 10, 1948–1998). Ann Thorac Surg 65:1809–1820
9. Harken DE, Ellis LB et al. (1948) The surgical treatment of mitral stenosis; valvuloplasty. N Engl J Med 239:801–809
10. Baker C, Brock RC, Campbell M (1950) Valvulotomy for mitral stenosis; report of six successful cases. Br Med J 1:1283–1293
11. Naef AP (2004) The mid-century revolution in thoracic and cardiovascular surgery: part 5. Interact Cardiovasc Thorac Surg 3:415–422
12. Sellors TH (1948) Surgery of pulmonary stenosis; a case in which the pulmonary valve was successfully divided. Lancet 1:988
13. Gibbon JH Jr (1954) Application of a mechanical heart and lung apparatus to cardiac surgery. Minn Med 37:171–185; passim
14. Starr A, Edwards ML (1961) Mitral replacement: clinical experience with a ball-valve prosthesis. Ann Surg 154:726–740
15. Harken DE, Soroff HS, Taylor WJ et al. (1960) Partial and complete prostheses in aortic insufficiency. J Thorac Cardiovasc Surg 40:744–762
16. Hufnagel CA, Harvey WP (1953) The surgical correction of aortic regurgitation: preliminary report. Bull Georgetown Univ Med Cent 6:60–61
17. Ross DN (1962) Homograft replacement of the aortic valve. Lancet 2:487
18. Barratt-Boyes BG (1964) Homograft aortic valve replacement in aortic incompetence and stenosis. Thorax 19:131–150
19. Binet JP, Duran CG, Carpenter A et al. (1965) Heterologous aortic valve transplantation. Lancet 2:1275
20. Carpentier A, Dubost C, Lane E et al. (1982) Continuing improvements in valvular bioprostheses. J Thorac Cardiovasc Surg 83:27–42

21. Murtra M (2002) The adventure of cardiac surgery. Eur J Cardiothorac Surg 21:167–180
22. Ross DN (1967) Replacement of aortic and mitral valves with a pulmonary autograft. Lancet 2:956–958
23. Bentall H, Bono A de (1968) A technique for complete replacement of the ascending aorta. Thorax 23:338–339
24. Carpentier A (1983) Cardiac valve surgery: the "French correction." J Thorac Cardiovasc Surg 86:323–337

Surgical Anatomy of the Heart Valves

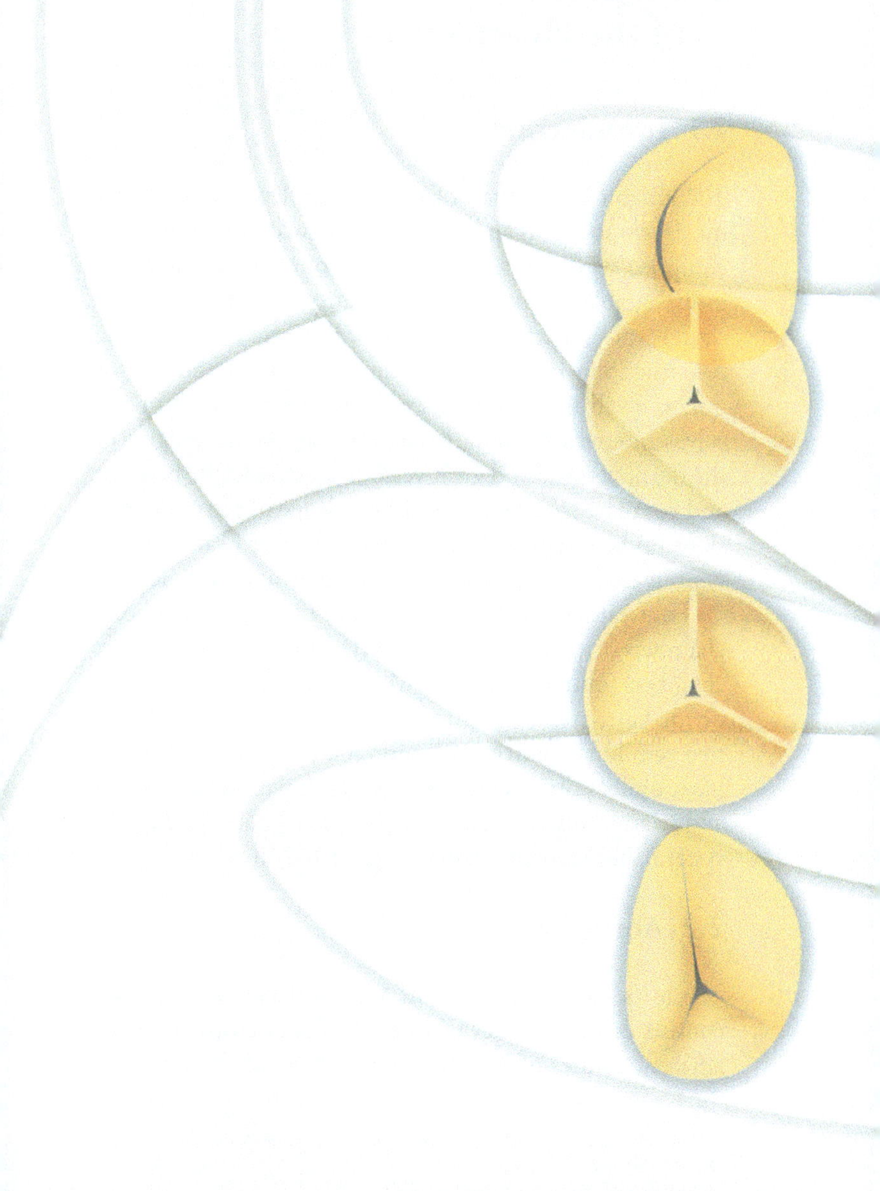

2 Surgical Anatomy of the Heart Valves

2.1 Introduction

The human heart, after a faultless completion of embryonic development, is an exquisitely designed pumping organ equipped with two working units. Four cardiac valves are indispensable components of this entity. Morphology of the cardiac valves merits admiration for its integration of subtle construction with perfect functionality and durability. Not only the valve architecture itself, but also the space-saving valves' interrelation in the heart center, and spiral wedging of the outflow tracts and great vessels, is a technically brilliant and compact solution. Perfect knowledge of the close relationship between the heart valves and other heart components is essential for both cardiac surgeons and cardiologists.

Four cardiac valves are situated in the right-sided heart chambers (tricuspid and pulmonary) and the left-sided heart chambers (mitral and aortic). Morphologically the valves are divided into two atrioventricular (mitral and tricuspid) and two semilunar (aortic and pulmonary) valves. The valves have, under normal circumstances, their typical localization and relationship to the central fibrous skeleton, conduction system, and coronary vessels (Figs. 2.1, 2.2).

2.2 Aortic Valve

The aortic valve situated in the left ventricular outflow tract consists of the complex of three semilunar cusps and their adjacent sinuses of Valsalva. Terminology of the sinuses is

J. Dominik and P. Zacek, *Heart Valve Surgery: An Illustrated Guide*,
DOI 10.1007/978-3-642-12206-4_2,

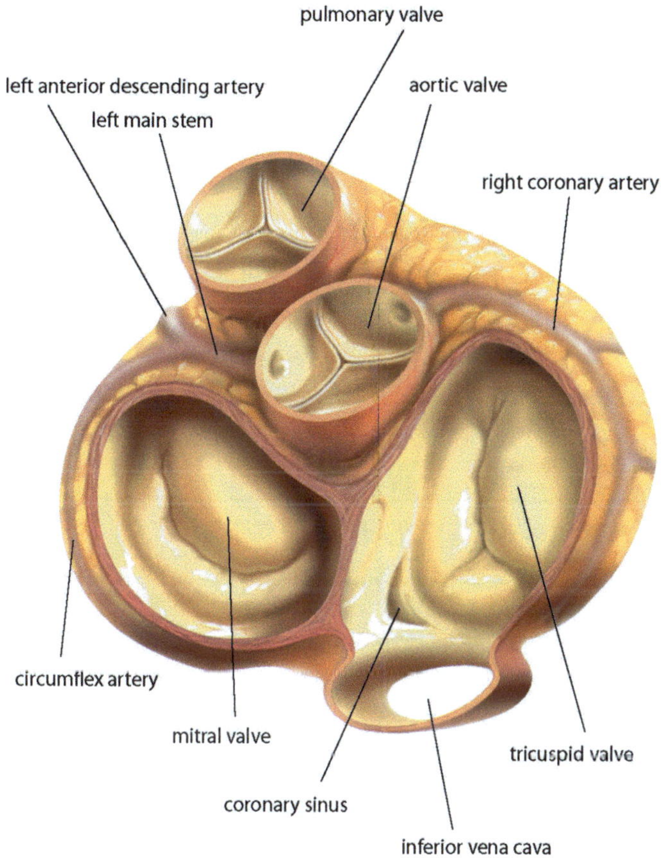

Fig. 2.1 Topographic interrelations of the heart valves

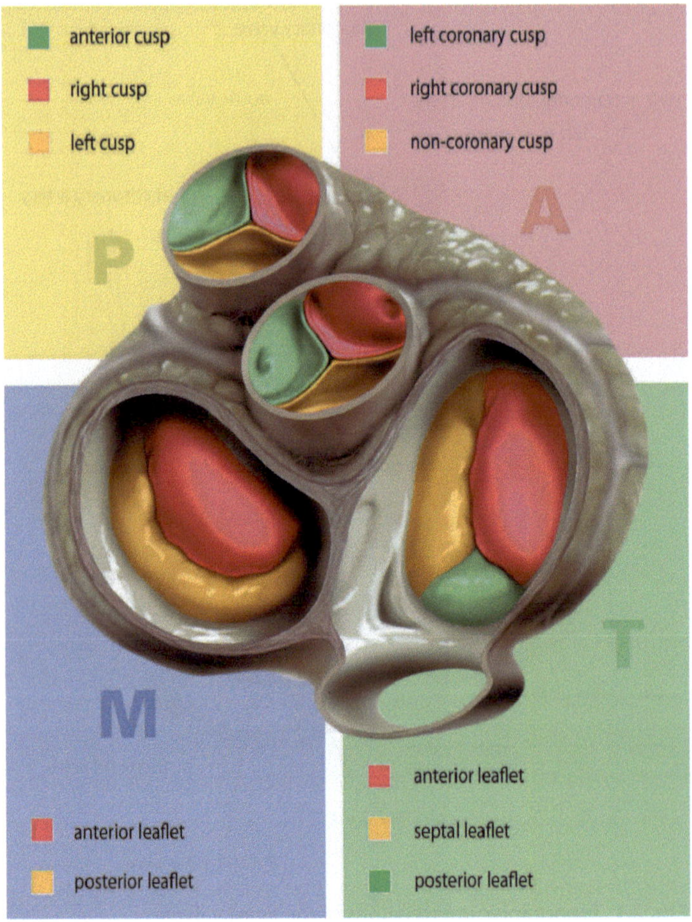

Fig. 2.2 Terminology of the valve cusps and leaflets. *P* pulmonary, *A* aortic, *M* mitral, *T* tricuspid

derived from the respective arising coronary arteries, i.e., left, right, and non-coronary (Figs. 2.3, 2.4). The aortic cusps coapt against each other in the center of the aortic orifice during diastole. The cusps display a mild thickening at the midpoint of its edge (nodulus Arantii), whereas near the commissure they are thinner or even contain small fenestrations.

The aortic valve does not have an anatomically defined annulus. The line of cusp insertion is crown-shaped with the highest points at the connection of the cusps (commissures) and the lowest points (nadir) in the middle between them (Fig. 2.5). The zone between the aortic root with bulging sinuses of Valsalva and the straight tubular ascending aorta is called the sinotubular junction. Aortic diameters at the level of aortic valve insertion ("annulus," ventriculoarterial junction) are important dimensions that characterize normal aortic root geometry and its pathological anomalies.

The aortic valve is located in the center of the heart close to other cardiac cavities. The non-coronary and left coronary cusps are directly connected to both fibrous trigones of the heart skeleton and in this way also to the anterior mitral leaflet. The triangular area below the right/non-coronary cusp commissure adjoins to the atrioventricular septum and the course of the bundle of His [1–4].

2.3 Mitral Valve

The mitral valve is a bileaflet atrioventricular valve between the left atrium and the left ventricle. The valve itself consists of the larger anterior (aortic, septal) leaflet and smaller posterior (mural, ventricular) leaflet (Figs. 2.6, 2.7). Clinical terminology divides both leaflets into respective thirds that are differentiated by small indentations (namely

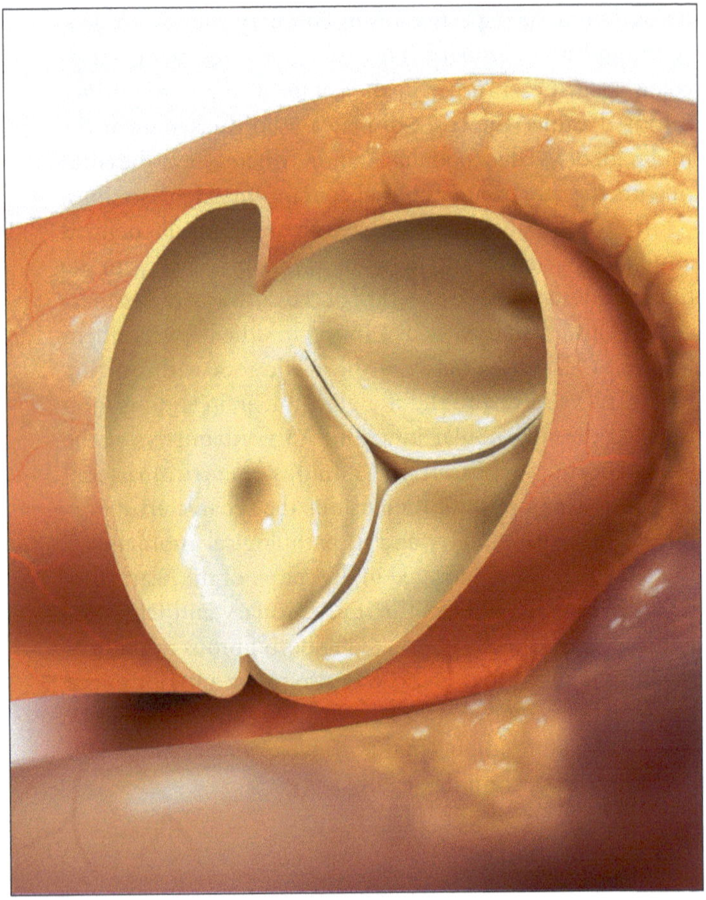

Fig. 2.3 Aortic valve viewed from transverse aortotomy

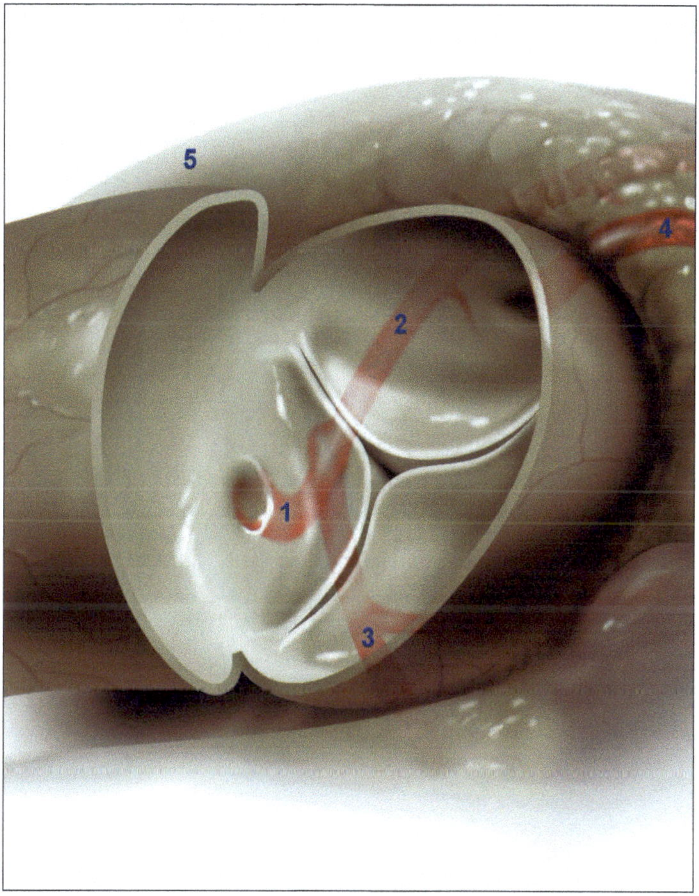

Fig. 2.4 Relation of the aortic valve to the coronary ostia. *1* Left main stem, *2* left anterior descending artery, *3* circumflex artery, *4* right coronary artery, *5* pulmonary artery trunk

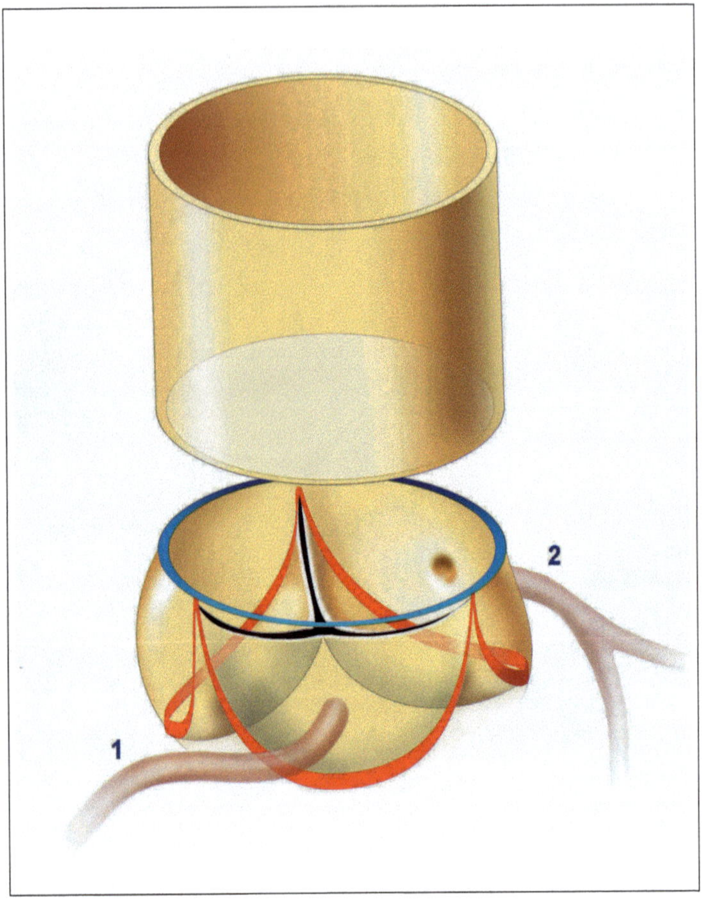

Fig. 2.5 Aortic root. *Red curve* attachment of aortic cusps, *blue curve* sinotubular junction, *1* right coronary artery, *2* left coronary artery

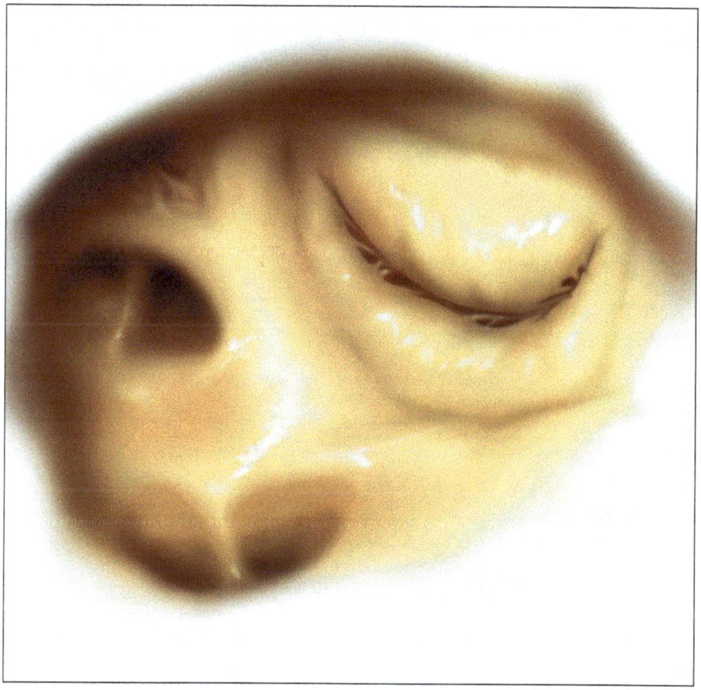

Fig. 2.6 Mitral valve viewed from the left atrium

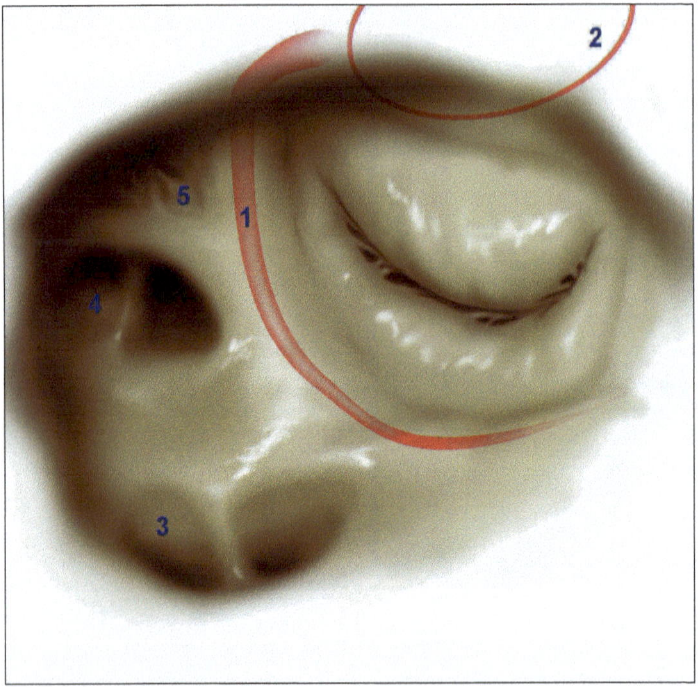

Fig. 2.7 Topographic interrelations of the mitral valve. *1* Circumflex artery, *2* aortic valve, *3* ostia of right-sided pulmonary veins, *4* ostia of left-sided pulmonary veins, *5* left atrial appendage

the posterior leaflet; Fig. 2.8). Both leaflets join together in the commissural areas. A sufficiently large zone of coaptation is necessary for proper competence of the valve.

Normal function of the valve depends not only on the morphology of the leaflets but also on the other components: the mitral annulus; the chordae; the papillary muscles; and the left ventricular geometry. Both mitral leaflets are connected by numerous chordae to both papillary muscles (anterolateral and posteromedial). The chordae of the first order are attached at the free margin of the leaflet, whereas the second-order chordae insert into the ventricular surface of the leaflet a short distance from the free edge. The chordae originating from the basal portion of the posterior leaflet are anchored directly to the left ventricular trabeculae (third-order chordae). The portion of the mitral annulus corresponding with the base of the anterior mitral leaflet is fixated within the fibrous heart skeleton and thus directly connects to the aortic valve (aortico-mitral continuity; Figs. 2.9, 2.10). The closely adjacent course of the circumflex artery is also of clinical relevance [1–3].

2.4 Tricuspid Valve

The tricuspid valve is between the right atrium and the right ventricle (Fig. 2.11). It consists of the anterior, posterior, and septal leaflets. The anterior leaflet is the largest leaflet, with eventual indentations. It is connected by the chordae to the medial and anterior papillary muscle. The posterior leaflet is the smallest leaflet and is connected to the anterior and posterior papillary muscles. The septal leaflet is slightly larger and its chordae are anchored to the posterior and septal papillary muscles. Close to the septal leaflet and the

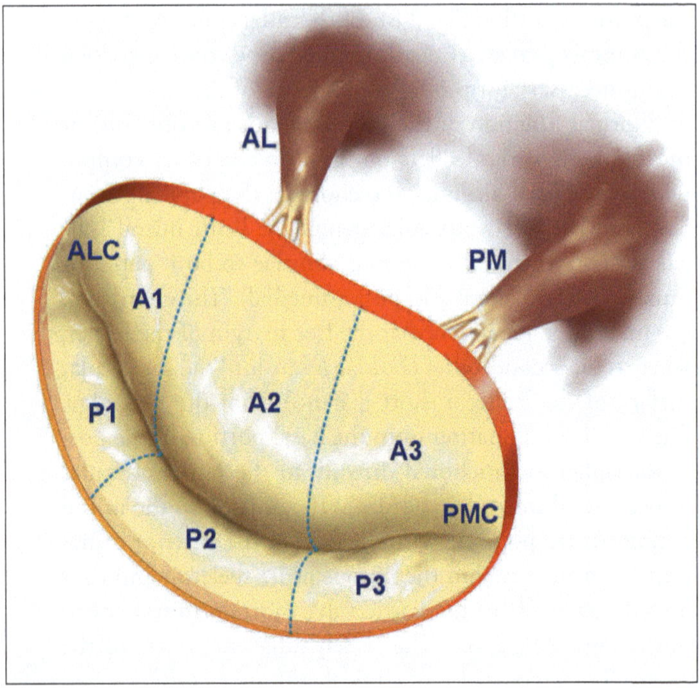

Fig. 2.8 Mitral valve. *A1–A3* anterior leaflet, *P1–P3* posterior leaflet, *ALC* anterolateral commissure, *PMC* posteromedial commissure, *AL* anterolateral papillary muscle, *PM* posteromedial papillary muscle

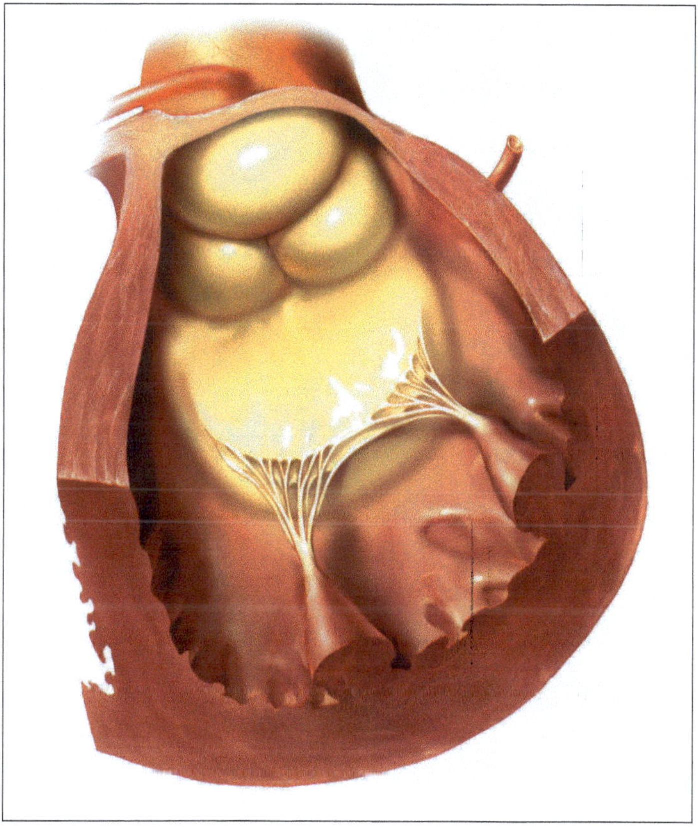

Fig. 2.9 Topographic interrelations of the aortic and mitral valve (aortico-mitral continuity)

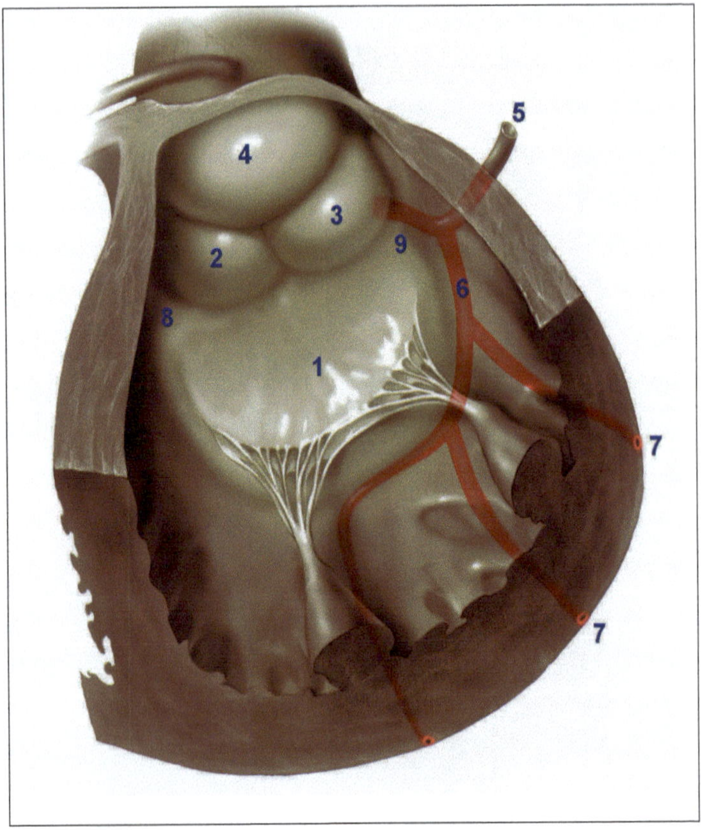

Fig. 2.10 Topographic interrelations of the aortic and mitral valve. *1* Anterior mitral leaflet, *2* non-coronary aortic cusp, *3* left coronary cusp, *4* right coronary cusp, *5* left anterior descending artery, *6* circumflex artery, *7* oblique marginal branches, *8* right fibrous trigone, *9* left fibrous trigone

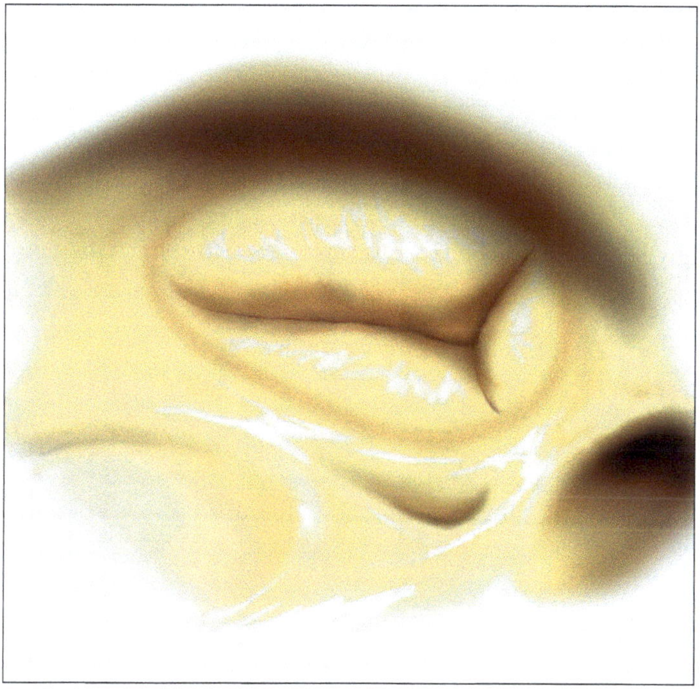

Fig. 2.11 Tricuspid valve viewed from the right atrium

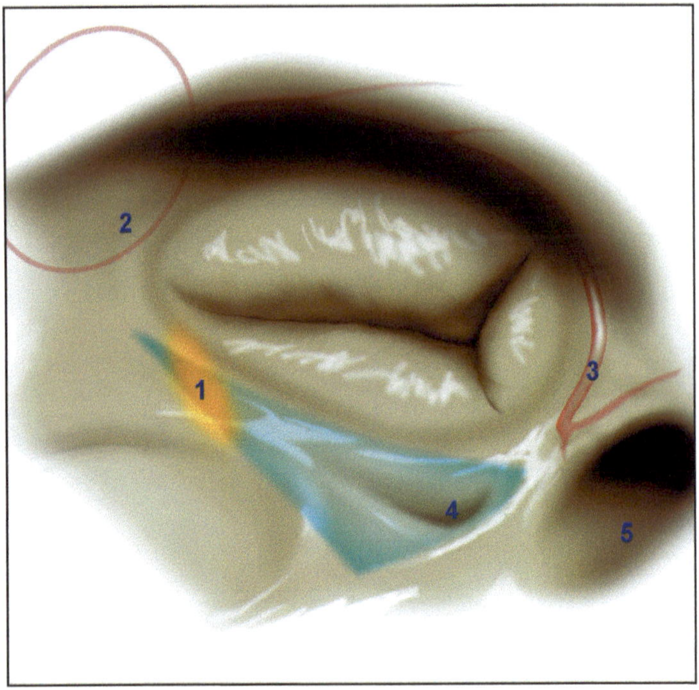

Fig. 2.12 Topographic interrelations of the tricuspid valve to adjacent structures. *1* atrioventricular node, *2* aortic valve, *3* right coronary artery, *4* coronary sinus, *5* inferior vena cava

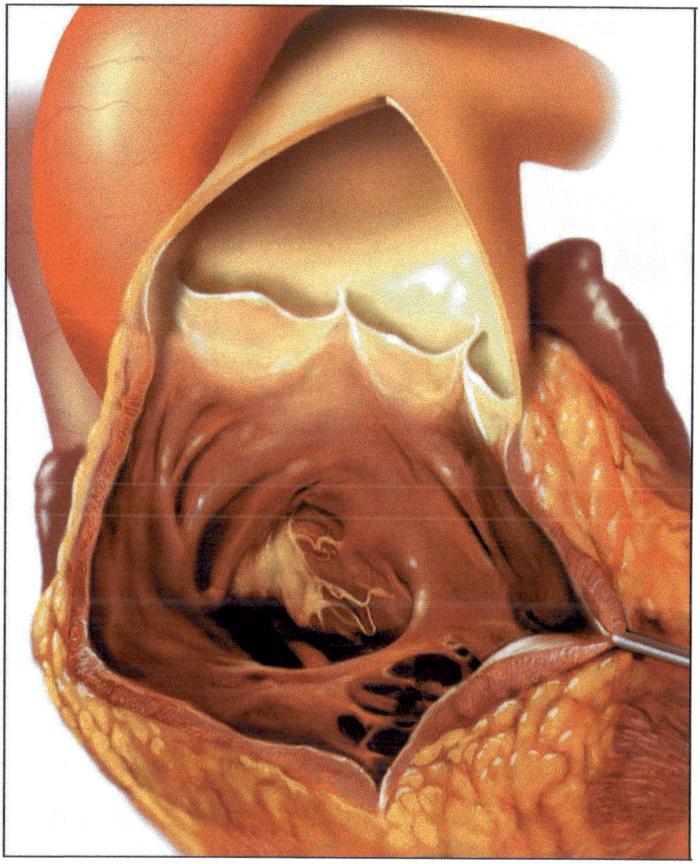

Fig. 2.13 View of the right ventricular outflow tract, pulmonary valve, and pulmonary artery trunk

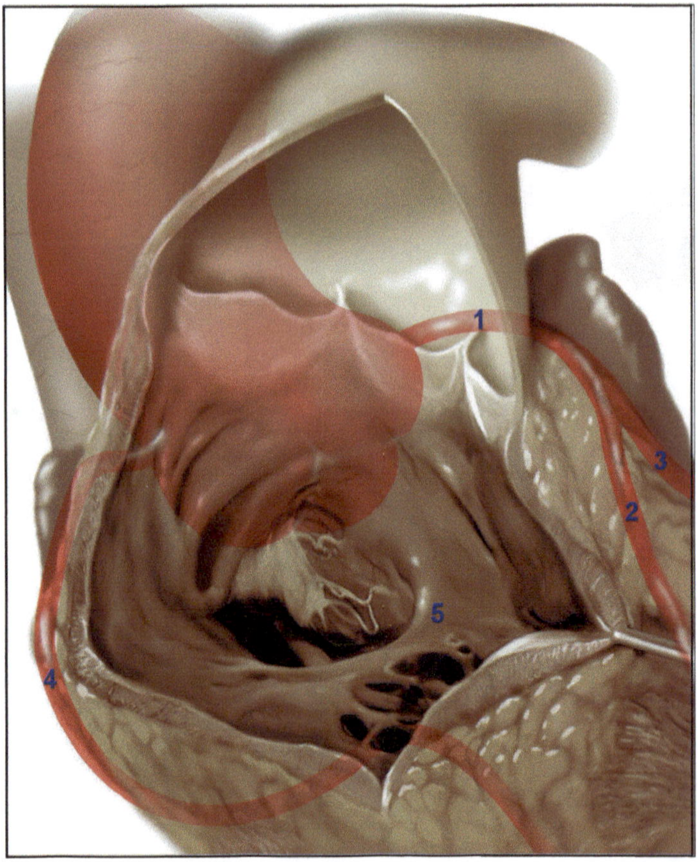

Fig. 2.14 Topographic interrelations of the great vessels and coronary arteries. *1* left main stem, *2* left anterior descending artery, *3* circumflex artery, *4* right coronary artery, *5* trabecula septomarginalis

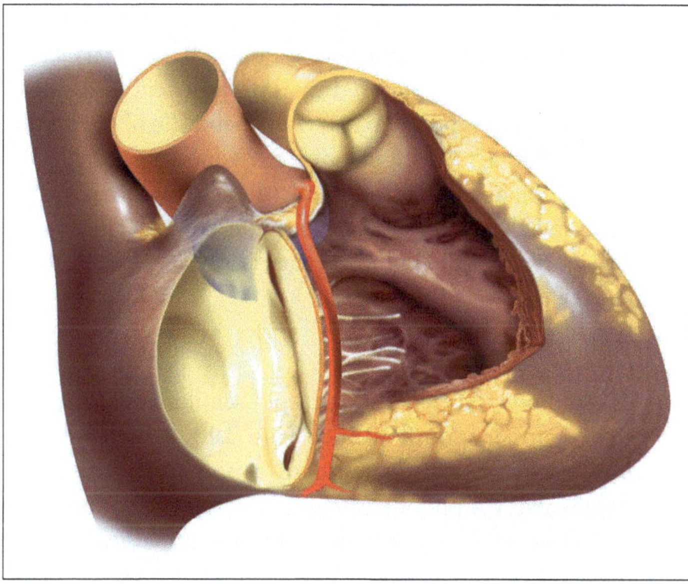

Fig. 2.15 Topographic interrelations of aortic, tricuspid, and pulmonary valves

anteroseptal commissure (the triangle of Koch, which is delineated by the septal leaflet annulus, the coronary sinus, and the tendon of Todaro) there is the atrioventricular node of the conduction system and the penetration of the bundle of His through the right fibrous trigone (Fig. 2.12). The area of the anteroseptal commissure is close to the aortic valve and the posterior leaflet annulus lies very close to the mid-portion of the right coronary artery [1–3].

2.5 Pulmonary Valve

The pulmonary valve is a tricuspid semilunar valve in the right ventricular outflow tract (Figs. 2.13, 2.14). The morphology of the sinuses and cusps is similar to that of the aortic valve; the pulmonary valve is, however, thinner. There are neither coronary ostia nor a fibrous continuity with the tricuspid valve (Fig. 2.15). The pulmonary valve cusps are usually termed the right, left, and anterior (non-septal) cusps.

References

1. Doty DB (ed) (1997) Cardiac anatomy. Cardiac surgery: operative technique. Mosby, St. Louis
2. Kirklin JW, Barratt-Boyes BG (1993) Anatomy, dimensions, and terminology. In: Kirklin JW, Barratt-Boyes BG (eds) Cardiac surgery, 2nd edn. Churchill Livingstone, London
3. Mill MR, Wilcox BR, Anderson RH (2008) Surgical anatomy of the heart. In: Cohn LH (ed) Cardiac surgery in the adult, 3rd edn. McGraw-Hill, New York
4. Sutton JP III, Ho SY, Anderson RH (1995) The forgotten interleaflet triangles: a review of the surgical anatomy of the aortic valve. Ann Thorac Surg 59:419–427

Overview of the Valve Replacement Devices

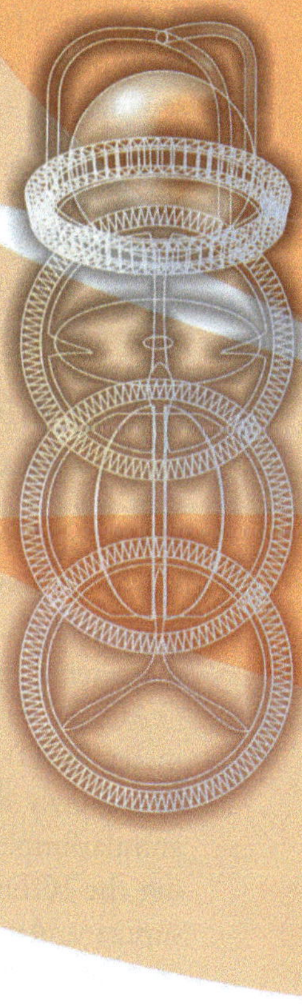

3 Overview of the Valve Replacement Devices

3.1 Introduction

Severely diseased heart valves that cause significant valvular disease, not amenable to repair due to extensive calcification, infection, or congenital malformation, have to be replaced by artificial or biological heart valves. Artificial heart valves (mechanical valves, prostheses) are constructed from plastic materials, titanium or metallic alloys with the sewing ring from various fabrics. In biological valves the valve itself is mostly a biological tissue from other animal species (xenograft) that is mounted on a stent equipped with a sewing ring (bioprosthesis). Less frequent options are the allografts (homografts) and autografts that are implanted without a stent or sewing ring.

3.2 Terminology of the Valve Replacement Devices Parameters

The label of mechanical and biological heart valves always consists of the trade name and a number indicating the valve size (in millimeters). This valve size represents the outer diameter of the valve housing/stent tissue annulus diameter (TAD, in millimeters; Fig. 3.1). The internal orifice diameter (IOD) of the valve is smaller than the labeled valve size. Newly developed bioprostheses designed for supraannular implantation have a different size labeling indicating the IOD (in millimeters). The reason is that in true supraannular implantation not only the sewing ring but

J. Dominik and P. Zacek, *Heart Valve Surgery: An Illustrated Guide*,
DOI 10.1007/978-3-642-12206-4_3,

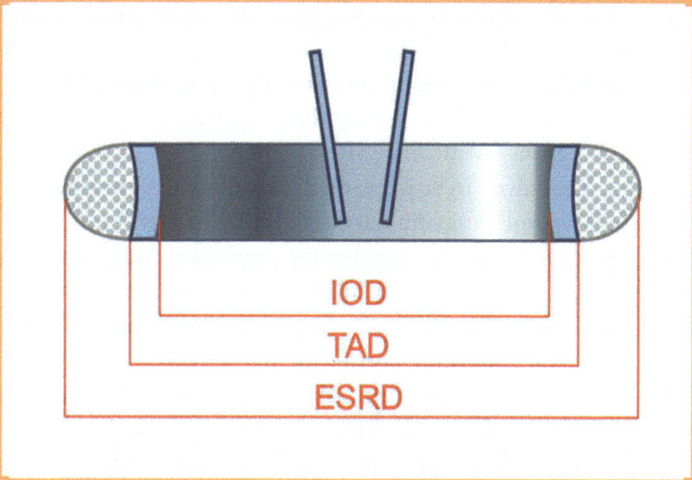

Fig. 3.1 Valve diameters. *IOD* internal orifice diameter, *TAD* tissue annulus diameter, *ESRD* external sewing ring diameter

also the housing/stent is placed above the patient's annulus and so the IOD is equal to the TAD (Fig. 3.2). The whole artificial valve diameter is then larger for several millimeters (the thickness of the sewing ring is added), i.e., the external sewing ring diameter (ESRD).

The valve can be implanted intraannulary, intrasupraannulary, and supraannulary (Fig. 3.2). In intraannular implantation ESRD is equal to the patient's annulus diameter (TAD). This is very disadvantageous in the case of a narrow annulus, because the valve housing and its sewing ring occlude an important portion of the patient's valve orifice; therefore, intrasupraannular implantation, in which the sewing ring is placed above the patient's annulus, is preferred. Modern bioprostheses and mechanical valves CarboMedics Top Hat, Sorin Bicarbon Overline, and Medtronic Advantage Supra are designed for completely supraannular implantation in which not only the sewing ring but also the valve housing/stent is located above the patient's annulus. In this way a valve with a much larger orifice area and therefore better hemodynamic parameters can be implanted into a given annulus.

Hemodynamically, the most important parameter of both mechanical valves and bioprostheses is their effective orifice area (EOA; Fig. 3.3). Effective orifice area has to be differentiated from geometric orifice area (GOA). Geometric orifice area is the whole inner area of the valve including the area occupied by the opened discs or leaflets, struts, and other mechanisms of the valve. Calculation of the GOA is simple; it is the calculation of the circular area, the radius of which is half of the IOD. By subtracting the area of opening components of the valve from GOA, the so-called clear orifice area (COA) is obtained, the value of which is, however,

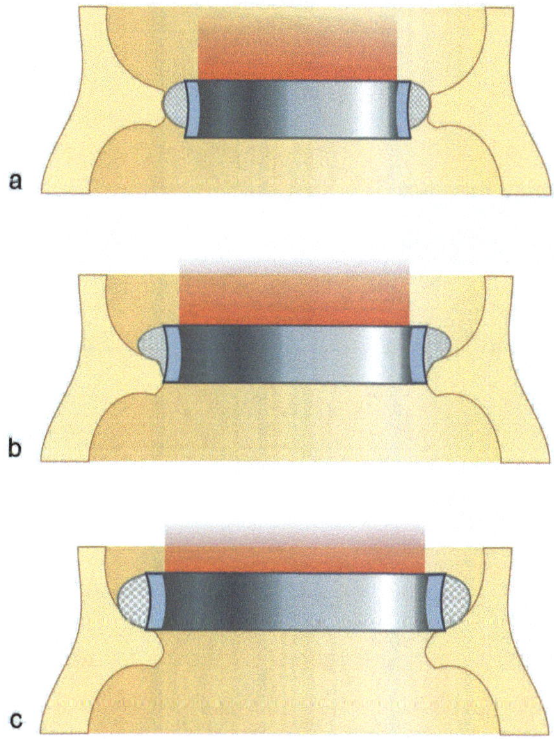

Fig. 3.2 Valve implanted **a** intraannulary (sewing ring inside of the aortic annulus), **b** intrasupraannulary (sewing ring is placed supraannulary, stent is located intraannulary), and **c** supraanulary (both sewing ring and stent are placed supraannulary)

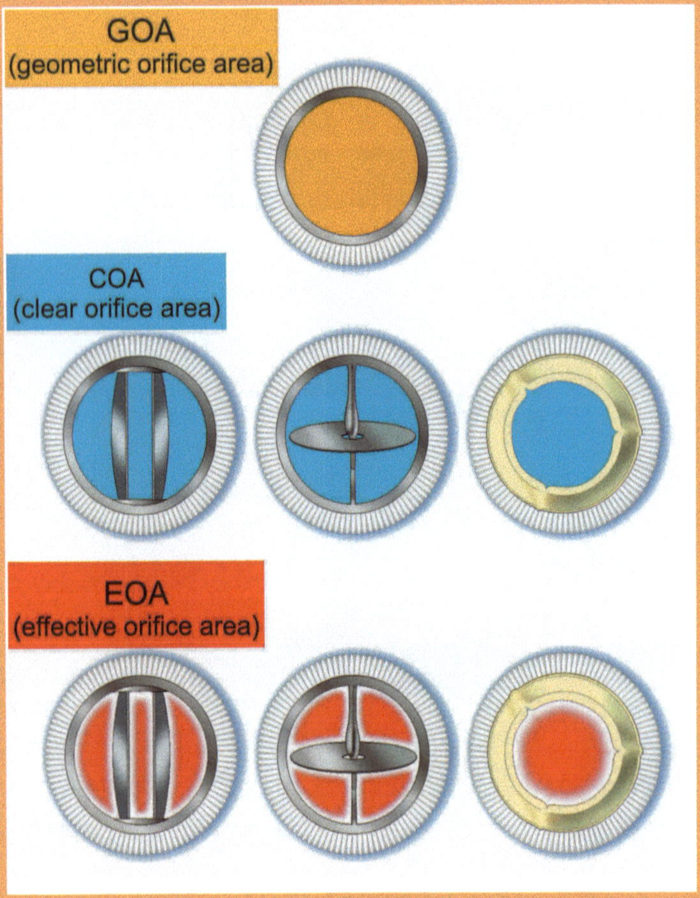

Fig. 3.3 GOA, COA, and EOA of bileaflet valves *(left column)*, tilting monodiscs *(center column)*, and bioprostheses *(right column)*

declared only seldom. The EOA is that portion of the valve orifice area through which the blood really flows. The EOA is usually one quarter or one third smaller than GOA. The size of EOA and GOA is measured in square centimeters. In a given patient, the most important parameter is the indexed value (IEOA), i.e., EOA related to 1 m^2 of the patient's body surface. It has to be kept in mind that values declared by the manufacturer used to look more optimistic (in vitro values) than post-implantation echocardiography values calculated on the basis of continuity equation (in vivo values).

The aim is to implant a valve large enough to avoid hemodynamically significant patient–prosthesis mismatch (PPM). It is important mainly in the aortic position where IEOA of the implanted valve should be greater than 0.85 cm^2/m^2. In the mitral valve the cut-off value for PPM is considered to be 1.2 cm^2/m^2. Severe patient–prosthesis mismatch occurs if IEOA is less than 0.65 cm^2/m^2 in the aortic position and less than 0.9 cm/m^2 in the mitral position [1, 2].

3.3 Mechanical Heart Valves

Mechanical heart valves (artificial valves, prostheses) have been implanted since the beginning of the 1960s. They have been subject to continuous development and refinement of technical, hemodynamic, and biocompatibility parameters. Mechanical valves can be divided into caged-ball, disc (monodisc), and bileaflet valves [3, 4].

3.3.1 Caged-Ball Valves

The Starr–Edwards valve is the best-known caged-ball valve. In the 1960s and 1970s it was the most-often implanted valve in the world. From a long development line of Starr–

Edwards valves, the successful mitral model 6120 has been manufactured without any modifications since 1966 [5, 6], as well as the aortic model 1260 since 1968 [7], and both valves are still being implanted at some centers [3, 8, 9]. The closing component of the valve is a silastic ball, which is held within a stellite alloy cage (opened position). In closed position the ball obturates the metallic ring equipped with a Teflon (DuPont, Wilmington, Del.) fabric sewing ring for implantation (Fig. 3.4).

Another well-known valve is the Smeloff–Cutter valve, which was introduced into clinical use in 1964 (but has not been implanted since 1988). In this model the silastic ball does not sit at the titanium alloy ring but is stopped by a second smaller cage. Three struts of the upper and lower cage are not connected (Fig. 3.5) [3].

After implantation of the caged-ball valves, patients experienced dramatic hemodynamic improvement but suffered from frequent thromboembolic complications. Effort to reduce these serious complications has led to development of the cloth-covered caged-ball valves. The best-known of these valves were the Braunwald–Cutter valve (Fig. 3.6), manufactured and implanted between 1968 and 1979 [3, 10, 11], and the cloth-covered Starr–Edwards valve, manufactured between 1967 and 1976 (Fig. 3.7). The struts and the ring were covered with polypropylene into which endothel grew within several weeks or months after implantation. Thereby, the whole housing of the artificial valve was endothelialized and, except for the ball, blood did not contact a foreign surface. Expected decrease in incidence of thromboembolic events and reduction of hemolysis were in fact achieved but remained limited to the first months or few years after implantation. Several years later, however,

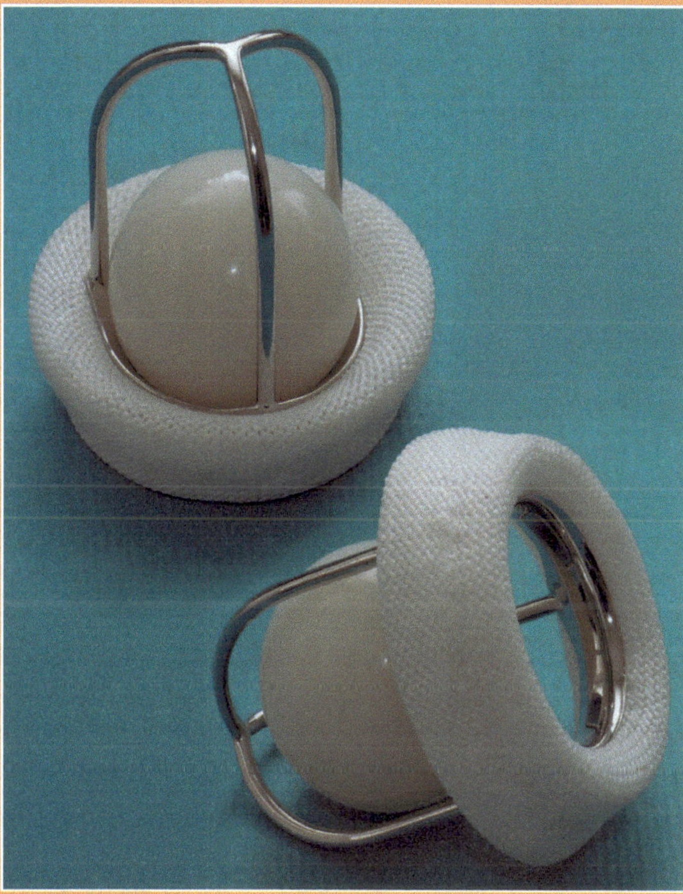

Fig. 3.4 Caged-ball valve Starr–Edwards (aortic model 1260)

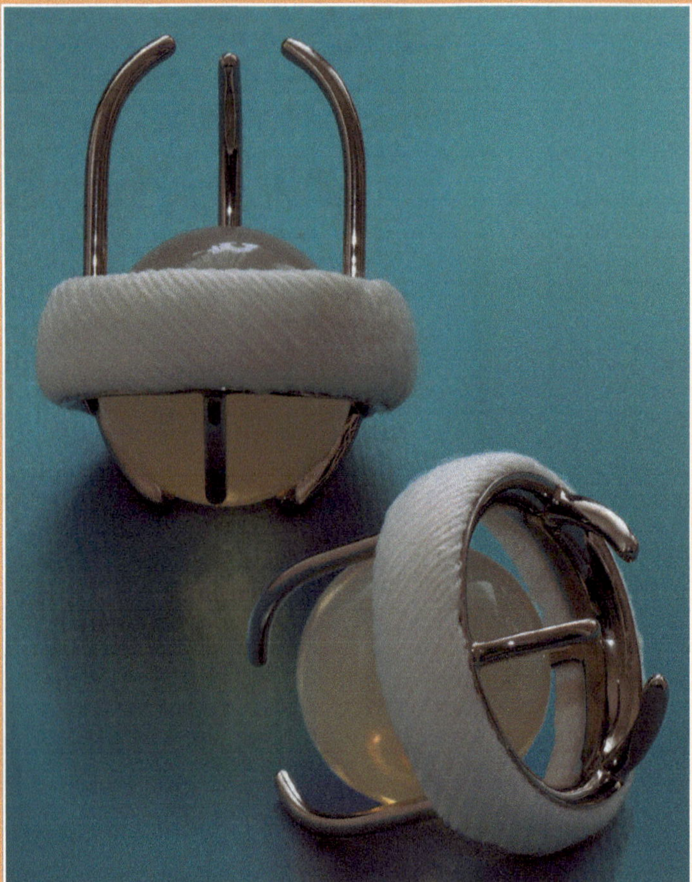

Fig. 3.5 Caged-ball valve Smeloff–Cutter

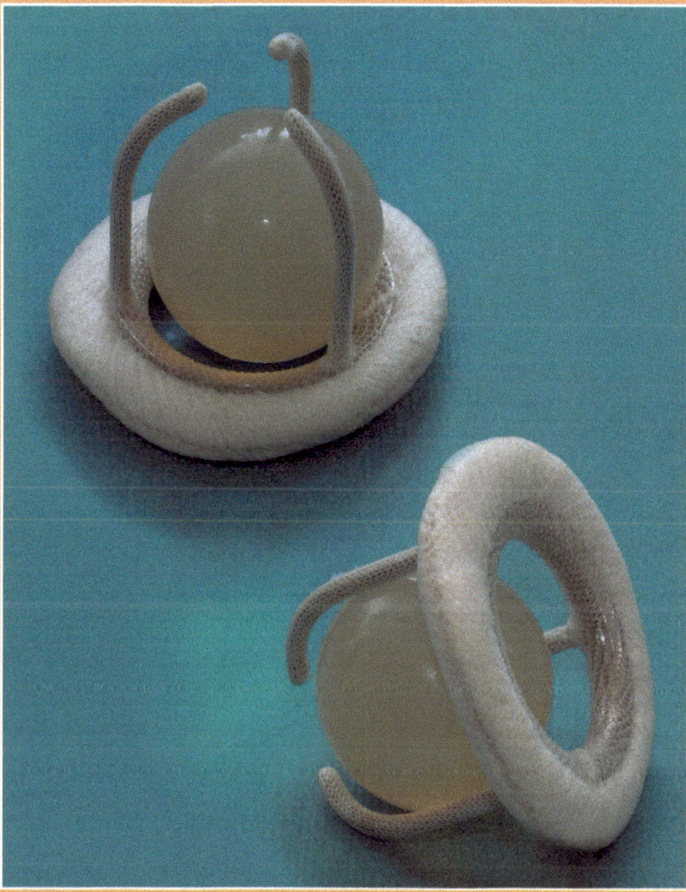

Fig. 3.6 Cloth-covered caged-ball valve Braunwald–Cutter

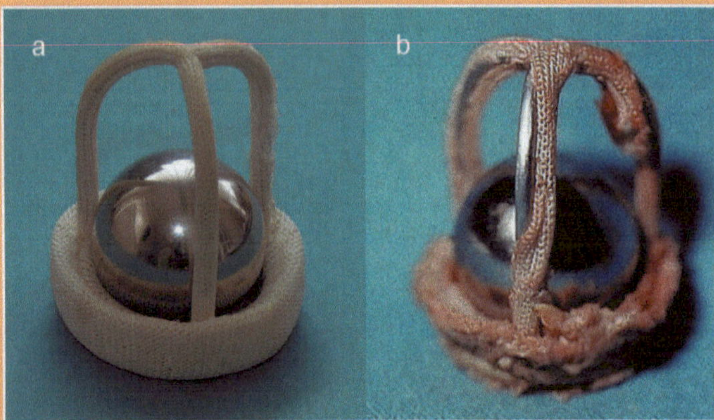

Fig. 3.7 **a** Cloth-covered caged-ball valve Starr–Edwards (aortic model 2320). **b** The valve was explanted due to tearing of the cloth 22 years after implantation

tearing of the cloth covering occurred as a result of hardness disparity between the ball and the endothelialized covering (Fig. 3.7). Torn covering initiated thrombus formation with subsequent thromboembolic events and also caused clinically significant hemolysis, which often prompted reoperation and valve reimplantation [12–14].

3.3.2 Disc Valves

In the late 1960s, non-tilting disc valves were introduced into clinical practice. The closing component was a poppet that was held in a cage (open position) or obturated the ring (closed position). A variety of these valves were manufactured and clinically implanted. In all of them the principle was identical, but they differed in the material of the disc, the housing, and the ring, and also in the cage design. The best-known valves were Beall (Fig. 3.8) [15, 16], Starr–Edwards (Fig. 3.8), and others (e.g., Kay–Shiley, Kay–Suzuki, Cooley–Cutter, and Cross–Jones). The advantages of non-tilting disc valves were low-profile design, easier implantation, very little opening resistance, and very short closure delay (and therefore very little regurgitation). On the other hand, the valves suffered from higher flow gradients, significant turbulence, frequent thromboembolic complications, and higher hemolysis. Due to these drawbacks, the non-tilting disc valves fell into disuse and were replaced by modern tilting disc valves.

Tilting monodiscs were the most-often implanted valves in the 1970s and 1980s. In Europe, the most commonly used valves were the Björk–Shiley valves. The first model of this valve was introduced into clinical practice in 1969. It had a flat delrin disc, which tilted up to 60° [17]. This type was soon replaced (in 1971) by a so-called standard

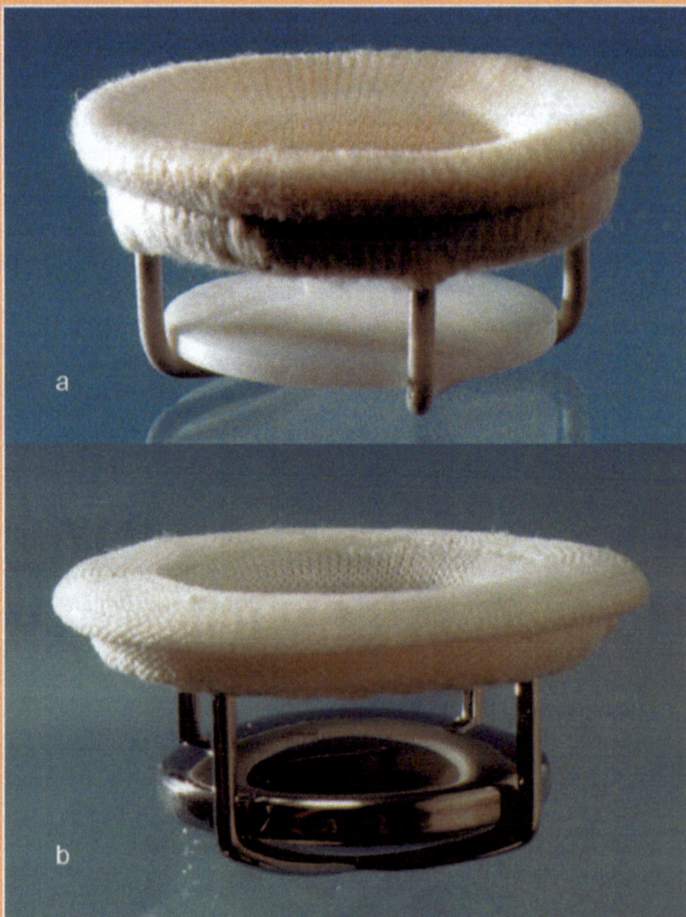

Fig. 3.8 Non-tilting disc valves **a** Beall and **b** Starr–Edwards

type (Fig. 3.9a) with pyrolytic carbon flat disc tilting up to 60°. In 1976, a convex–concave type valve (Fig. 3.9b) with significantly improved hemodynamic parameters was introduced. The hour-glass-shaped pyrolytic carbon disc was placed more centrally and tilted up to 60°. The latest Björk–Shiley developmental type, the monostrut (Fig. 3.9c), was introduced into clinical practice in 1982. The disc-housing system was changed and the angle of tilting was increased to 70° [18]. Hemodynamic characteristics of both, the convex–concave type and the monostrut, were very good; nonetheless, the convex–concave valves have not been marketed since the late 1980s. The reason for this was that the inflow bar broke in some of them after 2–3 years of perfect performance, causing escape of the disc and acute valve regurgitation [19–21]. This serious and mostly lethal complication (unless operated urgently) was related to convex–concave valves manufactured between 1981 and 1982. Risk of its incidence was estimated within a range of 2 promile to 2% per year with the implanted valve. Since then, the struts in all heart valves are not welded but manufactured from a single block of metal or alloy or from pyrolytic carbon.

A variety of heart valves have been designed on the principle of the tilting disc, with differences in the disc housing and the achieved angle of tilting. Precise knowledge of the tilting angle in monodisc and bileaflet valves is important for eventual diagnostics of the valve failure. Discs are radioopaque and therefore fluoroscopy imaging can confirm their normal mobility or diagnose restricted range of motion, or even complete occluder blockade.

Among the formerly used tilting monodisc valves, there are, for example, the Lillehei–Kaster valve, manufactured from 1970 to 1987 (pyrolytic carbon disc opening up to 80°

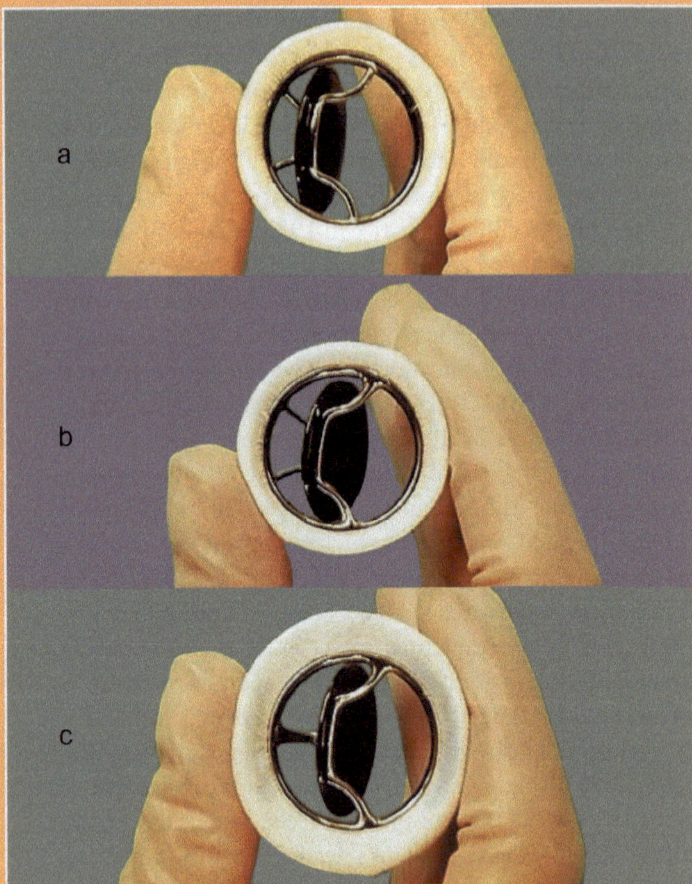

Fig. 3.9 Disc valve Björk–Shiley. **a** Standard type with flat disc. **b** Convex–concave type. **c** Monostrut

and closing at 18°), and Omniscience (Fig. 3.10), manufactured since 1978 and modified in 1984 under the name Omnicarbon. The Omnicarbon disc opens up to 80° and closes at 12°, thus achieving the tilting range of 68°. The latest model of Omnicarbon has the ring manufactured also from pyrolytic carbon. Among others, the disc valves of Sorin–Biomedica have been widely implanted. The developmental types Sorin–Monocast and Carbocast were followed by Allcarbon–Sorin, which has been in use since 1989 (Fig. 3.11). The pyrolytic carbon disc of this valve tilts up to 60° and all metallic components, together with the sewing ring, are carbon-film coated for better biocompatibility. The Ultracor–Aortech valves (developed in 1985), the tilting angle of which is 73° in the aortic model and 68° in the mitral model, have also been implanted.

Worldwide, the most frequently implanted disc valve is Medtronic–Hall (originally Hall–Kaster), which has been in clinical use without modification since 1977 (Fig. 3.12). The housing is made from titanium and the pyrolytic carbon disc opens up to 75° (aortic valve) and 70° (mitral valve) [22, 23].

3.3.3 Bileaflet Valves

Mechanical bileaflet valves have gained popularity since the mid-1980s and currently are the most frequently implanted valves in the world. There are a variety of bileaflet heart valves available. They are based on the same or similar principle but differ in the angle of tilting, design of the pivots, material and shape of the sewing ring, and also the depth of the leaflets in their open position. The best-known and most implanted mechanical bileaflet valve is the St. Jude Medical (SJM) valve (Fig. 3.13), which was introduced into

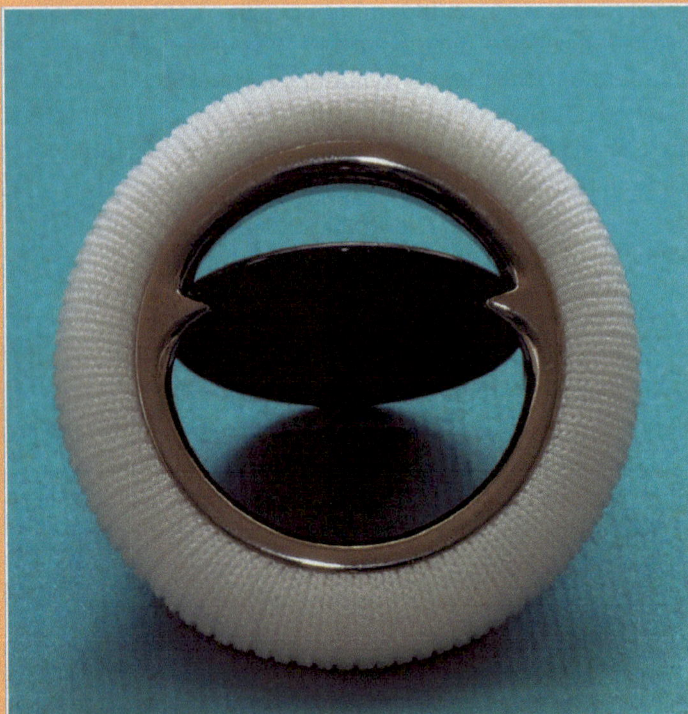

Fig. 3.10 Disc valve Omniscience

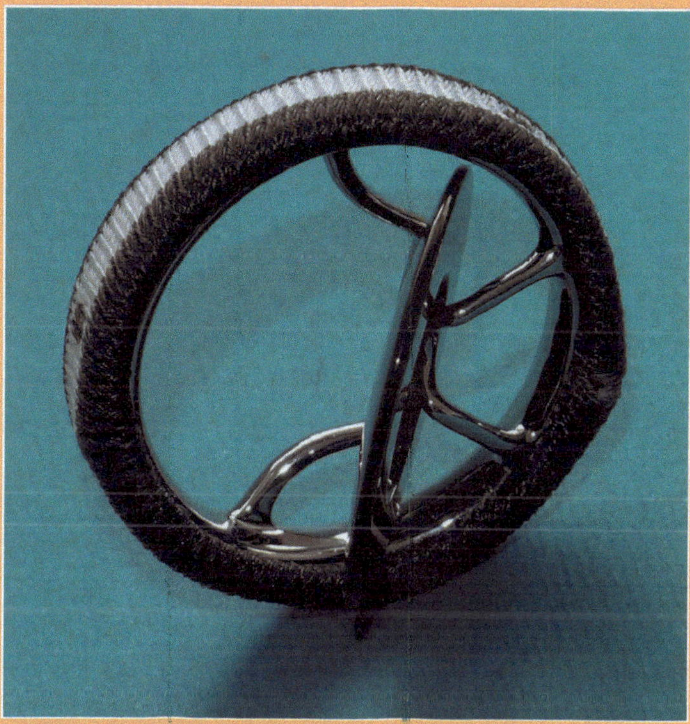

Fig. 3.11 Disc valve Allcarbon–Sorin

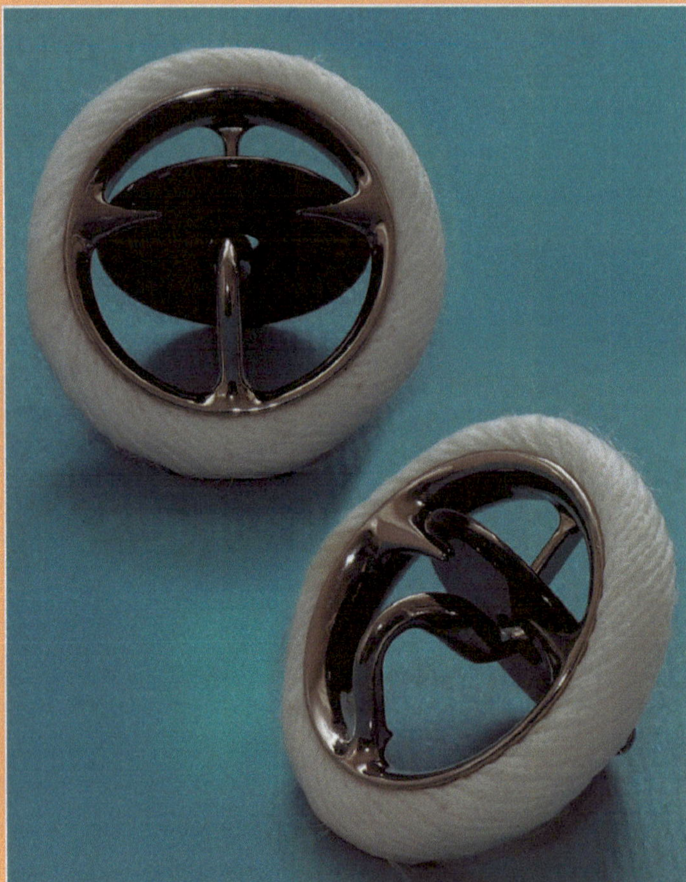

Fig. 3.12 Disc valve Medtronic–Hall

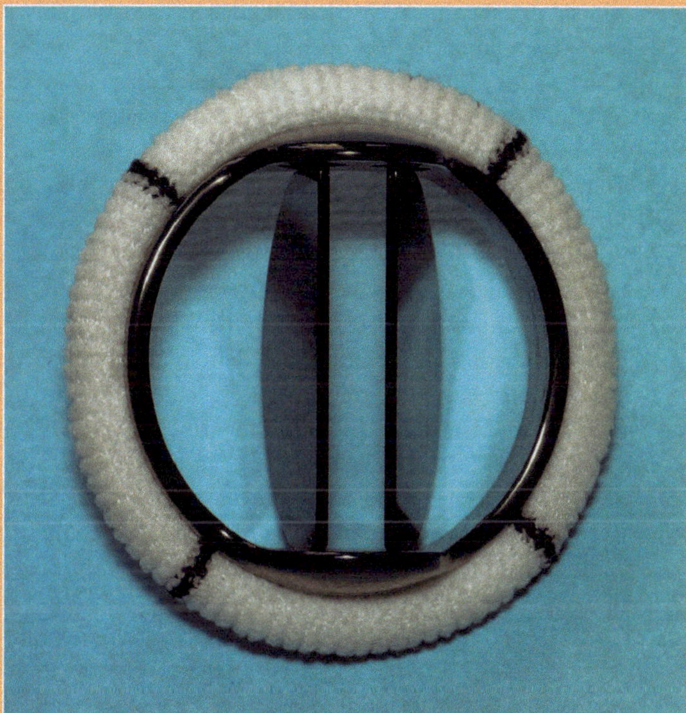

Fig. 3.13 Bileaflet valve St. Jude Medical

clinical practice in 1977 (SJM Standard). Its two pyrolytic carbon semilunar leaflets open up to 85° and close at 30°, which yields a tilting range of 55°. The valve mechanism has remained unchanged since its release, but a rotatable sewing cuff was added and other ring refinements were developed. The types SJM HP (hemodynamic plus, since 1992) and SJM Regent (since 1998) are equipped with a reduced sewing ring, which results in significant enlargement of the effective orifice area compared with the standard type [24, 25]. This important feature is very beneficial in avoiding patient-prosthesis mismatch in patients with small aortic annulus and large body-surface area. The standard SJM model size (21 mm) had an effective orifice area (EOA) of only 1.51 cm^2, the type HP 2.03 cm^2, and the latest model, Regent, 2.47 cm^2. Nonetheless, even a "small-size" SJM Regent 19-mm valve has an EOA of 1.84 cm^2, i.e., sufficient enough to prevent a significant patient–prosthesis mismatch in a patient with a body-surface area of 2 m^2.

Comparably excellent EOA is obtained with the second-most common bileaflet valve, Bicarbon–Sorin (manufactured since 1990). Its semilunar leaflets are convex–concave shaped and tilt up to 80° and close at 20° (Fig. 3.14). The valves are equipped with sewing rings Fitline or Slimline (suitable for small annuli) and Overline (intended solely for supraannular implantation). The same mechanism, but a different sewing-cuff material, is typical for the Edwards MIRA valve (since 1997).

Another known bileaflet valve is CarboMedics, which has been in clinical use since 1986. In 1991 the type CarboMedics R (with a significantly reduced sewing ring) was released in response to the problem of a narrow aortic annulus [26]. The model CarboMedics Top Hat was the first

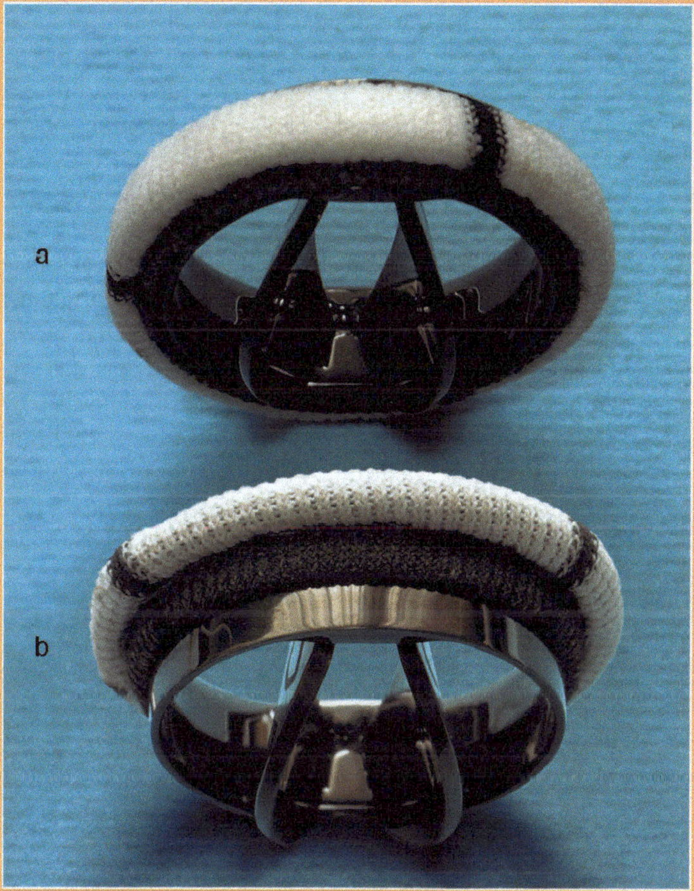

Fig. 3.14 Bileaflet valve Sorin–Bicarbon. **a** Slimline. **b** Overline

mechanical heart valve designed for totally supraannular implantation (both the housing and sewing ring are placed supraannulary) [27]. In 1994 a CarboMedics universal valve, Orbis, was launched, enabling implantation of the same valve either to the aortic or mitral position. The semilunar leaflets of CarboMedics valves tilt up to 78° and close at 25°, which gives a tilting range of 53°.

Two other bileaflet valves are the ATS Medical (since 1992), standard type and AP type (advanced performance) for small annuli [24], and OnX (since 1996), with different rings. An interesting feature of the OnX valve is that the pyrolytic carbon ring overtops the sewing ring and thereby prevents tissue from overgrowing into the valve mechanism.

Bileaflet valve Medtronic Advantage has, since 2003, a modification for supraannular implantation named Medtronic Advantage Supra. The most recent bileaflet valve introduced into clinical practice is the valve CardiaMed.

3.4 Biological Valves

The rationale for development of biological valves was to reduce the risk of serious complications related to the mechanical heart valves (thrombosis, embolism, bleeding complications due to anticoagulation therapy). The most frequently implanted tissue valves are xenografts manufactured as bioprostheses, whereas allografts and autografts are being implanted less often.

3.4.1 Bioprostheses

Bioprostheses are xenografts, i.e., valves prepared from tissues of other species. Xenografts are mounted on a cloth-covered stent, which is manufactured from stellite, titanium, or plastic (Fig. 3.15). Its slight flexibility is desirable, because it helps to absorb stress load and thereby prolong the xenograft's durability. The stent is covered with Teflon (DuPont, Wilmington, Del.) or polypropylene and adapted for tissue-valve mounting. The biological valve is either a porcine aortic valve (Fig. 3.16) or a valve assembled from bovine pericardium (Figs. 3.17, 3.18).

Bioprostheses are produced commercially, and a variety of models are currently available. The most commonly used porcine valve bioprostheses include, for example, SJM Epic and Epic Ultra (Fig. 3.16), Carpentier–Edwards, Hancock, Shelhigh, Medtronic–Mosaic, and Medtronic–Mosaic Ultra. Bioprostheses Sorin–Mitroflow, Sorin–Pericarbon More, Sorin–Soprano (Fig. 3.17), Sorin–Soprano Armonia, Edwards–Perimount Magna (Fig. 3.18), and Köhler Medical–Aspire are a few representatives of bovine pericardium xenografts [28].

Continuous development and intensive research has been aimed at creating a bioprosthesis with tissue leaflets that would exhibit long-term freedom from structural deterioration. A promising concept is detoxification (anticalcification, antidegenerative, antimineralization) treatment incorporated into the processing and storage of tissue valves. Different manufacturers have introduced their proprietary procedures, e.g., AoA (Medtronic), BiLinx AC (St. Jude Medical), XenoLogiX (Edwards), ThermaFix (Edwards), No-React (Shelhigh), and T6 (Hancock); however, only long-term results with implantations of valves processed in this way can bring the answer as to whether this modern treatment can result in delayed onset of structural degeneration of bioprostheses compared with classical valve preparation and 0.5% glutaraldehyde storage [29, 30].

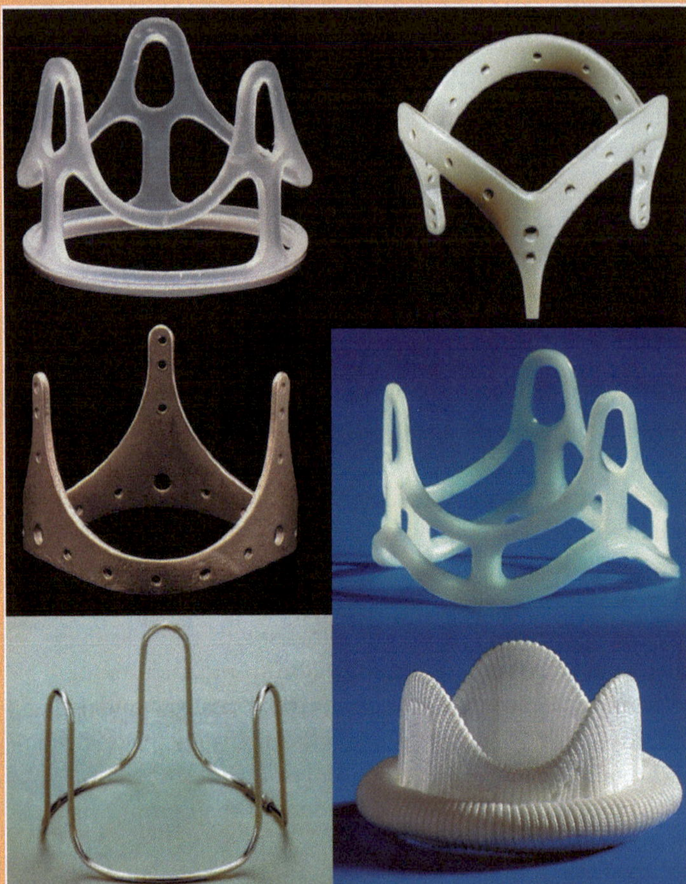

Fig. 3.15 Stents for bioprostheses

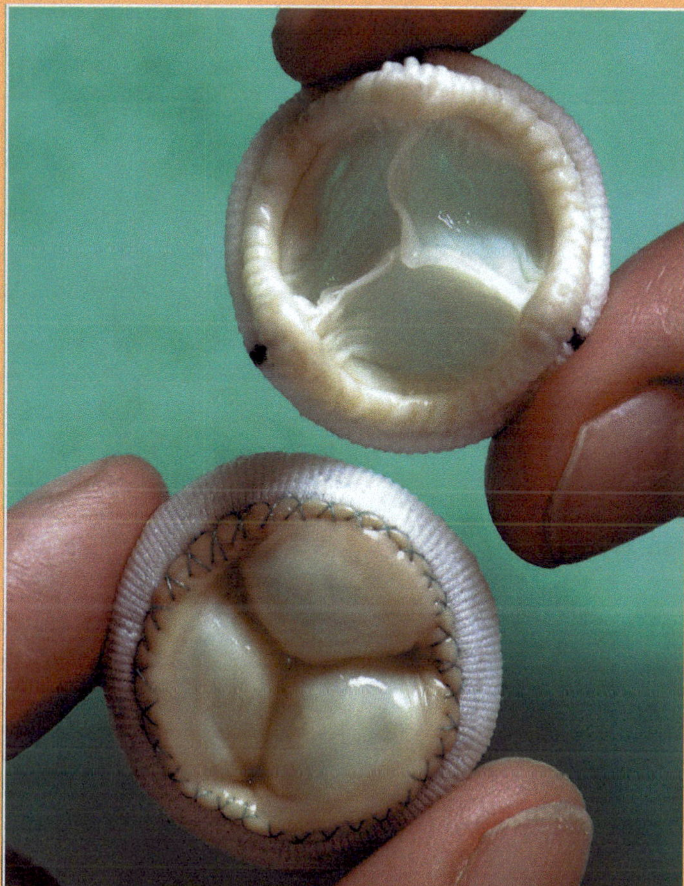

Fig. 3.16 Bioprosthesis St. Jude Medical–Epic

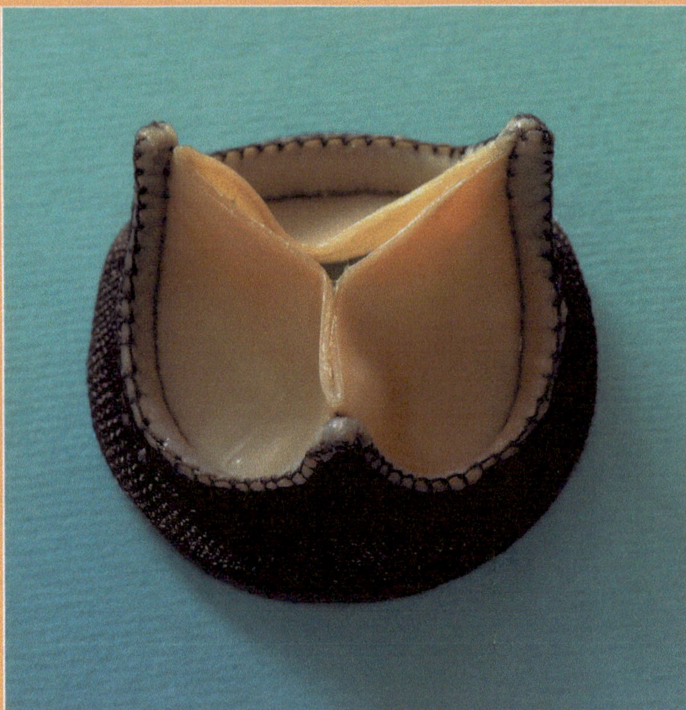

Fig. 3.17 Bioprosthesis Sorin–Soprano

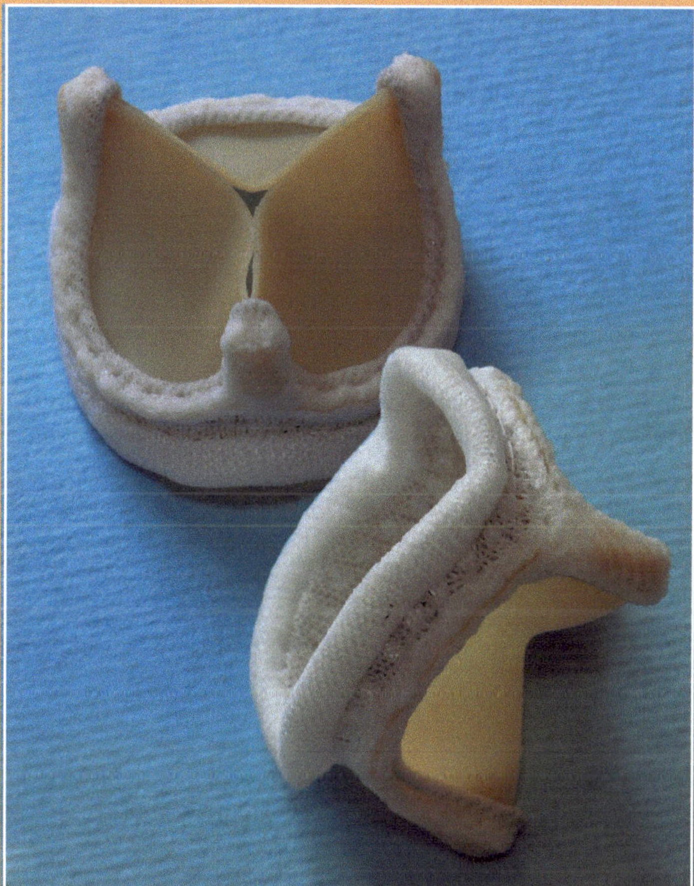

Fig. 3.18 Bioprosthesis Edwards–Perimount Magna

Stentless bioprostheses were introduced by Tirone David in Toronto and have been implanted into the aortic position since 1988. Stentless bioprostheses are xenografts, but they have neither stent nor sewing cuff. Into a given patient's aortic orifice, therefore, a stentless bioprosthesis that is larger than a stented bioprosthesis can be implanted (i.e., larger aortic EOA and lower transvalvular gradient). The best--known stentless bioprostheses are Toronto SPV (Fig. 3.19), Toronto Root, Edwards Prima (Fig. 3.20), Shelhigh Super-Stentless (Fig. 3.21), Sorin Freedom, Medtronic Freestyle, Elan, CryoLife-O'Brien, and others. Stentless bioprostheses have demonstrated superior hemodynamic features in terms of transvalvular gradients, EOA, and more complete regression of left ventricular hypertrophy [31–33]. A wave of enthusiasm for these valves, one that culminated in the mid- to late 1990s, has waned because research data proved no superiority of stentless bioprostheses over stented ones in long-term studies [34–41]. In addition to this, implantation of the stentless valves is technically more demanding and time-consuming. Moreover, the decline in use of stentless bioprostheses has also been caused by the development of bioprostheses designed for supraannular implantation. A supraannulary-seated sewing ring does not obstruct the aortic orifice area, and therefore the improved EOA is almost comparable to that of stentless bioprostheses.

3.4.2 Allografts

Allografts (homografts) represent another option for a tissue--valve implantation into the aortic (eventually pulmonary) orifice. Allografts, human cadaverous aortic valves, are harvested usually in the course of multiorgan donor explantations, and are dissected as an aortic root with the valve and the ascending

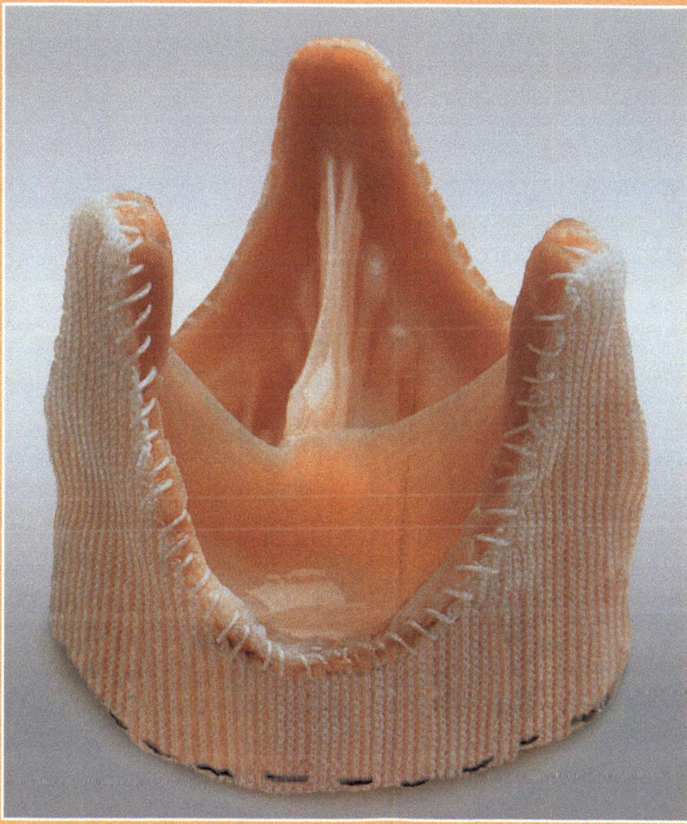

Fig. 3.19 Stentless bioprosthesis Toronto SPV

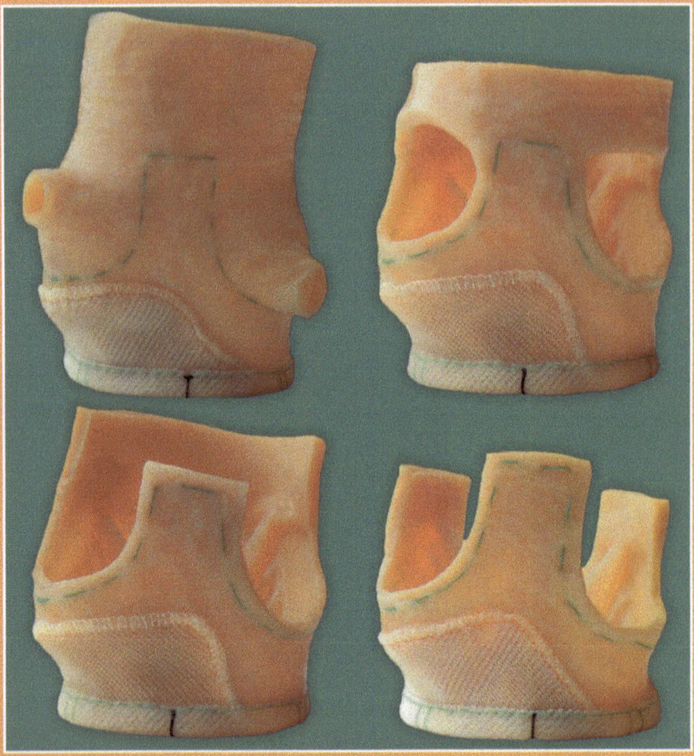

Fig. 3.20 Stentless bioprosthesis Edwards–Prima. Surgeons tailors its shape according to the technique of implantation

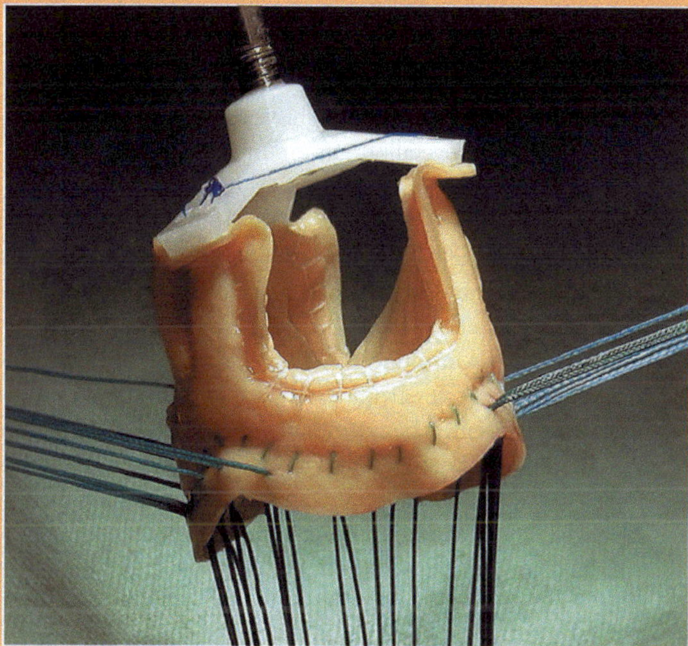

Fig. 3.21 Bioprosthesis Shelhigh SuperStentless

aorta (Figs. 3.22, 3.23). Pulmonary allograft was discontinued due to use of aortic valve replacement [42], but it still has its place in pediatric cardiac surgery and also in the Ross procedure for replacement of the right ventricular outflow tract.

Explanted valve allografts are first treated with antibiotic solution and then frozen (cryopreservation, cryoconservation) and stored in liquid nitrogen at 190°C for up to 5 years. After defrosting, the allografts' tissue still contains viable fibroblasts. Endothelium is not preserved, which turns out to be beneficial for reducing the allograft antigenicity, and thereby no immunosuppression is needed after implantation. Allografts are being used for aortic valve replacement quite infrequently, because their implantation is more difficult but rate of degeneration is the same as with bioprostheses. Allografts do not contain any fabric and are less susceptible to infection than bioprostheses and mechanical valves; therefore, they are used mostly for aortic valve replacement for infective endocarditis [43].

3.4.3 Autografts

An autograft is a biological tissue taken from the patient's body. In cardiac surgery, the pulmonary autograft is used for aortic valve replacement at the Ross procedure (and is itself, in its original place, substituted with a pulmonary allograft, replacing the right ventricular outflow tract with the pulmonary valve and the pulmonary trunk). The drawback of this procedure is its technical and time demands, as well as impending risk of failure of both implanted valves (autograft and allograft) in the long term. The advantages and disadvantages of mechanical valves, bioprostheses, allografts, and autografts, all of which influence decision making about the optimal valve selection for replacement, are discussed in Chap. 4.

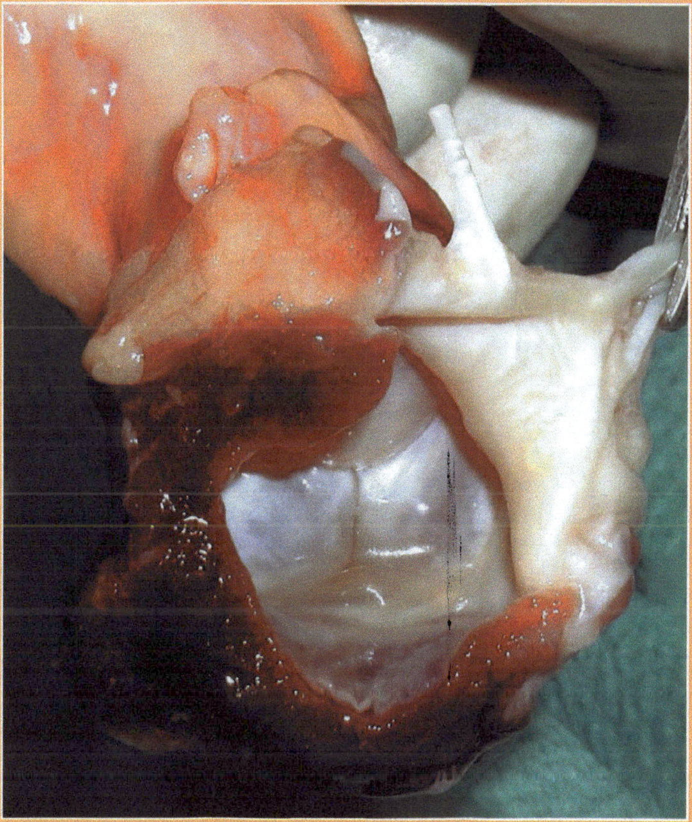

Fig. 3.22 Harvested allograft with anterior mitral leaflet, left ventricular muscle, and untrimmed aorta

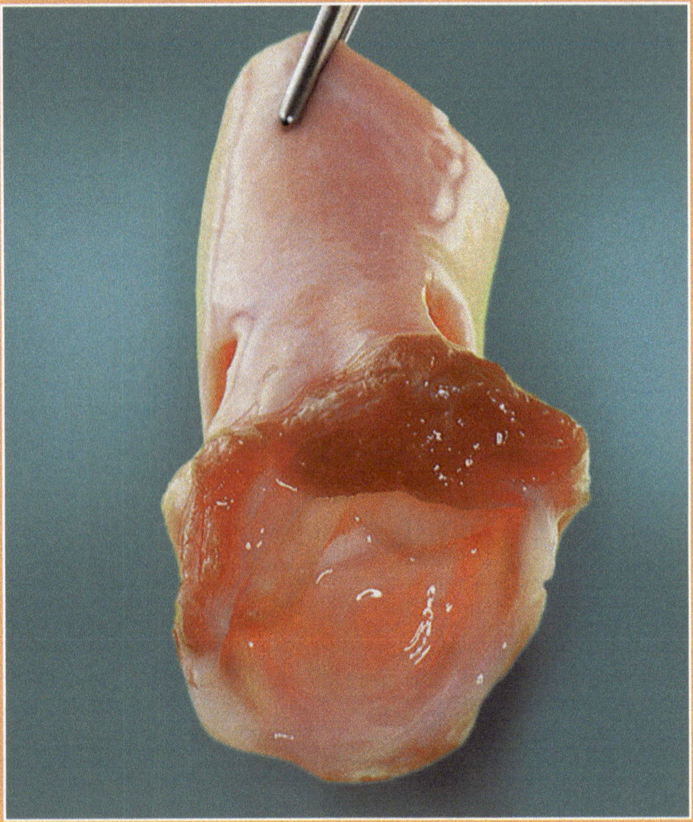

Fig. 3.23 Allograft prepared for root replacement

References

1. Magne J, Mathieu P, Dumesnil JG et al. (2007) Impact of prosthesis–patient mismatch on survival after mitral valve replacement. Circulation 115:1417–1425
2. Urso S, Sadaba R, Aldamiz-Echevarria G (2009) Is patient–prosthesis mismatch an independent risk factor for early and mid-term overall mortality in adult patients undergoing aortic valve replacement? Interact Cardiovasc Thorac Surg 9:510–518
3. Gott VL, Alejo DE, Cameron DE (2003) Mechanical heart valves: 50 years of evolution. Ann Thorac Surg 76:S2230–S2239
4. Unger F, Rainer WG, Horstkotte D et al. (2000) Standards and concepts in valve surgery. J Cardiovasc Surg (Torino) 41:585–593
5. Miller DC, Oyer PE, Stinson EB et al. (1983) Ten to fifteen year reassessment of the performance characteristics of the Starr–Edwards Model 6120 mitral valve prosthesis. J Thorac Cardiovasc Surg 85:1–20
6. Schoevaerdts JC, Buche M, el Gariani A et al. (1987) Twenty years' experience with the Model 6120 Starr–Edwards valve in the mitral position. J Thorac Cardiovasc Surg 94:375–382
7. Miller DC, Oyer PE, Mitchell RS et al. (1984) Performance characteristics of the Starr–Edwards Model 1260 aortic valve prosthesis beyond ten years. J Thorac Cardiovasc Surg 88:193–207
8. Godje OL, Fischlein T, Adelhard K et al. (1997) Thirty-year results of Starr–Edwards prostheses in the aortic and mitral position. Ann Thorac Surg 63:613–619
9. Murday AJ, Hochstitzky A, Mansfield J et al. (2003) A prospective controlled trial of St. Jude versus Starr–Edwards aortic and mitral valve prostheses. Ann Thorac Surg 76:66–74
10. Abdulali SA, Silverton NP, Schoen FJ et al. (1984) Late outcome of patients with Braunwald–Cutter mitral valve replacement. Ann Thorac Surg 38:579–585
11. Jonas RA, Garratt-Boyes BG, Kerr AR et al. (1982) Late follow-up of the Braunwald–Cutter valve. Ann Thorac Surg 33:554–561

12. Huber S, Burckhardt D, Raeder EA et al. (1980) Complications in patients with cloth-covered Starr–Edwards prostheses. J Cardiovasc Surg (Torino) 21:19–24
13. Sezai A, Hata M, Niino T et al. (2007) Prophylactic reoperation after mitral valve replacement with the Starr–Edwards ball valve: a report of four cases. Ann Thorac Cardiovasc Surg 13:316–321
14. Winter TQ, Reis RL, Glancy DL et al. (1972) Current status of the Starr–Edwards cloth-covered prosthetic cardiac valves. Circulation 45:I14–I24
15. Basta LL, Wolfson P, Kioschos JM et al. (1974) Clinical and angiographic features of Beall-valve-disc variance. J Cardiovasc Surg (Torino) 15:679–683
16. Joob AW, Kron IL, Craddock GB et al. (1985) A decade of experience with the model 103 and 104 Beall valve prostheses. J Thorac Cardiovasc Surg 89:444–447
17. Bjork VO (1969) A new tilting disc valve prosthesis. Scand J Thorac Cardiovasc Surg 3:1–10
18. Björk VO (1987) The Björk–Shiley tilting disc valve: past, present and future. Cardiac Surgery: state of the art reviews 1:183–202
19. Birkmeyer JD, Marrin CA, O'Connor GT (1992) Should patients with Bjork–Shiley valves undergo prophylactic replacement? Lancet 340:520–523
20. Blackstone EH, Kirklin JW (1992) Recommendations for prophylactic removal of heart valve prostheses. J Heart Valve Dis 1:3–14
21. van der Graaf Y, de Waard F, van Herwerden LA et al. (1992) Risk of strut fracture of Bjork–Shiley valves. Lancet 339:257–261
22. Butchart EG, Li HH, Payne N et al. (2001) Twenty years' experience with the Medtronic Hall valve. J Thorac Cardiovasc Surg 121:1090–1100
23. Kleine P, Hasenkam MJ, Nygaard H et al. (2000) Tilting disc versus bileaflet aortic valve substitutes: intraoperative and postoperative hemodynamic performance in humans. J Heart Valve Dis 9:308–312
24. Bernet FH, Baykut D, Grize L et al. (2007) Single-center outcome analysis of 1,161 patients with St. Jude medical and

ATS open pivot mechanical heart valves. J Heart Valve Dis 16:151–158
25. Emery RW, Krogh CC, Arom KV et al. (2005) The St. Jude Medical cardiac valve prosthesis: a 25-year experience with single valve replacement. Ann Thorac Surg 79:776–783
26. Chambers J (1997) Editorial comment on hemodynamic evaluation of the CarboMedics, St. Jude Medical HP and Sorin–Bicarbon valve in patients with small aortic anulus: Noera et al. Eur J Cardiothorac Surg 11:477–478
27. Roedler S, Czerny M, Neuhauser J et al. (2008) Mechanical aortic valve prostheses in the small aortic root: Top Hat versus standard CarboMedics aortic valve. Ann Thorac Surg 86:64–70
28. Jamieson WR, Koerfer R, Yankah CA et al. (2009) Mitroflow aortic pericardial bioprosthesis: clinical performance. Eur J Cardiothorac Surg 36:818–824
29. Clark JN, Ogle MF, Ashworth P et al. (2005) Prevention of calcification of bioprosthetic heart valve cusp and aortic wall with ethanol and aluminum chloride. Ann Thorac Surg 79:897–904
30. Schoen FJ, Levy RJ (2005) Calcification of tissue heart valve substitutes: progress toward understanding and prevention. Ann Thorac Surg 79:1072–1080
31. Borger MA, Preston M, Ivanov J et al. (2004) Should the ascending aorta be replaced more frequently in patients with bicuspid aortic valve disease? J Thorac Cardiovasc Surg 128:677–683
32. Jin XY, Pepper JR (2002) Do stentless valves make a difference? Eur J Cardiothorac Surg 22:95–100
33. Westaby S, Horton M, Jin XY et al. (2000) Survival advantage of stentless aortic bioprostheses. Ann Thorac Surg 70:785–791
34. Ali A, Halstead JC, Cafferty F et al. (2007) Early clinical and hemodynamic outcomes after stented and stentless aortic valve replacement: results from a randomized controlled trial. Ann Thorac Surg 83:2162–2168
35. Bove T, Van Belleghem Y, Francois K et al. (2006) Stentless and stented aortic valve replacement in elderly patients: factors affecting midterm clinical and hemodynamical outcome. Eur J Cardiothorac Surg 30:706–713

36. Cohen G, Christakis GT, Joyner CD et al. (2002) Are stentless valves hemodynamically superior to stented valves? A prospective randomized trial. Ann Thorac Surg 73:767–778
37. Desai ND, Merin O, Cohen GN et al. (2004) Long-term results of aortic valve replacement with the St. Jude Toronto stentless porcine valve. Ann Thorac Surg 78:2076–2083
38. Doss M, Martens S, Wood JP et al. (2003) Performance of stentless versus stented aortic valve bioprostheses in the elderly patient: a prospective randomized trial. Eur J Cardiothorac Surg 23:299–304
39. Chambers JB, Rimington HM, Hodson F et al. (2006) The subcoronary Toronto stentless versus supra-annular Perimount stented replacement aortic valve: early clinical and hemodynamic results of a randomized comparison in 160 patients. J Thorac Cardiovasc Surg 131:878–882
40. Kallikourdis A, Jacob S (2007) Is a stentless aortic valve superior to conventional bioprosthetic valves for aortic valve replacement? Interact Cardiovasc Thorac Surg 6:665–672
41. Risteski PS, Martens S, Rouhollahpour A et al. (2009) Prospective randomized evaluation of stentless vs. stented aortic biologic prosthetic valves in the elderly at five years. Interact Cardiovasc Thorac Surg 8:449–453
42. Harringer W, Loose R, Guha M et al. (1998) Long term results of aortic valve replacement with allografts: thirteen years follow-up. Cor Europaeum 7:29–32
43. O'Brien MF, Harrocks S, Stafford EG et al. (2001) The homograft aortic valve: a 29-year, 99.3% follow up of 1,022 valve replacements. J Heart Valve Dis 10:334–344

Choice of the Optimal Valve for Replacement

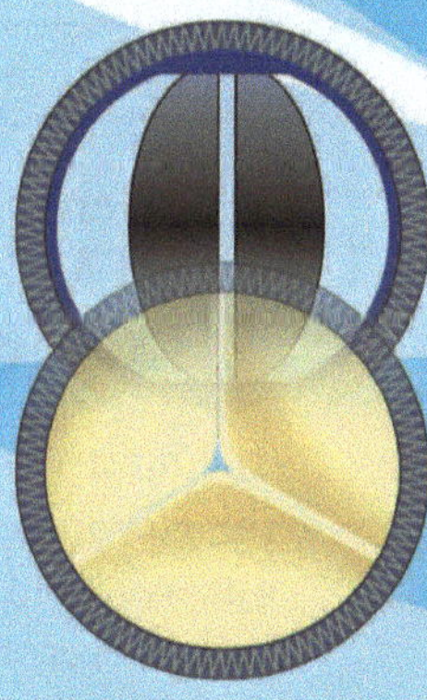

4 Choice of the Optimal Valve for Replacement

4.1 Introduction

There is a plenitude of mechanical and biological valve prostheses available for surgeons' use. Choice of the optimal valve replacement device may not always be easy, because there does not exist a single valve considered to be the best and most suitable for all patients and situations; however, there always exists a valve that is optimal for a given patient.

The fundamental step is to decide between a mechanical or a tissue valve [1, 2]. The choice of some type of mechanical prosthesis or biological valve is of lesser importance. The decision-making process has to reflect the general advantages and drawbacks of mechanical valves, bioprostheses, allografts, and autografts in relation to the particular patient planned for heart valve replacement.

4.2 General Advantages and Drawbacks of Mechanical Prostheses, Bioprostheses, Allografts, and Autografts

The most valuable feature of modern mechanical valves is the guarantee of their lifelong functional durability without wear and structural dysfunction. The main drawback is, however, the necessity of permanent anticoagulation. Anticoagulation therapy is associated with constant risk of bleeding complications and grossly complicates traumatic events, inevitable operation, or onset of disease contraindicating anticoagulation. The incidence of bleeding compli-

J. Dominik and P. Zacek, *Heart Valve Surgery: An Illustrated Guide*,
DOI 10.1007/978-3-642-12206-4_4,

cations has decreased slightly in comparison with previous studies. The reason is that a lower value of international normalized ratio (INR) is required in aortic valve replacement. Safer anticoagulation drugs may also be expected in the future as well as wider spread of self-monitoring and self-management, which will make anticoagulation therapy even safer [3, 4].

The main advantage of the bioprostheses is the fact that after operation, patients do not need permanent anticoagulation therapy. Anticoagulation is discontinued 3 months after implantation of aortic bioprosthesis (if no other reasons for anticoagulation exist) and patients are left on antiaggregation medication only. In recent years the inevitability of this short-term anticoagulation therapy has been widely debated. Many cardiac surgeons already do not administer anticoagulation after implantation of bioprosthesis into aortic position and an increasing number of studies give evidence of its needlessness; therefore, presently postoperative heparinization during hospital stay followed by antiaggregation medication only (in absence of other reasons for anticoagulation) can be accepted as a correct treatment [2, 5–14].

The main and most serious drawback of bioprotheses is the uncertainty about their long-term proper function. Dysfunction is a result of gradual development of degenerative changes that cause stiffness of calcified bioprosthetic cusps (Fig. 4.1). The cusp may sometimes even tear away from the bioprosthetic stent (Fig. 9.5). In this way the bioprosthesis develops hemodynamically significant stenosis, regurgitation, or a combination of both. Clinically relevant bioprosthesis dysfunction then necessitates relatively demanding reoperation in, as a rule, elderly and comorbid patients.

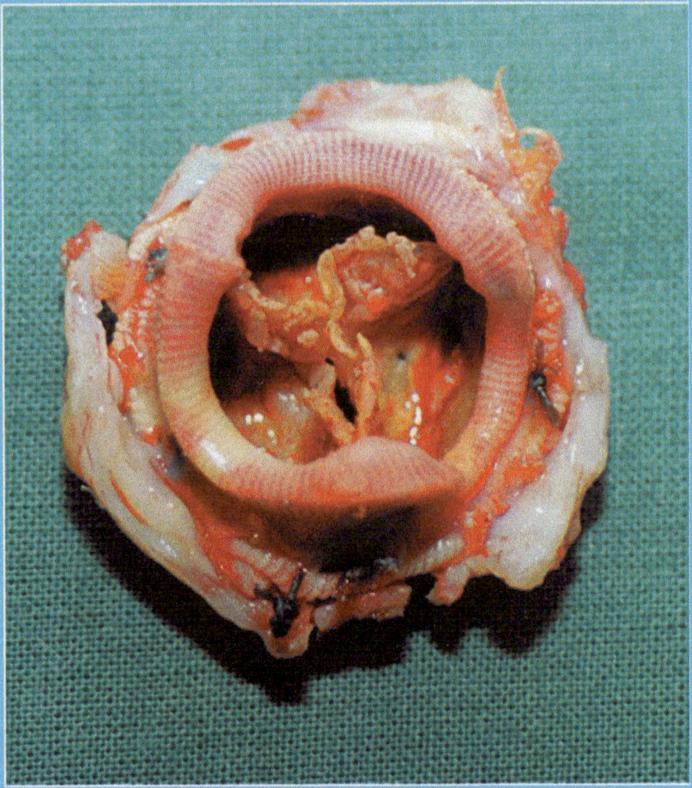

Fig. 4.1 Degenerative changes in the cusps of bioprosthesis (calcifications). Bioprosthesis explanted 8 years after implantation

The rate of development of bioprosthesis degeneration depends above all on the recipient's age and stress load of the valve cusps [15]. In childhood the onset of degeneration is rapid; valve failure occurs in almost 50% of the operated children after 4 years and in 80% at 6 years.

In adults below the age of 60 years bioprosthesis failure is reported in approximately 5% of cases within 5 years, 20% within 8 years, 30% within 10 years, and 50% within 15 years, respectively. In patients under 65 years of age the risk for structural valve deterioration began to increase 7 years postoperatively [16]. At the age between 60 and 70 years the incidence of bioprosthesis failure is 15% in first 15 years, and in patients over 70 years bioprosthesis failure occurs in 3–10% of cases within 15 years after operation [16–19].

Since the process of implanting bioprostheses with anticalcification treatment is just over 10 years old, in the near future research data will answer the question as to whether modern tissue-processing techniques in bioprostheses manufacturing will delay the onset of degeneration [15].

The allograft degeneration rate is similar to that of bioprostheses [20, 21]. Allograft implantation is, however, technically more demanding and time-consuming, and also expected reoperation due to degeneration is more difficult compared with reoperation after bioprosthesis implantation [3, 22]. The need for reoperation is reported to be 50% within 12–16 years in patients with a mean age 45 years [21, 23]. The younger the recipient is, the sooner the allograft degenerates. In addition, increasing donor's age, male donor's gender, and larger allograft diameter also negatively affect freedom from degeneration [21, 23–25]. Allografts do not require antithrombotic medication and display lower pressure gradient compared with stented bioprostheses. Lesser susceptibility to infection is another important advantage of allografts, which are therefore useful in aortic valve endocarditis, namely in periannular spread of infection [21, 22, 25].

The balance between the advantages and drawbacks of the Ross procedure (aortic valve replacement with pulmonary autograft) in selected young patients with aortic valve disease has been debated for more than 30 years. An unquestionable advantage is that after the Ross procedure, patients do not need anticoagulation or even antiaggregation medication and therefore avoid the risk of bleeding and thromboembolic complications. The risk of endocarditis is also substantially lower compared with bioprostheses. Durability of autografts at the aortic position in these young patients is unparalleled to xenografts or allografts. On the other hand, the Ross procedure is technically very demanding operation with approximately three times longer duration of cardiopulmonary bypass than at prosthesis implantation. Operative mortality of this extensive surgery is significantly higher than mortality of aortic valve replacement with mechanical prosthesis, which in this young age group should range below 1% [26]. According to the international Ross procedure registry, the mortality rate in recent years has oscillated between 3 and 4% (some authors report lower and higher mortality rates as well) [27–31]. Long-term results of the Ross procedure are as important as the early results. The largest cohort is the Ross procedure registry containing data from 5000 operated patients. According to this registry, extensive reoperation is required in 20% of the patients within the first 10 years (11% for autograft failure, 9% for allograft failure) [32]. Other articles report the need for reoperation in 16–30% in the first decade [28–31, 33–35]. The Ross procedure can be perceived as an irreplaceable operation in children (autograft has a growth potential) [27, 31] and a possible, but very controversial, alternative for young and active patients who wish to avoid anticoagulation therapy [36]. The Ross procedure is not suitable for young patients with rheumatic heart disease [30, 37]. After accurate information about the operative risks and expectations of difficult reoperation, if the patient still wishes to have this procedure, it should be performed. The operation should be carried out by a surgeon who is very experienced in the procedure and performs it frequently.

4.3 Factors that Affect the Choice of the Valve Replacement Device

In a given patient planned for valve replacement, all the abovementioned advantages and drawbacks of mechanical and biological valves have to be carefully evaluated. In some patients the choice is straightforward, because the relevant factors clearly indicate either mechanical or biological valve. Other patients have conflicting factors, and careful evaluation is needed to choose a valve with maximum benefits and minimum drawbacks for each individual. The patient's own preference, after receiving accurate information, also has to be taken into consideration.

The most important factor is the age of the patient and his attitude toward the anticoagulation therapy. Anticoagulation influences almost all factors. Other factors are the size and quality of the annulus, the presence or absence of thromboembolism risk factors, gender, comorbidities, life expectancy, and in cases of valve reoperation, the cause.

Correct and deliberate choice of the valve for replacement contributes positively to the patient's quality of life, reduction of complications in the long term, and prolongation of life span. It is one of the ways to improve the long-term results of heart valve replacement.

4.3.1 Age

The recommended age limit after which a tissue valve should be preferred over the mechanical one is considered to be 60–75 years (majority of the guidelines report 65 years) [2, 20, 38–46]. Shifting of the age limit above 65 years originates from duly justified concerns of high-risk tissue-valve reoperations in octogenarians and elderly polymorbid patients [43, 47]. On the contrary, setting the age limit below 65 years is based on the belief that currently performed antidegenerative processing will ensure much longer durability of the modern tissue valves. The exact data will be available in a few years, because the bioprostheses with antidegenerative processing have been implanted only since the mid-1990s; therefore, the long-term results will soon answer the question as to whether enthusiasm for such processed tissue valves is justified. Currently, the prevailing opinion, in accordance with the majority of the guidelines, is to implant tissue valves in the patients older than 65 years in case of aortic position, and in those above 70 years in case of mitral position [18].

Improved myocardial protection and even more sophisticated perioperative care resulted in reduced risk of heart reoperation when required for tissue-valve failure. For example, the estimated risk of death at reoperation for a 73-year--old man without significant comorbidities is 5% (additive Euroscore) and 9% (logistic Euroscore). This may trigger a debate regarding why not to implant modern tissue valves with antidegenerative processing, even in the patients over 50 years, and accept the fact of probable reoperation after 15–20 years. Questions remain to be answered as to whether this given risk of reoperation exceeds the accumulated risk of 15–20 years of the life with mechanical valve and with inevitable anticoagulation. Reoperation in many of these patients would, however, be more risky due to polymorbidity acquired in the interim [1].

4.3.2 Attitude to the Anticoagulation Therapy

The patient's attitude to the anticoagulation therapy is crucial in decision making. Patients with contraindication for anticoagulation therapy and those in whom effectively controlled anticoagulation therapy cannot be guaranteed (e.g., undisciplined patients, alcoholics, patients refusing medication, patients from developing countries, troublesome or unavailable medical care) should be offered tissue valves. On the other hand, mechanical valve is a proper choice for patients already on chronic anticoagulation for other medical reasons [2, 38].

4.3.3 Size and Quality of the Annulus

The size and quality of the patient's annulus also affects the choice of the optimal valve for replacement. For heavily calcified, rigid, and rough annulus it is advantageous to choose the valve with a wide and soft sewing ring that can comply with uneven surface of the annulus. If the annulus is damaged due to native-valve endocarditis or prosthetic endocarditis, the optimal choice for the aortic orifice is allograft because of documented lesser susceptibility to infection compared with mechanical valve or bioprosthesis [17].

On the other hand, numerous authors report very similar results obtained with prostheses and bioprostheses. Actually, allografts are being implanted in only 5% of patients operated for endocarditis. In case the annulus is not severely affected by endocarditis, it is possible to implant prosthesis or bioprosthesis after excision of the valve with vegetations, careful debridement of all infected tissues, and disinfection of the annulus [48–53]. If infection, however, damages the annulus, spreads beyond it, and forms periannular abscesses, allograft implantation is the optimal choice for aortic position [21, 22, 38, 54]. A good alternative to allografts for valve replacement in active endocarditis complicated by annular abscess is implantation of stentless bioprosthesis [55].

The size of the aortic annulus plays an important role in patients with small aortic annulus and simultaneously large body-surface area in whom a valve with the largest possible effective orifice area has to be chosen to avoid patient–prosthesis mismatch. Patient–prosthesis mismatch is a clinical condition characterized by too small an effective orifice area with regard to the patient's body-surface area. Hemodynamically, this situation results in increased gradient at the correctly implanted valve, slower postoperative left ventricular hypertrophy regression, and higher operative mortality (in particular in patients with severe left ventricular hypertrophy) [56–59].

A cut-off value stated usually for a significant patient–prosthesis mismatch is indexed effective orifice area of the implanted valve less than 0.85 cm^2/m^2, whereas the value below 0.65 cm^2/m^2 represents severe patient–prosthesis mismatch [56, 60]. Effort is therefore aimed at implanting such a valve into the aortic position to avoid patient–prosthesis mismatch [56, 60–63]. Since modern mechanical aortic valves designed for small aortic annuli have larger orifice area compared with stented bioprostheses, they sometimes have to be implanted even in those elderly patients with small annulus who should otherwise receive a bioprosthesis. This strategy has been supported by two recent articles that document surprisingly superior early- and long-term results after implantation of mechanical prostheses in octogenarians [64, 65]. In recent years, however, bioprostheses designed for supraannular implantation are available with an effective orifice area that almost equals that of mechanical valves. As a result, implantations of stentless bioprostheses that increase the operative risk in elderly and polymorbid patients by 1–2% (longer and technically more demanding implantation) are becoming less frequent.

4.3.4 Risk of Thromboembolism

Risk factors for thromboembolism are atrial fibrillation, large left atrium (>55 mm), history of thromboembolism, presence of thrombi in the left atrium, and postinfarction left ventricular dyskinesis with thrombus. The presence of these risk factors dictates the necessity of long-term anticoagulation therapy, and therefore such patients should be given a mechanical valve. If only atrial fibrillation is present, it can be abolished surgically (with 75% success rate) (radiofrequency or cryosurgical ablation) and then a bioprosthesis can be implanted in patients 65–70 years and older.

4.3.5 Pregnancy

The most problematic issue is the choice of valve for women who wish to get pregnant subsequently. Implantation of a bioprosthesis enables relatively problem-free pregnancy but is hampered by two drawbacks. Firstly, the mother is at inevitable risk of reoperation for early bioprosthesis degeneration. Secondly, in some instances the planned pregnancy may not occur immediately but later, at the time of already developed severe valve disease caused by bioprosthesis degeneration.

In case of the aortic valve, the Ross procedure may also be chosen. The Ross procedure, however, carries a higher operative risk together with the risk of reoperation (although reoperations after the Ross procedure are necessary much later than after bioprosthesis implantation and are, in fact, generally required for late pulmonary allograft degeneration rather than for autograft failure).

The role of the allograft at the aortic position in young women does not differ greatly from a bioprosthesis, except for a more demanding technique of implantation and more difficult reoperation.

Implantation of a mechanical valve is a definitive solution for the mother and perhaps the most reasonable option. Difficulties, however, arise with the anticoagulation therapy during pregnancy [38, 66]. Administration of warfarin during the 6–12 weeks of pregnancy may cause in 5–10% of cases the so-called fetal warfarin syndrome (embryopathy). To avoid this serious complication, warfarin administration should be stopped within 6–12 weeks (eventually during the first trimester) of pregnancy and replaced by heparin [2, 38]. Warfarin is safe again from the second trimester, and later, in the 36th week, it has to be replaced again by heparin. If the required level of INR can be maintained by warfarin in a daily dose not exceeding 5 mg, then the risk of warfarin syndrome is minimal [67]. In such a case warfarin can be administered throughout the whole pregnancy until its replacement by heparin in the 36th week.

Heparin anticoagulation throughout the whole pregnancy is safe for the fetus but dangerous for the mother (thromboembolic complications) and therefore not recommended [2, 38].

The decision between the abovementioned treatment options is always problematic and depends on the informed patient's preference. The safest alternative is the implantation of a mechanical valve, which will also enable pregnancy after several years.

4.3.6 Other Factors

Concomitant diseases may, by their nature, require or contraindicate chronic anticoagulation. This directly affects the decision between mechanical and biological valve. Among other comorbidities, chronic renal failure accelerates the development of degenerative changes at the tissue-valve cusps, and therefore mechanical valves should be implanted to these patients (unless their life expectancy is short) [2, 44–45, 68].

Site of implantation has a significant impact on choice of the valve. The rate of degeneration of bioprostheses is influenced most of all by the patient's age, but amount of stress load also plays a role [15, 69]. Maximum stress load occurs at the mitral valve, and therefore age-limit recommendation for tissue-valve implantation should be at least 5 years higher for the mitral position than for the aortic position [20]. Least stress load is at the pulmonary and tricuspid valves. Though replacement of these valves is performed relatively rarely, it is generally recommended to implant bioprostheses into the tricuspid orifice [70–74] and bioprostheses or homografts into pulmonary position. Bioprosthesis in the tricuspid orifice allows later introduction of the pacemaker lead into the right ventricle (contrary to mechanical valves). Detrimental for mechanical valves is also their susceptibility to thrombosis in the low-pressure right-heart circulation.

Life expectancy affects the choice of the valve for patients whose life prognosis is limited to less than 10 years due to age or serious comorbidities. In such cases implantation of a bioprosthesis should be preferred [2, 44, 75].

At reoperation required for surprisingly early bioprosthesis failure, it is recommended to replace it with a mechanical valve. On the other hand, mechanical valve thrombosis during properly maintained anticoagulation therapy may be a reason for considering a bioprosthesis, which has a very low risk of thrombosis. If the patient already has one mechanical valve implanted and is on chronic anticoagulation therapy, the second valve (aortic or mitral) should also be a mechanical one [2, 38, 45].

References

1. El Oakley R, Kleine P, Bach DS (2008) Choice of prosthetic heart valve in today's practice. Circulation 117:253–256
2. Vahanian A, Baumgartner H, Bax J et al. (2007) Guidelines on the management of valvular heart disease: The Task Force on the Management of Valvular Heart Disease of the European Society of Cardiology. Eur Heart J 28:230–268
3. Dagenais F, Cartier P, Voisine P et al. (2005) Which biologic valve should we select for the 45- to 65-year-old age group requiring aortic valve replacement? J Thorac Cardiovasc Surg 129:1041–1049
4. Herijgers P, Verhamme P (2007) Improving the quality of anticoagulant therapy in patients with mechanical heart valves: What are we waiting for? Eur Heart J 28:2424–2426

5. Colli A, Verhoye JP, Heijmen R et al. (2008) Antithrombotic therapy after bioprosthetic aortic valve replacement: ACTION Registry survey results. Eur J Cardiothorac Surg 33:531–536
6. Colli A, Verhoye JP, Leguerrier A et al. (2007) Anticoagulation or antiplatelet therapy of bioprosthetic heart valves recipients: an unresolved issue. Eur J Cardiothorac Surg 31:573–577
7. Marco F di, Meneghetti G, Gerosa G (2005) Early anticoagulation after aortic valve replacement with bioprostheses: Time to abandon it? J Thorac Cardiovasc Surg 130:1482–1483
8. Dunning J, Versteegh M, Fabbri A et al. (2008) Guideline on antiplatelet and anticoagulation management in cardiac surgery. Eur J Cardiothorac Surg 34:73–92
9. El-Husseiny M, Salhiyyah K, Raja SG et al. (2006) Should warfarin be routinely prescribed for the first three months after a bioprosthetic valve replacement? Interact Cardiovasc Thorac Surg 5:616–623
10. Gherli T, Colli A, Fragnito C et al. (2004) Comparing warfarin with aspirin after biological aortic valve replacement: a prospective study. Circulation 110:496–500
11. Goldsmith I, Turpie AG, Lip GY (2002) Valvar heart disease and prosthetic heart valves. Br Med J 325:1228–1231
12. Nowell J, Wilton E, Markus H et al. (2007) Antithrombotic therapy following bioprosthetic aortic valve replacement. Eur J Cardiothorac Surg 31:578–585
13. Sundt TM, Zehr KJ, Dearani JA et al. (2005) Is early anticoagulation with warfarin necessary after bioprosthetic aortic valve replacement? J Thorac Cardiovasc Surg 129:1024–1031
14. Vaughan P, Waterworth PD (2005) An audit of anticoagulation practice among UK cardiothoracic consultant surgeons following valve replacement/repair. J Heart Valve Dis 14:576–582
15. Schoen FJ, Levy RJ (2005) Calcification of tissue heart valve substitutes: progress toward understanding and prevention. Ann Thorac Surg 79:1072–1080
16. Eichinger WB, Hettich IM, Ruzicka DJ et al. (2008) Twenty-year experience with the St. Jude medical Biocor bioprosthesis in the aortic position. Ann Thorac Surg 86:1204–1210

17. Aazami M, Schafers HJ (2003) Advances in heart valve surgery. J Interv Cardiol 16:535–541
18. Jamieson WR, Gudas VM, Burr LH et al. (2009) Mitral valve disease: if the mitral valve is not reparable/failed repair, is bioprosthesis suitable for replacement? Eur J Cardiothorac Surg 35:104–110
19. Jamieson WR, Koerfer R, Yankah CA et al. (2009) Mitroflow aortic pericardial bioprosthesis: clinical performance. Eur J Cardiothorac Surg 36:818–824
20. Rahimtoola SH (2003) Choice of prosthetic heart valve for adult patients. J Am Coll Cardiol 41:893–904
21. Takkenberg JJ, Klieverik LM, Bekkers JA et al. (2007) Allografts for aortic valve or root replacement: insights from an 18-year single-center prospective follow-up study. Eur J Cardiothorac Surg 31:851–859
22. Joudinaud TM, Baron F, Raffoul R et al. (2008) Redo aortic root surgery for failure of an aortic homograft is a major technical challenge. Eur J Cardiothorac Surg 33:989–994
23. Sadowski J, Kapelak B, Bartus K et al. (2003) Reoperation after fresh homograft replacement: 23 years' experience with 655 patients. Eur J Cardiothorac Surg 23:996–1001
24. Harringer W, Loose R, Guha M et al. (1998) Long-term results of aortic valve replacement with allografts: thirteen years follow--up. Cor Europaneum 7:29–32
25. O'Brien MF, Harrocks S, Stafford EG et al. (2001) The homograft aortic valve: a 29-year, 99.3% follow up of 1,022 valve replacements. J Heart Valve Dis 10:334–444
26. Brown JM, O'Brien SM, Wu C et al. (2009) Isolated aortic valve replacement in North America comprising 108,687 patients in 10 years: changes in risks, valve types, and outcomes in the Society of Thoracic Surgeons National Database. J Thorac Cardiovasc Surg 137:82–90
27. Al-Halees Z, Pieters F, Qadoura F et al. (2002) The Ross procedure is the procedure of choice for congenital aortic valve disease. J Thorac Cardiovasc Surg 123:437–442

28. Brown JW, Ruzmetov M, Shahriari A et al. (2009) Midterm results of Ross aortic valve replacement: a single-institution experience. Ann Thorac Surg 88:601–608
29. Kouchoukos NT, Masetti P, Nickerson NJ et al. (2004) The Ross procedure: long-term clinical and echocardiographic follow-up. Ann Thorac Surg 78:773–781
30. Kumar AS, Talwar S, Mohapatra R et al. (2005) Aortic valve replacement with the pulmonary autograft: mid-term results. Ann Thorac Surg 80:488–494
31. Pasquali SK, Shera D, Wernovsky G et al. (2007) Midterm outcomes and predictors of reintervention after the Ross procedure in infants, children, and young adults. J Thorac Cardiovasc Surg 133:893–899
32. Blauth C (2003) The Ross procedure in 2003. Cardiac Surgery Today 1:60–67
33. de Kerchove L, Rubay J, Pasquet A et al. (2009) Ross operation in the adult: long-term outcomes after root replacement and inclusion techniques. Ann Thorac Surg 87:95–102
34. Elkins RC, Thompson DM, Lane MM et al. (2008) Ross operation: 16-year experience. J Thorac Cardiovasc Surg 136:623–630
35. Luciani GB, Favaro A, Casali G et al. (2005) Ross operation in the young: a ten-year experience. Ann Thorac Surg 80:2271–2277
36. Jonas RA (2005) The Ross procedure is not the procedure of choice for the teenager requiring aortic valve replacement. Semin Thorac Cardiovasc Surg Pediatr Card Surg Annu:176–180
37. Sampath Kumar A, Talwar S, Saxena A et al. (2006) Ross procedure in rheumatic aortic valve disease. Eur J Cardiothorac Surg 29:156–161
38. Bonow RO, Carabello BA, Kanu C et al. (2006) ACC/AHA 2006 guidelines for the management of patients with valvular heart disease. A report of the American College of Cardiology/American Heart Association Task Force on Practice Guidelines (writing committee to revise the 1998 Guidelines for the Management of Patients With Valvular Heart Disease); developed in collaboration with the Society of Cardiovascular Anesthesiologists; endorsed by the Society for Cardiovascular Angiography

and Interventions and the Society of Thoracic Surgeons. Circulation 114:e84–e231
39. Brown ML, Schaff HV, Lahr BD et al. (2008) Aortic valve replacement in patients aged 50 to 70 years: improved outcome with mechanical versus biologic prostheses. J Thorac Cardiovasc Surg 135:878–884
40. Doss M, Martens S, Wood JP et al. (2003) Performance of stentless versus stented aortic valve bioprostheses in the elderly patient: a prospective randomized trial. Eur J Cardiothorac Surg 23:299–304
41. Chan V, Jamieson WR, Germann E et al. (2006) Performance of bioprostheses and mechanical prostheses assessed by composites of valve-related complications to 15 years after aortic valve replacement. J Thorac Cardiovasc Surg 131:1267–1273
42. Kulik A, Bedard P, Lam BK et al. (2006) Mechanical versus bioprosthetic valve replacement in middle-aged patients. Eur J Cardiothorac Surg 30:485–491
43. Logeais Y, Langanay T, Corbineau H et al. (1998) Aortic valve replacement in the elderly: Bioprosthesis or mechanical valve? Ann Thorac Surg 66:S77–S81
44. Peterseim DS, Cen YY, Cheruvu S et al. (1999) Long-term outcome after biologic versus mechanical aortic valve replacement in 841 patients. J Thorac Cardiovasc Surg 117:890–897
45. Unger F, Rainer WG, Horstkotte D et al. (2000) Standards and concepts in valve surgery. J Cardiovasc Surg (Torino) 41:585–593
46. Prasongsukarn K, Jamieson WR, Lichtenstein SV (2005) Performance of bioprostheses and mechanical prostheses in age group 61–70 years. J Heart Valve Dis 14:501–511
47. Ninet J, Tronc F, Robin J et al. (1998) Mechanical versus biological isolated aortic valvular replacement after the age of 70: equivalent long-term results. Eur J Cardiothorac Surg 13:84–89
48. Bauernschmitt R, Vahl CF, Lange R et al. (1996) Surgical treatment of acute endocarditis of the aortic valve with paravalvular abscess: considerations justifying the use of mechanical replacement devices. Eur J Cardiothorac Surg 10:741–747

49. Baumgartner FJ, Omari BO, Robertson JM et al. (2000) Annular abscesses in surgical endocarditis: anatomic, clinical, and operative features. Ann Thorac Surg 70:442–447
50. Gaudino M, Filippo C de, Pennestri F et al. (1997) The use of mechanical prostheses in native aortic valve endocarditis. J Heart Valve Dis 6:79–83
51. Klieverik LM, Yacoub MH, Edwards S et al. (2009) Surgical treatment of active native aortic valve endocarditis with allografts and mechanical prostheses. Ann Thorac Surg 88:1814–1821
52. Moon MR, Miller DC, Moore KA et al. (2001) Treatment of endocarditis with valve replacement: the question of tissue versus mechanical prosthesis. Ann Thorac Surg 71:1164–1171
53. Renzulli A, Carozza A, Romano G et al. (2001) Recurrent infective endocarditis: a multivariate analysis of 21 years of experience. Ann Thorac Surg 72:39–43
54. David TE, Regesta T, Gavra G et al. (2007) Surgical treatment of paravalvular abscess: long-term results. Eur J Cardiothorac Surg 31:43–48
55. Siniawski H, Lehmkuhl H, Weng Y et al. (2003) Stentless aortic valves as an alternative to homografts for valve replacement in active infective endocarditis complicated by ring abscess. Ann Thorac Surg 75:803–808
56. Blais C, Dumesnil JG, Baillot R et al. (2003) Impact of valve prosthesis–patient mismatch on short-term mortality after aortic valve replacement. Circulation 108:983–988
57. Fuster RG, Montero Argudo JA, Albarova OG et al. (2005) Patient–prosthesis mismatch in aortic valve replacement: Really tolerable? Eur J Cardiothorac Surg 27:441–449
58. Ruel M, Al-Faleh H, Kulik A et al. (2006) Prosthesis–patient mismatch after aortic valve replacement predominantly affects patients with preexisting left ventricular dysfunction: effect on survival, freedom from heart failure, and left ventricular mass regression. J Thorac Cardiovasc Surg 131:1036–1044
59. Tasca G, Brunelli F, Cirillo M et al. (2005) Impact of valve prosthesis–patient mismatch on left ventricular mass regression following aortic valve replacement. Ann Thorac Surg 79:505–510

60. Urso S, Sadaba R, Aldamiz-Echevarria G (2009) Is patient–prosthesis mismatch an independent risk factor for early and mid-term overall mortality in adult patients undergoing aortic valve replacement? Interact Cardiovasc Thorac Surg 9:510–518
61. David TE (2005) Is prosthesis–patient mismatch a clinically relevant entity? Circulation 111:3186–3187
62. Dumesnil JG, Pibarot P (2006) Prosthesis–patient mismatch and clinical outcomes: the evidence continues to accumulate. J Thorac Cardiovasc Surg 131:952–955
63. Pibarot P, Dumesnil JG (2000) Hemodynamic and clinical impact of prosthesis–patient mismatch in the aortic valve position and its prevention. J Am Coll Cardiol 36:1131–1141
64. de Vincentiis C, Kunkl AB, Trimarchi S et al. (2008) Aortic valve replacement in octogenarians: Is biologic valve the unique solution? Ann Thorac Surg 85:1296–1301
65. Vicchio M, Della Corte A, Santo LS de et al. (2008) Tissue versus mechanical prostheses: quality of life in octogenarians. Ann Thorac Surg 85:1290–1295
66. Al-Lawati AA, Venkitraman M, Al-Delaime T et al. (2002) Pregnancy and mechanical heart valves replacement: dilemma of anticoagulation. Eur J Cardiothorac Surg 22:223–227
67. Santo LS de, Romano G, Della Corte A et al. (2005) Mitral mechanical replacement in young rheumatic women: analysis of long-term survival, valve-related complications, and pregnancy outcomes over a 3707-patient-year follow-up. J Thorac Cardiovasc Surg 130:13–19
68. Chan V, Jamieson WR, Fleisher AG et al. (2006) Valve replacement surgery in end-stage renal failure: mechanical prostheses versus bioprostheses. Ann Thorac Surg 81:857–862
69. David TE, Armstrong S, Sun Z (1998) The Hancock II bioprosthesis at 12 years. Ann Thorac Surg 66:S95–S98
70. Guenther T, Noebauer C, Mazzitelli D et al. (2008) Tricuspid valve surgery: a thirty-year assessment of early and late outcome. Eur J Cardiothorac Surg 34:402–409
71. Kawano H, Oda T, Fukunaga S et al. (2000) Tricuspid valve replacement with the St. Jude Medical valve: 19 years of experience. Eur J Cardiothorac Surg 18:565–569

72. Kunadian B, Vijayalakshmi K, Balasubramanian S et al. (2007) Should the tricuspid valve be replaced with a mechanical or biological valve? Interact Cardiovasc Thorac Surg 6:551–557
73. Peterffy A, Szentkiralyi I (2001) Mechanical valves in tricuspid position: cause of thrombosis and prevention. Eur J Cardiothorac Surg 19:735–736
74. Rizzoli G, Vendramin I, Nesseris G et al. (2004) Biological or mechanical prostheses in tricuspid position? A meta-analysis of intra-institutional results. Ann Thorac Surg 77:1607–1614
75. Birkmeyer NJ, Birkmeyer JD, Tosteson AN et al. (2000) Prosthetic valve type for patients undergoing aortic valve replacement: a decision analysis. Ann Thorac Surg 70:1946–1952

Aortic Valve Surgery

5 Aortic Valve Surgery

5.1 Introduction

Hemodynamically significant aortic valve disease – both stenosis and regurgitation, regardless of its etiology – can be treated surgically. Adult patients with aortic stenosis require valve replacement with either mechanical or tissue valves. In patients with aortic regurgitation the valve can in some instances be repaired.

Aortic stenosis in infancy and childhood is usually not operated but treated with percutaneous balloon valvuloplasty. Balloon valvuloplasty of the aortic valve may, however, be chosen for elderly and polymorbid patients who would not tolerate cardiac surgery. The first balloon dilation of a calcified aortic valve was performed by Alain Cribier in Rouen in 1985. The increase in stenotic aortic valve area is followed by immediate decrease of afterload, decrease of the left ventricular filling pressure, decrease of pulmonary hypertension, and improvement of left ventricular ejection fraction. Formerly, the clinical improvement was only temporary due to early restenosis and therefore this method was only seldom employed. Continuous technological and procedural refinement has led to improvement of midterm results and to a certain renaissance of balloon valvuloplasty. It is beginning to be performed as a palliative alternative to valve replacement in elderly and comorbid patients contraindicated for surgery and also in patients with critical aortic stenosis who require vital major extracardiac surgery. The procedure can be repeated upon restenosis.

J. Dominik and P. Zacek, *Heart Valve Surgery: An Illustrated Guide*,
DOI 10.1007/978-3-642-12206-4_5,

The aortic valve can presently be implanted via a catheter from a transfemoral approach or transapically via the surgical left minithoracotomy. Since the first implantation by Cribier in 2002 the initial encouraging results have been built-upon in more than 10,000 patients. This costly procedure is at present reserved for those patients in whom the standard surgical procedure was contraindicated, usually on the basis of advanced age and serious comorbidities. Growing interest in this technique nevertheless suggests its dissemination to other cardiac centers. Future technical improvements and evidence of good long-term results will probably lead to more liberal indications for this method.

5.2 Aortic Stenosis

Aortic stenosis is the most common acquired valve disease in adults and the elderly in developed countries, and hence, the valve disease most frequently indicated for surgical treatment. Obstruction of the aortic valve orifice presents a long-term pressure overload of the left ventricle. During each myocardial contraction the systolic volume is ejected across the obstacle created by the stenotic aortic valve. As a result of adaptation to the permanent pressure overload, the left ventricle gradually develops concentric hypertrophy. This compensatory mechanism has, however, a negative impact: the decrease of coronary flow reserve and the development of left ventricular diastolic dysfunction. Clinical manifestation of the negative impact of ventricular hypertrophy is the classic triad of symptoms of significant aortic stenosis: (a) shortness of breath on effort; (b) angina pectoris; and (c) syncope. The concentric left ventricular hypertrophy is an independent risk factor for operative mortality at aortic valve replacement. In advanced state of aortic stenosis the left ventricular ejection fraction (EF) decreases, the cardiac output decreases, the pulmonary hypertension increases, and symptoms of the congestive heart failure appear.

Efficient medical treatment of aortic stenosis does not exist. Life expectancy of the patients with clinical manifestation of some of the classic symptoms is reported to be approximately 3 years, and only 1 year in those after the onset of congestive heart failure. Surgical treatment (valve replacement), with an average hospital mortality rate of 3% and excellent long-term results, presents a prominent therapeutic option.

5.2.1 Etiology of Aortic Stenosis

There are two leading etiological causes of aortic stenosis: congenital and degenerative stenosis. A third cause, rheumatic aortic stenosis, is much less prevalent in developed countries, and other causes remain very rare.

Congenital aortic stenosis is a relatively common disease with an incidence of 1–2%. Its hemodynamic severity varies. Clinical symptoms may appear immediately after birth at critical stenosis; or the stenosis remains hemodynamically insignificant for a long time and first signs appear only in adulthood. Congenital aortic stenosis is most frequently a valvular stenosis. Subvalvular stenosis is rare and supravalvular stenosis is extraordinarily rare.

Congenital valvular aortic stenosis is bicuspid [1, 2] or, rarely, unicuspid (Figs. 5.1, 5.2) [2]. Clinically important is the fact that the congenitally bicuspid aortic valve (stenosis and regurgitant) is frequently accompanied by

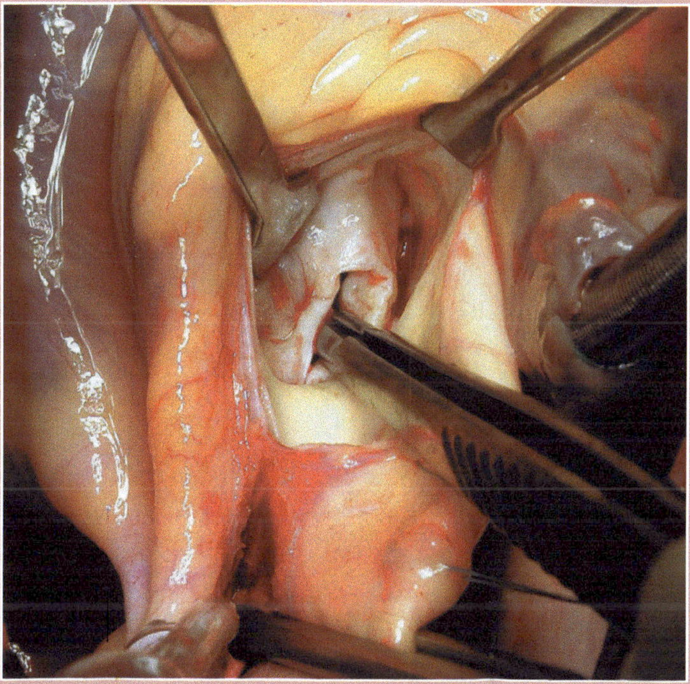

Fig. 5.1 Congenital unicuspid aortic valve

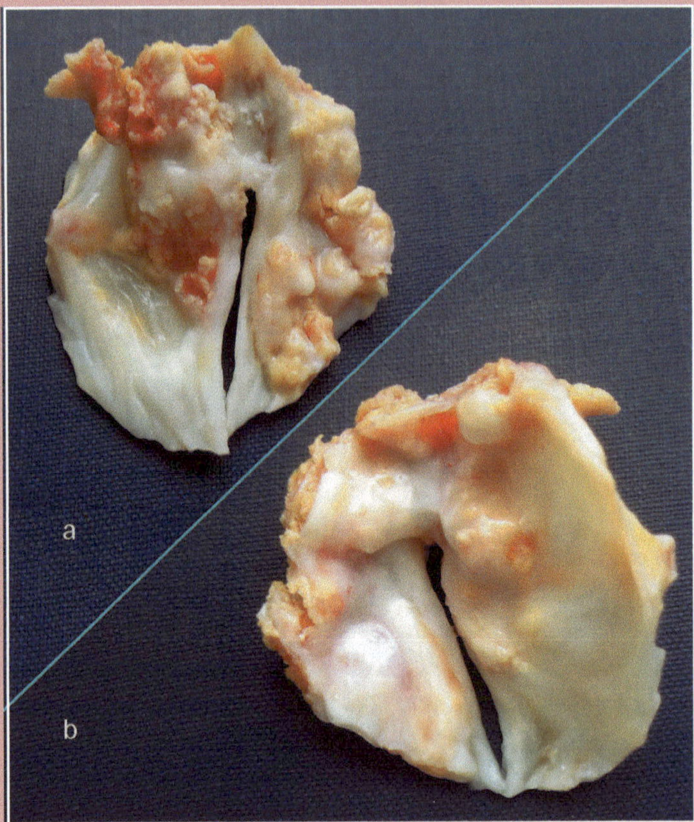

Fig. 5.2 Unicuspid unicommissural congenital aortic stenosis. Stenotic slit-like orifice and cusps penetrated by calcifications. **a** View from aorta. **b** View from left ventricle

gradually developing ascending aortic dilation (Fig. 5.3). The course of the aortic dilation is slow but constant and continues even after aortic valve replacement. Dilated ascending aorta at the bicuspid aortic valve carries a high risk of aortic dissection.

Senile degenerative calcific aortic stenosis has become the most frequent cause of aortic valve replacement. There is much similarity between the atheromatous plaque and the initial phase of development of the degenerative aortic stenosis, which is also called aortic sclerosis. Similar pathogenetic features of both aortic valvular disease and atherosclerosis favor the hypothesis that the main known risk factors for atherosclerosis are also risk factors for degenerative aortic stenosis. The advanced stage of the disease is characterized by the presence of extensive dystrophic calcifications in the aortic valvular cusps, which causes the rigidity of the valve. Often the calcifications grow in the annulus, the aortic root, and the anterior mitral leaflet. The commissures, however, are not fused (Figs. 5.4a, 5.5, 5.6).

Rheumatic aortic stenosis results in rigid stenotic or steno-incompetent orifice. In contrast to degenerative etiology, this calcified aortic stenosis typically has fused commissures (Figs. 5.4b, 5.7, 5.8). Rheumatic aortic stenosis gradually starts to become a rare valvular disease. It does not occur as an isolated aortic valve disease but only in cases of simultaneous involvement of the mitral valve (rheumatic aortic–mitral disease).

Other causes of aortic stenosis are extremely rare and only exceptionally may require surgery (e.g., rheumatoid heart disease, familiar hypercholesterolemia, lupus erythematosus, and ochronosis).

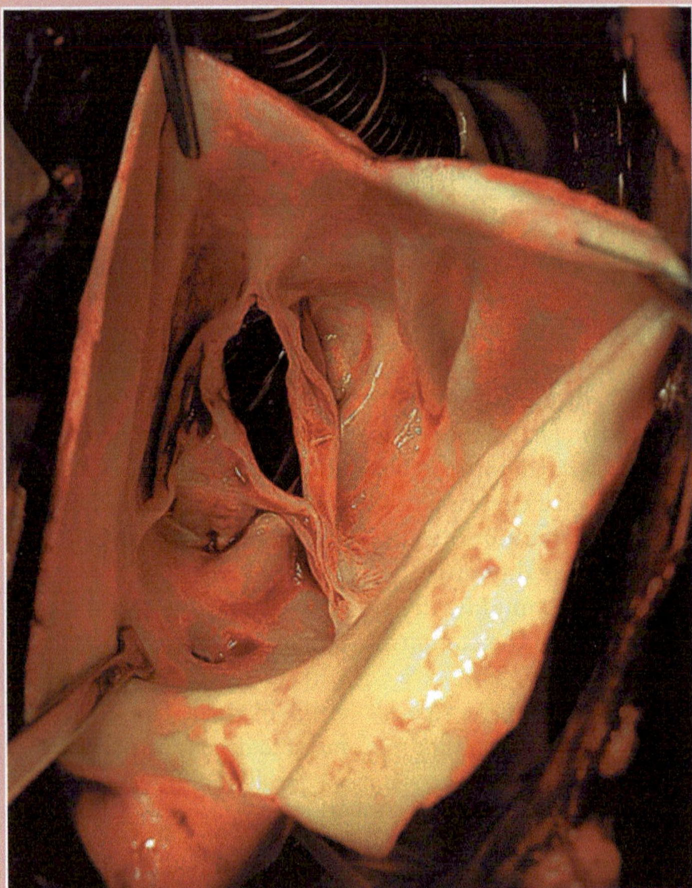

Fig. 5.3 Congenital bicuspid aortic valve with ascending aortic dilation

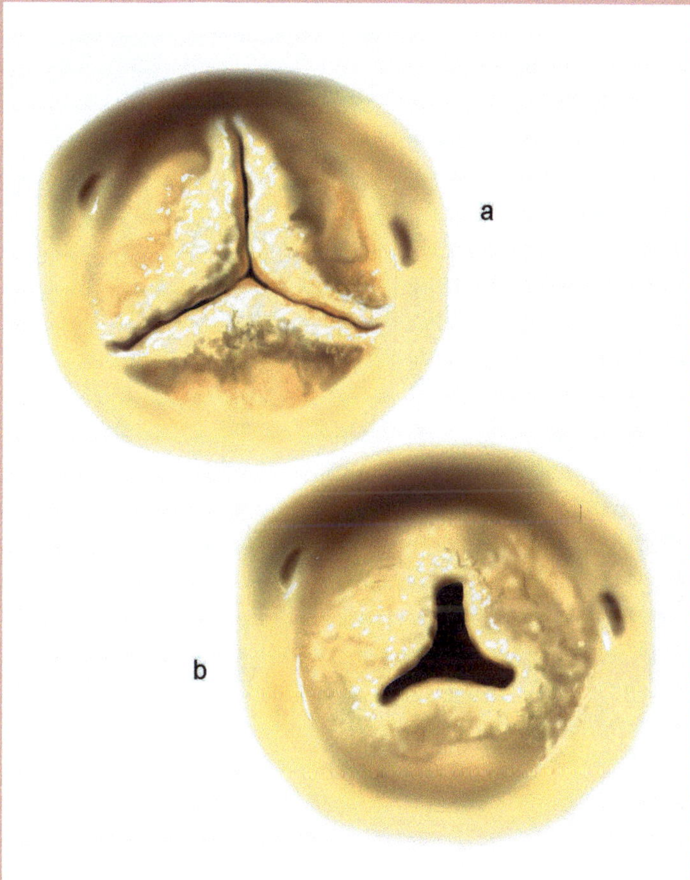

Fig. 5.4 Calcified aortic stenosis. **a** Degenerative etiology. **b** Rheumatic etiology

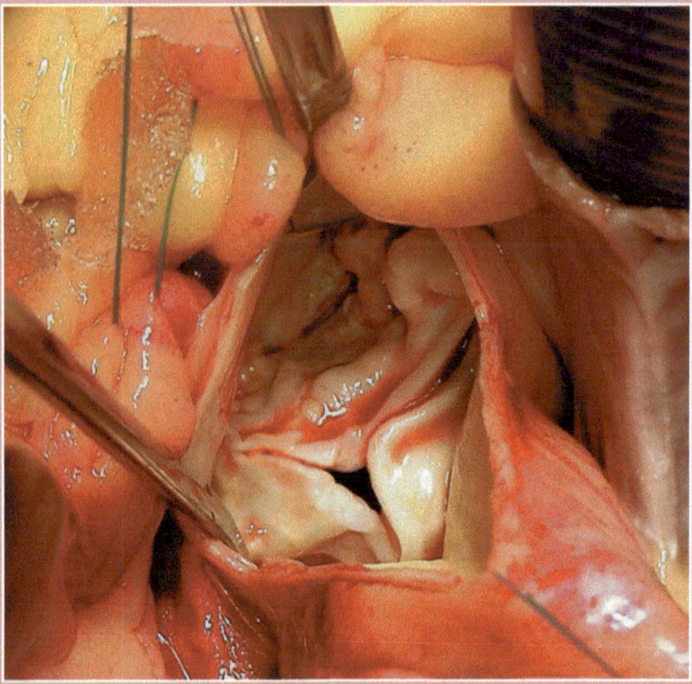

Fig. 5.5 Senile degenerative calcified aortic stenosis. Cusps penetrated by calcifications and commissures are not fused

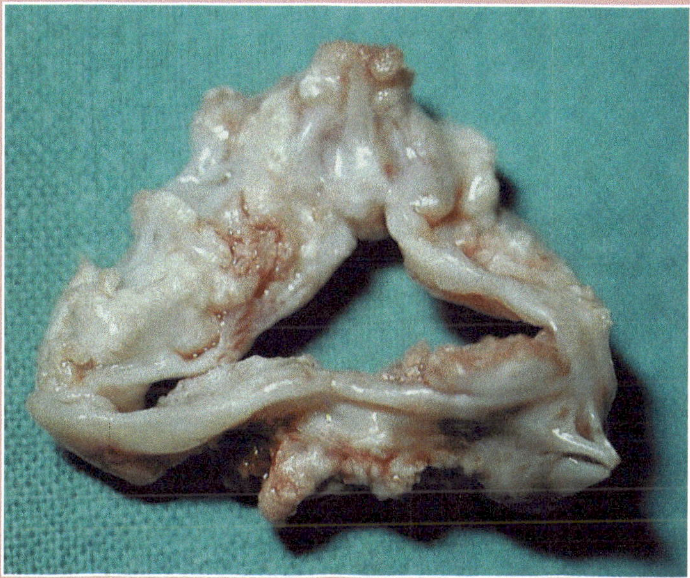

Fig. 5.6 Aortic valve excised for extensive calcifications in all cusps (degenerative etiology). Combined valve disease (stenosis and regurgitation)

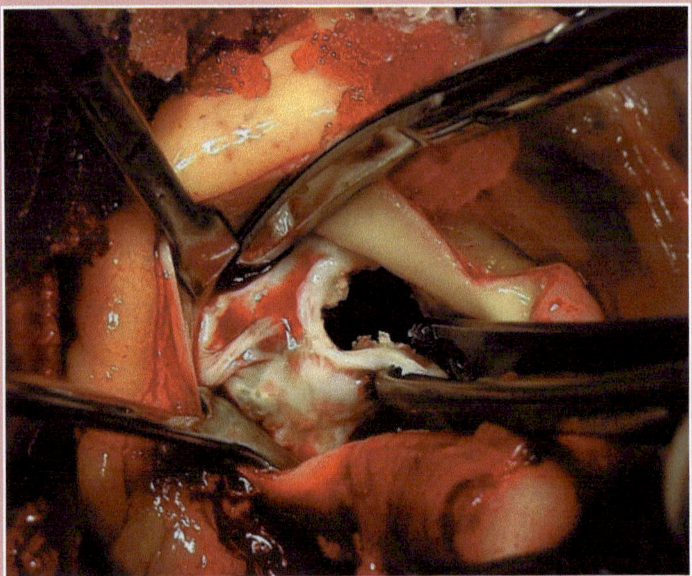

Fig. 5.7 Rheumatic aortic stenosis

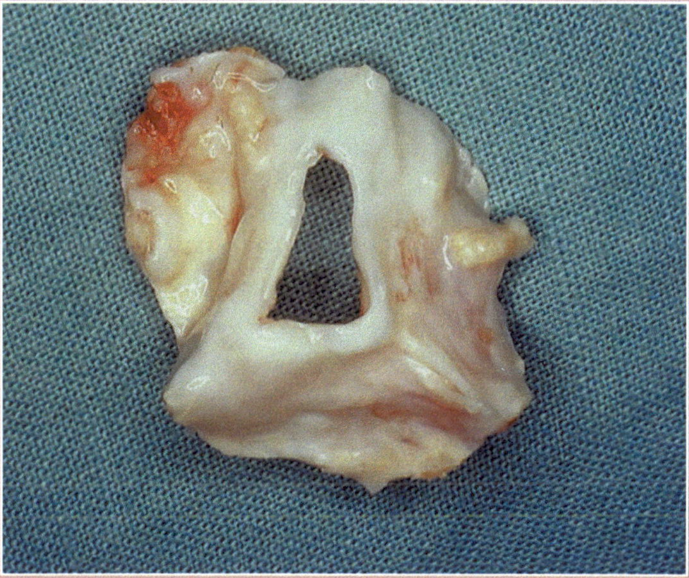

Fig. 5.8 Aortic valve excised for rheumatic aortic valve disease. Dominance of stenosis and concomitant regurgitation through a narrow rigid orifice. Calcified cusps and fused commissures

5.2.2 Indications for Surgery

In deciding whether the patient with aortic stenosis should be operated, one has to take into consideration:

1. If the patient is symptomatic or asymptomatic
2. What the degree of severity of the aortic stenosis is
3. Whether there is an isolated aortic valve procedure planned or a combined procedure [coronary artery bypass graft (CABG), mitral valve procedure, etc.]
4. What the left ventricular function and dimensions are
5. What the comorbidities are

Clinical symptoms of severe aortic stenosis present in a well-known triad: (a) dyspnea; (b) angina; and (c) syncope. Parameters of severe aortic stenosis are: (a) orifice area <0.5 cm^2/m^2 (the updated U.S. and European guidelines recommend the value of 0.6 cm^2/m^2, which, however, includes a lot of asymptomatic patients); (b) mean gradient >40 mmHg; and (c) maximum flow velocity (V_{max}) on aortic valve V_{max} >4 m/s [3, 4]. Gradients are significantly influenced by the cardiac output and therefore the aortic valve orifice area should be taken into consideration in preference.

5.2.2.1 Symptomatic Severe Aortic Stenosis

Symptomatic severe aortic stenosis is a straightforward indication for surgery [3, 4]. More difficult is the decision making in symptomatic aortic stenosis with low ejection fraction (EF <35%) and low gradient (mean gradient <30 mmHg) simultaneously. In these patients the myocardial contractile reserve has to be tested, usually by means of dobutamine stress echocardiography [3]. During this test the patients with myocardial contractile reserve display an increase of left ventricular EF of at least 10%, stroke volume of 20%, and an increase of mean gradient over 30 mmHg. The patients with proven myocardial contractile reserve are unequivocally indicated for operation [5, 6]. This population has very good early and long-term operative results. The patients without myocardial contractile reserve, however, have high operative mortality, and even those who survive have poor life expectancy similar to the patients on medication only; therefore, operation in these patients is not indicated or remains a dubious option, and the final decision is strictly individual. Young age, large annulus, absence of comorbidities, etc., may facilitate the decision to replace the aortic valve [7]; otherwise, heart transplantation is the only solution. Destination therapy (permanent mechanical assistance to the failing heart) has not been introduced routinely. Mechanical ventricular assistance devices are currently employed mostly like a bridge to transplant or to overcome otherwise untreatable phases of reversible heart failure.

5.2.2.2 Asymptomatic Severe Aortic Stenosis

Patients whose hemodynamic parameters correspond with severe aortic stenosis may occasionally be asymptomatic. Stress testing is mandatory in such patients to detect if they are truly asymptomatic. Pathological response to stress testing is blood pressure decrease, occurrence of arrhythmia, or ischemia. In cases of positive stress test, the operation is indicated even in these subjectively asymptomatic patients. If the patients with severe aortic stenosis are really asymptomatic, the aortic valve operation is indicated if the left ventricular systolic dysfunction is already present (EF <50%), if the patient is indicated for another cardiac procedure (e.g., CABG, other valve procedure) or other major non-cardiac operation, and in cases of planned pregnancy in women [3, 4].

If the patient with parameters of a severe aortic stenosis has excessive calcifications in the valve, his aortic valve orifice area is below 0.4 cm^2/m^2, and mean gradient exceeds 60 mmHg, the operation should not be delayed until the onset of symptoms. In cases of already heavily calcified aortic stenosis, the estimated rate of progression can be quantified by reduction of the aortic valve orifice to 0.14 cm^2 and increase of the mean gradient to 7 mm for each year [8].

Asymptomatic moderate aortic stenosis (valve orifice area 0.8–0.6 cm^2/m^2, mean gradient 25–40 mmHg, V_{max} 3–4 m/s) is indicated for valve replacement only as a concomitant procedure to coronary or other valve surgery [3, 4].

5.2.3 Surgical Treatment of Aortic Stenosis

Congenital valvular aortic stenosis may clinically manifest in early infancy with symptoms of critical cardiac defect, and in such a case percutaneous balloon valvuloplasty is the treatment of choice. The same strategy is applied in severe aortic stenosis in childhood. In older children and adolescents a more precise surgical solution, commissurotomy with use of cardiopulmonary bypass, should be preferred. Nevertheless, after percutaneous balloon valvuloplasty or surgical commissurotomy, all children are probable candidates for aortic valve surgery for valve restenosis, regurgitation, combined valve disease, or infective endocarditis within several years or several decades. Reoperation occurs in almost 50% of these children within 25 years after the primary intervention.

Congenital subvalvular aortic stenosis is caused by a membraneous or fibromuscular ring localized in the left ventricular outflow tract, usually 5–10 mm beneath the aortic annulus. Surgical treatment is resection of the ring via aortotomy through the aortic valve on an arrested heart with use of cardiopulmonary bypass. Indications for surgery should be earlier than in valvular stenosis to prevent damage of the leaflets from turbulent blood flow (Fig. 5.9).

Congenital subvalvular aortic stenosis is very rare in adults, contrary to congenital valvular aortic stenosis (i.e., bicuspid calcified aortic valve), which is relatively common.

The adult patients indicated for operation for aortic stenosis have the aortic valve damaged to such a degree that it does not allow any valve-sparing procedure; therefore, should the etiology of aortic valve stenosis be degenerative, congenital, or rheumatic, the treatment is always replacement of the valve. The aortic valve can be replaced with a mechanical valve, stented or stentless bioprosthesis, allograft (homograft), autograft (Ross procedure), or valved conduit (Bentall procedure). The advantages and drawbacks of the specific replacement devices, as well as the factors that go into decision making, are the topics of Chaps. 3 and 4.

5.2.3.1 Aortic Valve Replacement with a Prosthesis

Aortic valve replacement for senile degenerative calcified aortic stenosis is currently the most frequent valve operation. Other reasons for aortic valve replacement are congenital aortic valve stenosis and rheumatic aortic valve stenosis. Replacement of the aortic valve is indicated also for acute infective endocarditis if failure of antibiotic treatment is documented or after successful antibiotic treatment when endocarditis results in an incompetent aortic valve.

Non-infective aortic regurgitation, congenital or acquired, is mostly an indication for valve replacement as

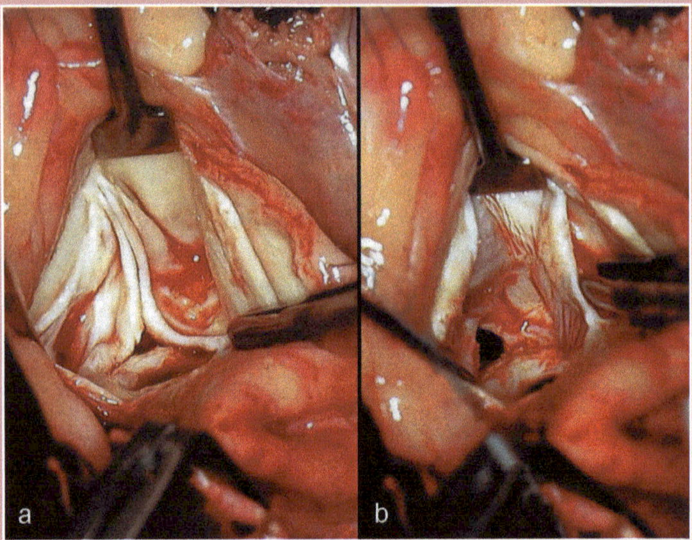

Fig. 5.9 Subvalvular aortic stenosis. **a** Thickened aortic cusps with mild retraction caused by turbulent flow above the subvalvular stenosis. **b** Subvalvular membranous aortic stenosis

well, though there is growing interest in saving the valve by means of various valve-sparing procedures (e.g., valve repair, remodelation, and reimplantation; see Sect. 5.3.3), and such efforts are being made.

The operation is usually performed using the classic median sternotomy approach. Less invasive approaches can also be used, preferably the upper partial sternotomy (upper hemisternotomy). In this technique a partial upper longitudinal sternotomy is carried to a level of third or fourth rib interspace where the right half of the sternum is transsected into the rib interspace (Fig. 5.10). The right internal thoracic artery should be salvaged; if injured, it is ligated. The right pleural cavity is left unopened. The supposed benefit of lesser invasiveness remained, however, unproven in several randomized studies. Moreover, a certain discomfort of the smaller approach did not result in an increase of complications. Technical disadvantages are the potential difficulties with insertion of the venous cannula, limited de-airing of the heart, difficult placement of the pacing wires and pericardial drains, absence of a visual control of the heart filling and contractility during weaning from cardiopulmonary bypass, and the need for application of the external defibrillation electrodes; thus, the only benefit consists of better cosmetic appearance (shorter incision) and impossibility of the postoperative sternal dehiscence [9–14]. Other less frequently used approaches are right-sided parasternal incision with transsection of the second, third, and fourth rib cartilage, and internal thoracic artery ligation, short right anterior thoracotomy, reversed Z-sternotomy, upper V-type ministernotomy, and the probably least used transverse sternotomy, necessitating ligation of both internal thoracic arteries [15–17].

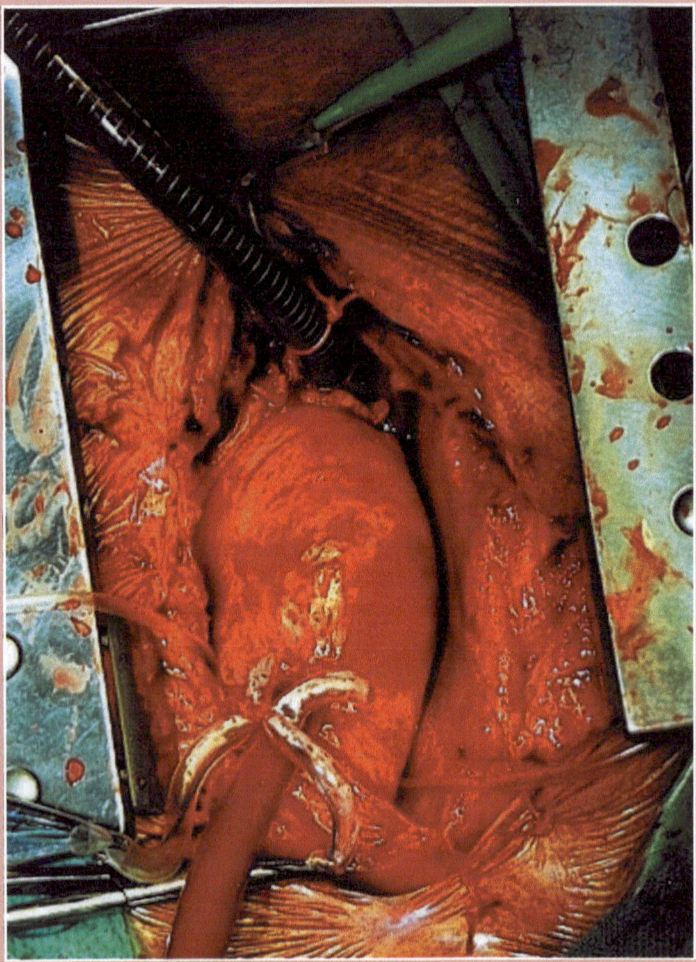

Fig. 5.10 Less-invasive approach for aortic valve replacement via upper hemisternotomy. Aortic cannula is inserted in the ascending aorta and venous cannula through the right atrial appendage into the inferior vena cava

Aortic valve procedure is performed in a standardized manner regardless of the chosen approach. The arterial cannula of the cardiopulmonary bypass is inserted into the ascending aorta and the venous drainage is accomplished by means of a single "two-stage" cannula introduced via the right atrial appendage into the right atrium and the inferior vena cava. The same technique of cannulation is used in less invasive approaches or, alternatively, the vessels in the groin or the axillary artery may be used. Vent, a cannula for de-airing, unburdening of the left ventricle, and suction of the blood from the operative field, is introduced most frequently via the right superior pulmonary vein into the left ventricle. Alternatively, the vent may be placed via the pulmonary trunk or, occasionally, into the left ventricle through the aortic annulus and later through the implanted valve.

After aortic cross-clamping, the myocardial protection against ischemia is provided by the administration of a cold crystalloid or blood cardioplegia that leads to asystole and hypothermia of the myocardium. The superiority of the blood cardioplegia over the crystalloid one has become widely accepted. At our unit we formerly used blood cardioplegia only for demanding, combined procedures or in patients with severe left ventricular dysfunction. At present we use blood cardioplegia exclusively. Administration of the cold cardioplegic solution is repeated in combined procedures in 20- to 30-min intervals or immediately in case of reappearance of ECG activity. In cases of isolated aortic valve replacement with external cooling of the heart, assumed there is no activity on ECG and aortic de-clamping will take place within 40 min, repeating of the cardioplegia is not necessary. The initial dose of 1000 ml of the cardioplegic solution is administered in the ascending aorta and later a smaller amount is instilled directly into the coronary ostia. In extensive combined procedures we also use the technique of retrograde cardioplegia application via the coronary sinus. Maintenance of constant myocardial hypothermia is facilitated by repeated rinsing of the heart by ice-cold saline solution. After excision of the aortic valve, the left ventricular cavity is washed out by the cold saline solution. This maneuver not only helps to maintain hypothermia in the subendocardial layer of the myocardium, which is most vulnerable to ischemia, but also washes out potentially present calcium debris after removal of the heavily calcified valve.

The aortic valve is accessed through a transverse aortotomy carried close above the sinotubular junction. The valve is excised, which may sometimes be difficult when extensive and severely dystrophic calcifications grow into the aortic annulus (Fig. 5.11). A meticulous debridement and decalcification of the annulus (Fig. 5.12) has to be performed followed sometimes by the removal of continuous calcium from the anterior mitral leaflet. A thorough decalcification of the annulus is of utmost importance in prevention of the paravalvular leak, and in addition it creates a pliable annulus and thus enables implantation of a bigger valve. A careful inspection of the annulus and the area of coronary ostia is mandatory to exclude any mobile calcifications. Then the size of the aortic orifice is measured by means of sizers specific for the concrete type of the valve prosthesis (Fig. 5.13). An effort is made to implant the biggest possible valve to avoid patient–prosthesis mismatch.

The stitches are anchored in the annulus and the sewing ring of the implanted prosthesis at a distance (Fig. 5.14). After insertion of all the stitches, the implanted prosthesis

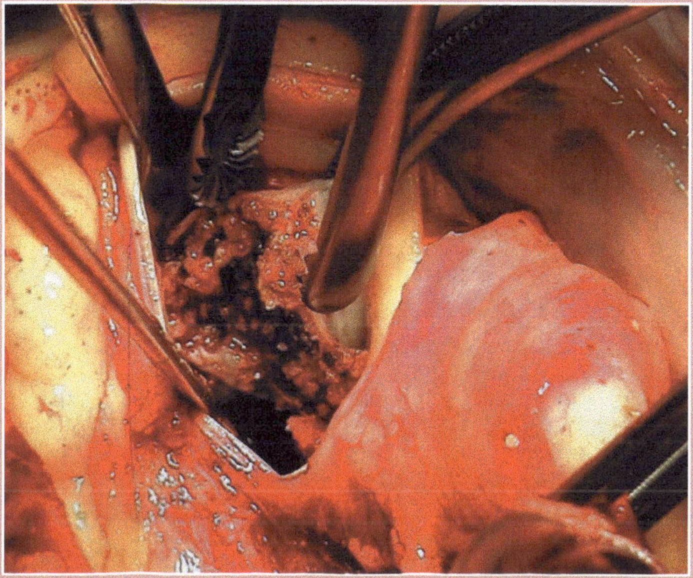

Fig. 5.11 Extensive calcifications in the area of commissure between right and non-coronary aortic cusp

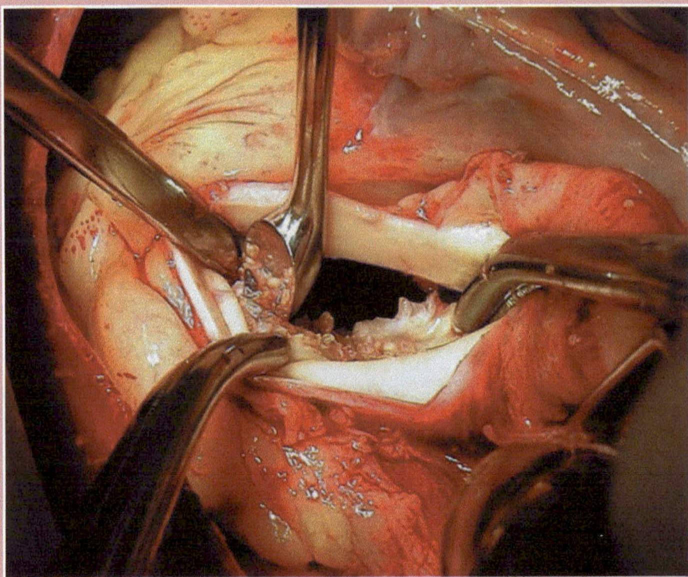

Fig. 5.12 Debridement and decalcination of aortic annulus after excision of stenotic aortic valve

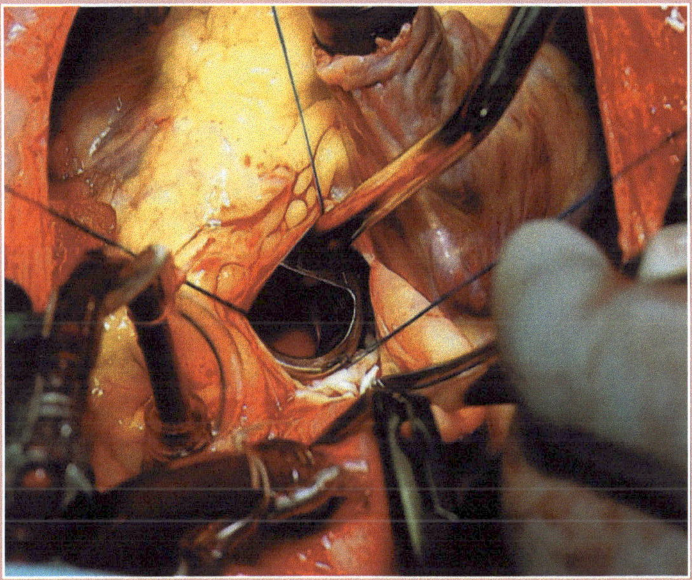

Fig. 5.13 Sizing of the aortic annulus

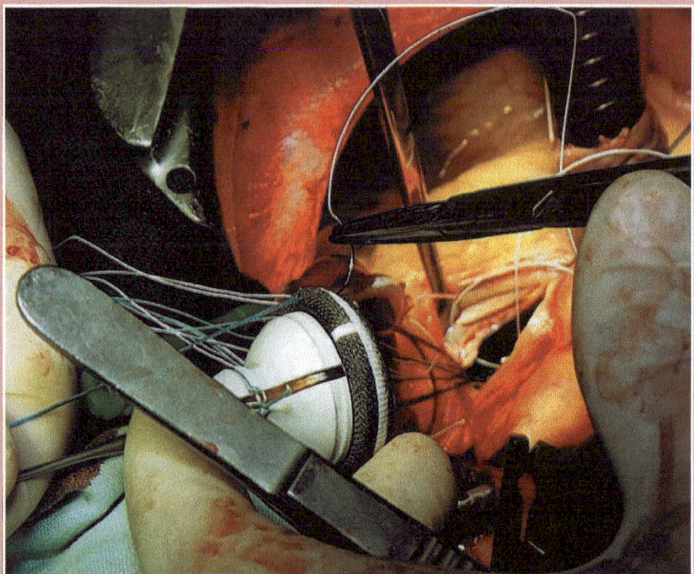

Fig. 5.14 Placement of sutures into the sewing ring of aortic prosthesis

is run down along the stitches into the aortic annulus (Fig. 5.15). In the case of today's most frequently implanted valve, St. Jude Medical, the sutures tied first are those adjacent to the pivot guards to secure their correct position inside the annulus. When all the sutures are tied, the unrestricted mobility of the disc, or leaflets of the mechanical valves, has to be controlled (Figs. 5.16, 5.17), and in case of any uncertainty the prosthesis has to be rotated to a better position. All the currently used models of the mechanical valves allow device rotation.

The technique for implantation of mechanical valves and that for stented bioprostheses (Fig. 5.18) is basically the same. It is based on fixation of the valve sewing ring into the patient's annulus. The fixation can be achieved by means of various modifications of single or continuous sutures. Isolated single stitches (Fig. 5.19a) and figure-of-eight stitches were used at our unit in the past. This technique enabled good intraannular implantation of the valve. Pledgeted stitches were introduced in mid-1980s, and since then we use almost exclusively mattress stitches with pledgets placed supraannulary (Fig. 5.19b) or subannulary (Fig. 5.19c), or continuous stitches (Fig. 5.19d). The use of continuous stitches is faster and cheaper. In the opinion of the present authors, these stitches are not optimal in poor-quality annulus due to the risk of cutting through, and also in cases of suboptimal exposure of the annulus because of difficult control of proper tightening of all the loops. Continuous stitches do not enable the suprannular implantation currently offered by modern bioprostheses since the implantation obtained with continuous stitches is intraannular (see Fig. 3.2a) or intra-supraannular (see Fig. 3.2b). The author prefers implantation of bioprostheses

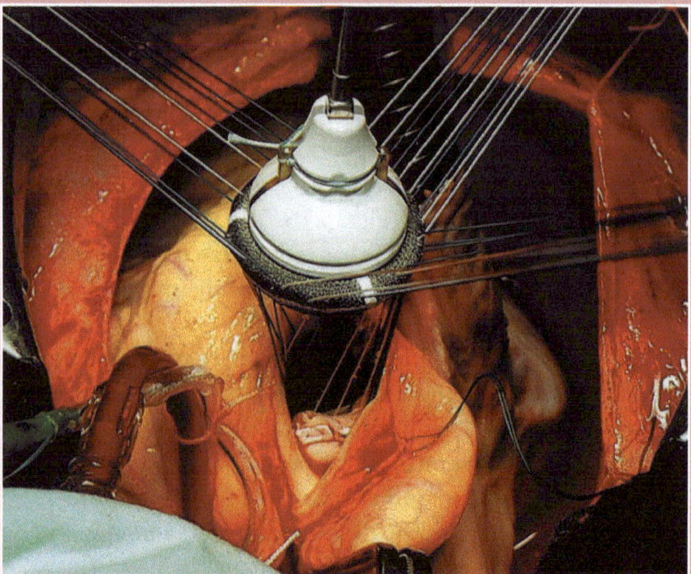

Fig. 5.15 Aortic valve prosthesis after placement of all sutures before running down into the aortic annulus

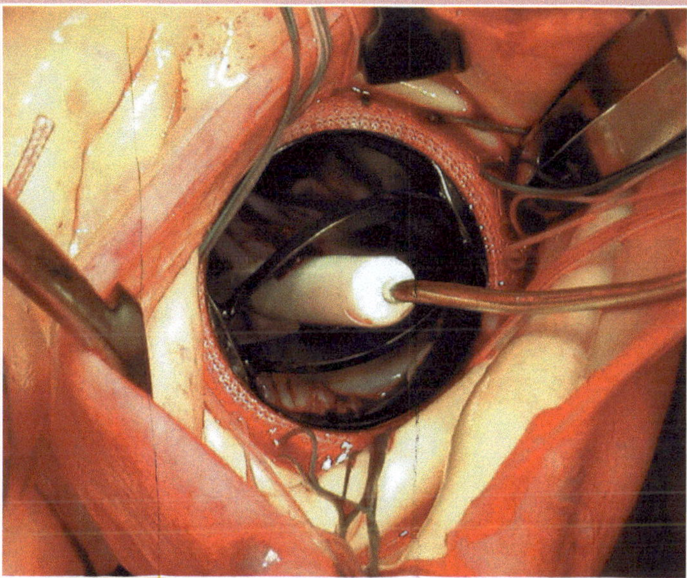

Fig. 5.16 Control of free mobility of semilunar leaflets of implanted bi-leaflet valve Sorin–Bicarbon

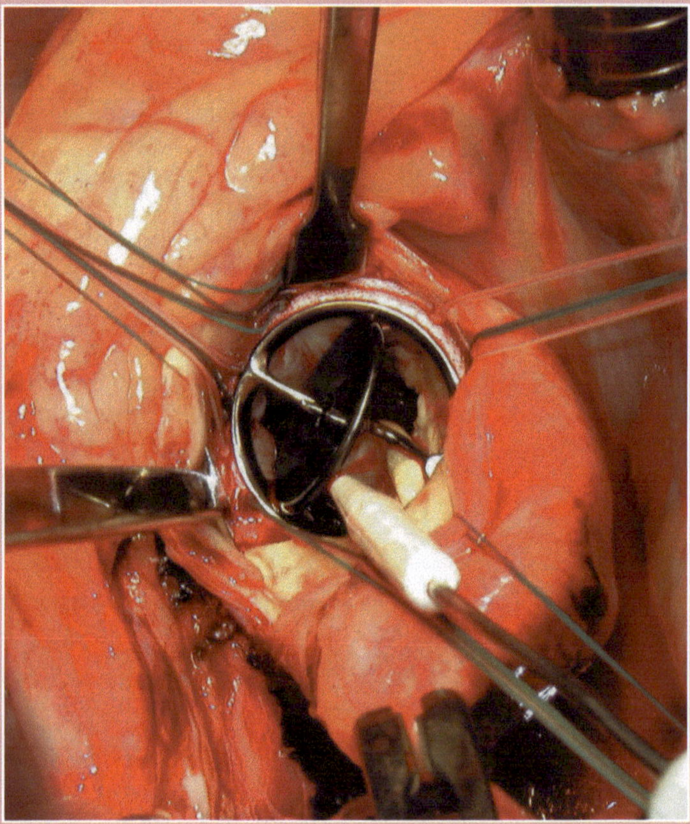

Fig. 5.17 Disc valve Medtronic–Hall implanted into aortic orifice: control of free mobility of the tilting disc

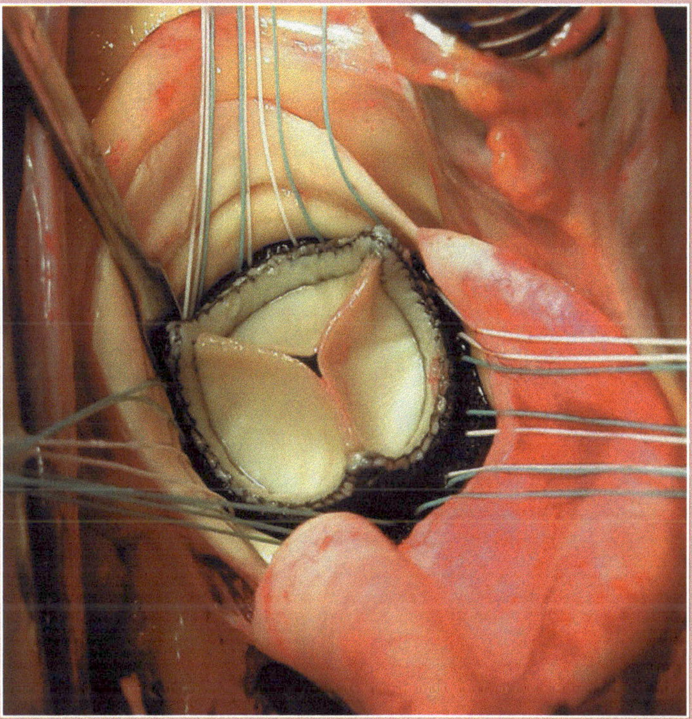

Fig. 5.18 Bioprosthesis Sorin–Soprano implanted into aortic orifice

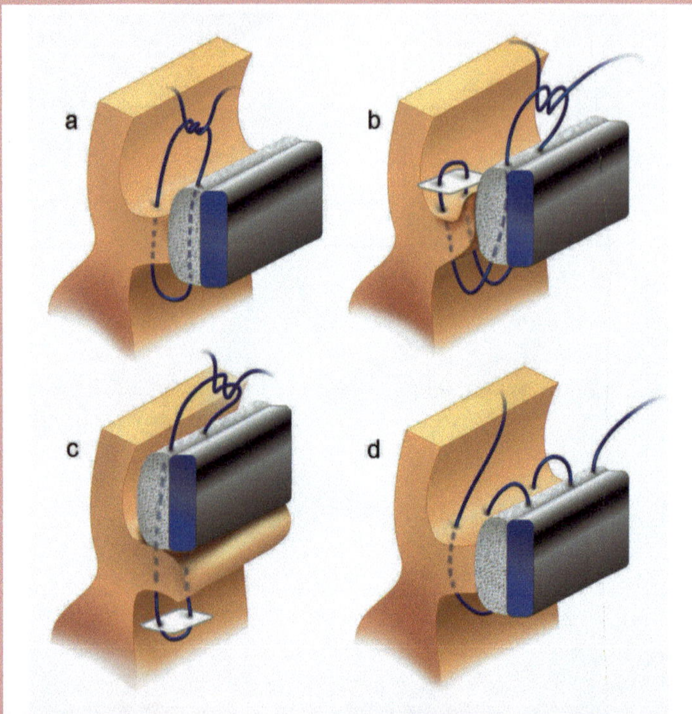

Fig. 5.19 Basic techniques of valve suturing to the patient's annulus. **a** Single interrupted suture. **b** Mattress suture with pledget placed supra-annulary. **c** Mattress suture with pledget placed subannulary. **d** Continuous suture

with mattress stitches with pledgets placed subannulary, which results in a true supraannular position of the bioprosthesis (see Fig. 3.2c). For mechanical valves in large annuli we use mattress stitches with pledgets placed supraannulary. In a narrow aortic annulus the subannular placement of the pledgets facilitates the decision for a bigger valve in case the sewing ring enables this type of implantation. Great care has to be taken, however, to avoid impressing the annulus tissue into the valve orifice (reduction of the effective orifice area and also the risk of interference with the tilting disc). Globally, the choice of the fixation technique depends on the expertise and personal preferences of a given surgeon.

Precise placement of the stitches in the sewing ring of the mechanical valve is very important as well as the precise length of the cut-off threads after knotting to exclude the risk of their interposition with the closing mechanism of the valve.

Proper valve orientation is required in order to get optimal hemodynamic results (lowest gradient and minimal turbulence). The optimal valve orientation has to respect the asymmetric blood flow pattern through the aortic root, which curves into the 140–150° angle between the longitudinal axis of the left ventricle and aorta so that the peak flow velocity and maximum flow output is directed toward the non-coronary sinus (Fig. 5.20). The lowest gradient on the mechanical tilting disc valve is obtained when the larger orifice of the valve is oriented toward the non-coronary sinus. In bileaflet valves the lowest gradient is obtained when the longitudinal gap between the semilunar discs is again oriented toward the non-coronary sinus [18, 19].

After valve implantation, the aortotomy is sutured with a continuous monofilamentous stitch, usually in two layers

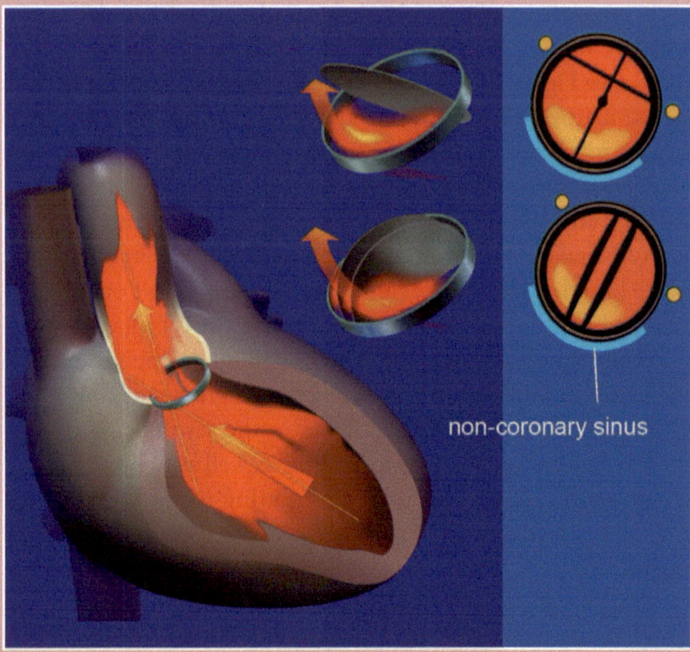

Fig. 5.20 Correct orientation of mechanical disc and bileaflet valves in aortic position

in the "over-and-over" manner or, alternatively, the first layer with the everting continuous stitch and then the second layer "over-and-over." The presence of a firm aortic wall enables performance of the aortotomy suture in one layer only, whereas in the case of a "paper-like" weak wall it is advisable to reinforce the suture with several pledgeted mattress stitches. After careful de-airing, the aortic cross-clamp is released. The onset of the heart rhythm is usually spontaneous; if ventricular fibrillation occurs, it is terminated by defibrillation. Temporary pacing wires are implanted during the reperfusion period.

5.2.3.2 Aortic Valve Replacement with Enlargement of the Aortic Annulus

Narrow aortic annulus in patients with a large body-surface area disables implantation of a valve large enough (sufficient effective orifice area) to avoid patient–prosthesis mismatch. All the manufacturers of mechanical valves have developed specially modified valve models suitable for this specific situation. The effective orifice area of these modified valve types was increased through reduction and reshaping of the sewing ring (eventually also of the housing of the valve) without changing the mechanism of the valve. In bioprostheses that generally display less favorable effective orifice area values compared with mechanical valves, the sewing rings were reshaped to fit for suprannular implantation [20]. The stentless bioprostheses that do not have sewing ring and stent have larger effective orifice area than the stented bioprostheses. As a result of these new options (modified mechanical valves, supraannulary implanted bioprostheses, and stentless bioprostheses) the necessity to enlarge the aortic annulus occurs rarely [21–23].

A simple surgical technique enables implantation of disc prostheses 2–4 mm larger than the narrow aortic annulus. The prosthesis is sutured in the area corresponding to the non-coronary sinus in a supraannular position. Pledgeted horizontal mattress sutures are passed from outside through the aortic wall a few millimeters above the annulus and through the sewing ring of the aortic valve prosthesis (Fig. 5.21) [24, 25]. It is important to orient the opening of the disc toward the non-coronary sinus.

In case the aortic annulus enlargement is inevitable, the procedure described by Nicks et al. [26] in 1970 or by Manouguian and Seybold-Epting [28] in 1979 may be used. If the narrow annulus is suspected already preoperatively based on echocardiography data correlated with the body-surface area and estimated physical activity of the patient, the aortotomy is carried obliquely into the non-coronary sinus. Once the unacceptable narrow annulus is confirmed, the incision is prolonged deep into the non-coronary sinus, cuts the aortic annulus, and stops at the base of the anterior mitral leaflet (Nicks procedure; Fig. 5.22) [26, 27]. Should even this enlargement be insufficient, the incision can be carried farther across the fibrous mitral annulus into the anterior mitral leaflet. With the Manouguian technique the aortotomy is extended into the commissure between the left and non-coronary sinus and then into the anterior mitral leaflet (Fig. 5.23). A patch from the pericardium or vascular graft is sutured into the incision and the resulting enlargement of the annulus makes the implantation of a one- to two-size-bigger valve feasible. The valve is sutured to the neoannulus in the patch area by mattress stitches with pledgets placed externally [28].

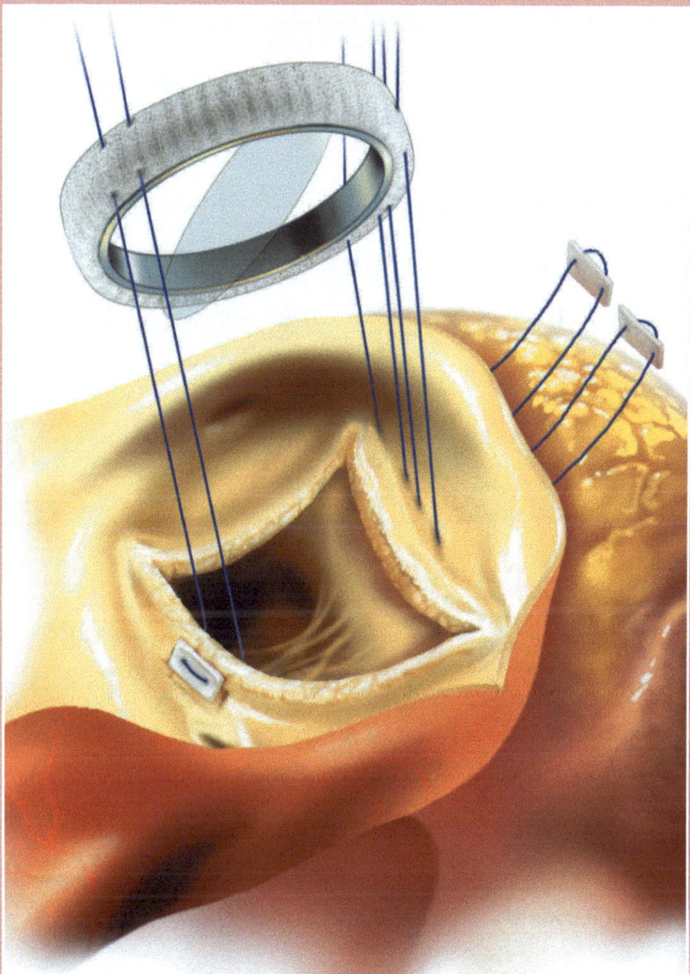

Fig. 5.21 Partial supraannular valve implantation (in the area of non-coronary sinus)

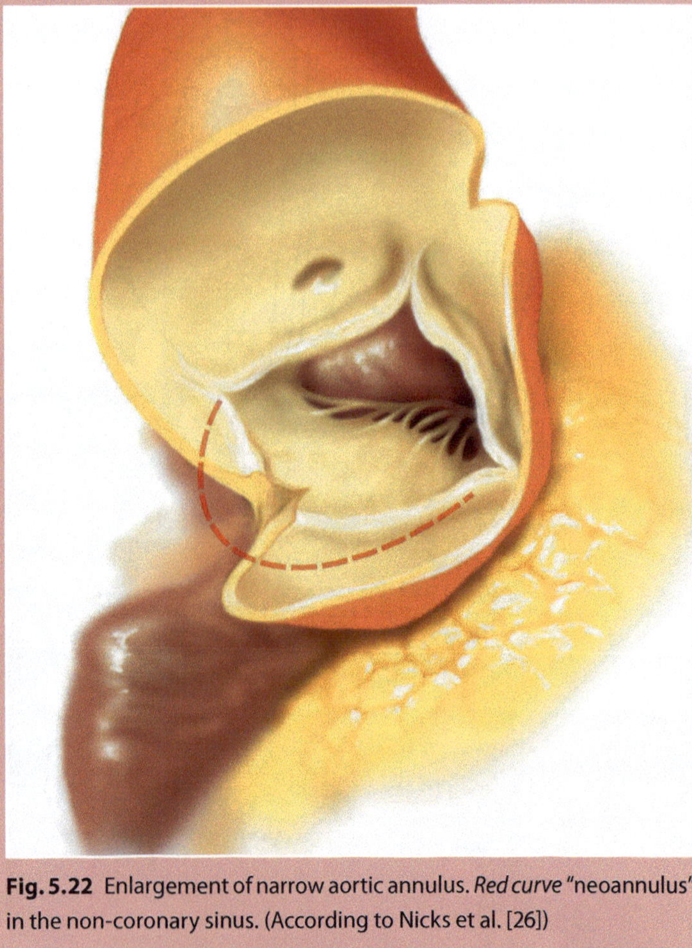

Fig. 5.22 Enlargement of narrow aortic annulus. *Red curve* "neoannulus" in the non-coronary sinus. (According to Nicks et al. [26])

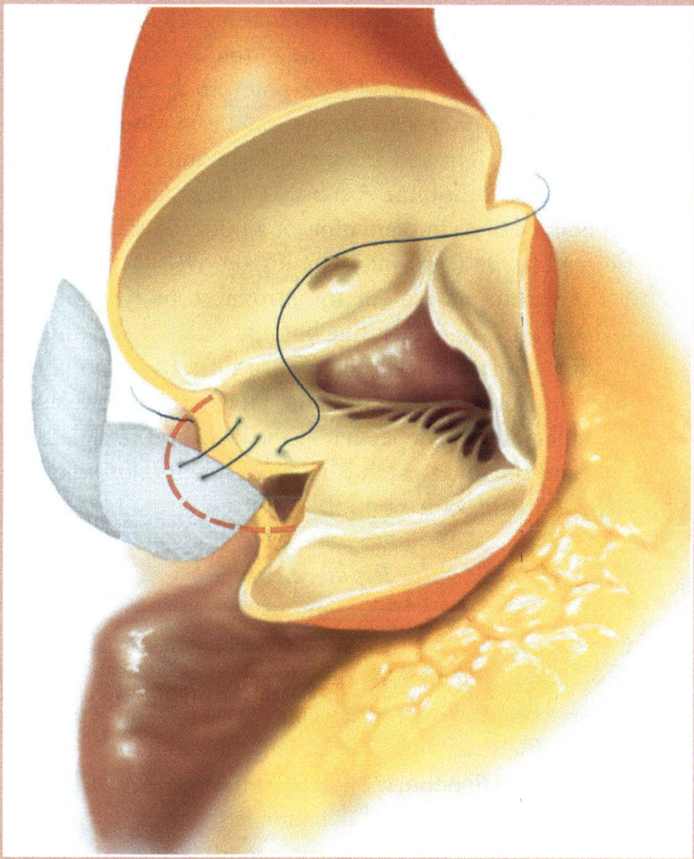

Fig. 5.23 Enlargement of narrow aortic annulus according to Manouguian and Seybold-Epting [28]. *Red curve* "neoannulus" in the commissure between left and non-coronary sinus

In 1997 Otaki et al. [29] described the bidirectional aortic annulus enlargement. The aortotomy has the shape of an inversed Y. One arm of the Y points to the non-coronary sinus and the other arm cuts the annulus in the commissure between the right and left aortic cusps and continues into the septal myocardium. A substantial annulus enlargement is obtained after implantation of a butterfly-shaped patch from a Dacron (DuPont, Wilmington, Del.) graft [29].

The aortoventriculoplasty introduced by Konno et al. in 1975 [30] is a demanding but unavoidable procedure in children with a tunnel fibromuscular subaortic stenosis with a hypoplastic aortic annulus. The aortic annulus is enlarged by implantation of a patch into the incised ventricular septum and the other patch is required for the closure of the right ventricular incision [30].

5.2.3.3 Aortic Valve Replacement with the Septal Myectomy

Concentric left ventricular hypertrophy in some patients with aortic stenosis leads to the echocardiography signs of hypertrophic obstructive cardiomyopathy. In these patients asymmetric septal hypertrophy is localized in the subaortic area. This small population of patients is jeopardized by the occurrence of functional dynamic left ventricular outflow tract obstruction once the aortic stenosis is relieved. The left ventricular outflow tract obstruction is caused by systolic anterior motion (SAM), which is simultaneously also responsible for hemodynamically significant mitral regurgitation. Relief of afterload (resolution of the aortic stenosis), decrease of preload (hypovolemia), and inotropic medication (catecholamines) are three elementary factors contributing to the onset of this serious complication in selected patients.

Treatment consists of rapid volume replenishment simultaneously with catecholamine withdrawal and administration of negative chronotropic and inotropic agents (betablockers, calcium blockers). If no response appears, reoperation is necessary. Mitral valve replacement seems to be the safest strategy, or, alternatively, Alfieri repair, provided the mitral annulus is large enough.

To avoid this rare but very serious complication, septal myectomy according to Morrow and Brockenbrough [31] is to be performed as an adjunct to aortic valve replacement. This procedure should be undertaken in patients indicated for aortic valve replacement in whom the preoperative echocardiography displays hypertrophic and hypercontractile left ventricle and a narrow left ventricular outflow tract resulting from asymmetric septal hypertrophy. After excision of the stenotic aortic valve and debridement of the annulus, the septal myectomy is performed. The principle of the procedure is excision of myocardium from the hypertrophic subvalvular bulk (Figs. 5.24, 5.25). A rare but serious complication of the septal myectomy is perforation of the ventricular septum (surgeon has to be aware of the actual septum thickness) and also the risk of complete atrioventricular block. (The extent of incision in the rightward direction must not get beyond the midpoint of the right coronary cusp so that the bundle of His is not jeopardized.) On the other hand, insufficient extent of the incision in both length and depth may lead to failure of the procedure.

5.2.3.4 Aortic Valve Replacement with the Stentless Bioprosthesis

Aortic valve replacement with the stentless bioprosthesis differs technically from the use of a mechanical valve or stented

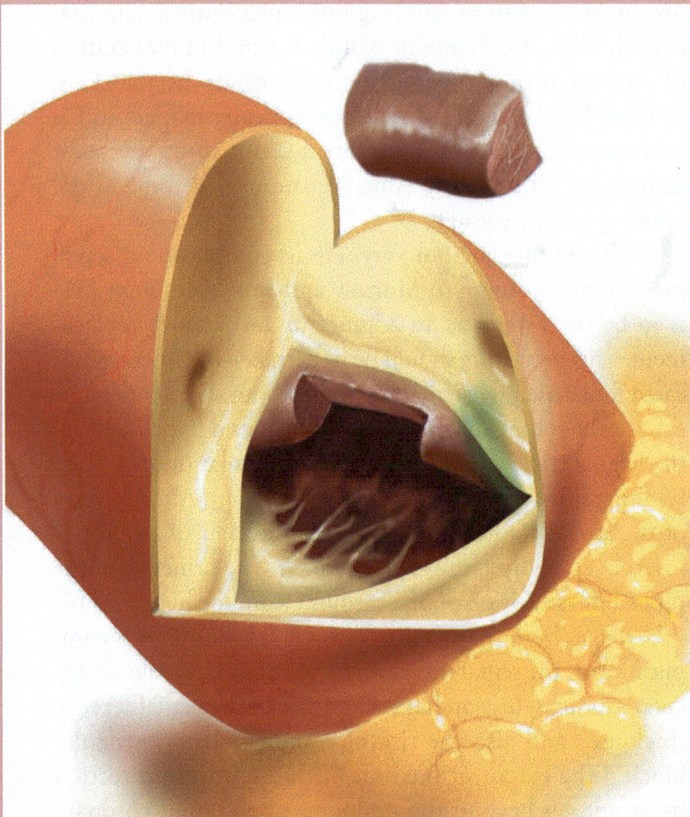

Fig. 5.24 Septal myectomy. Marked in *green* is the expected course of bundle of His. (According to Morrow and Brockenbrough [31])

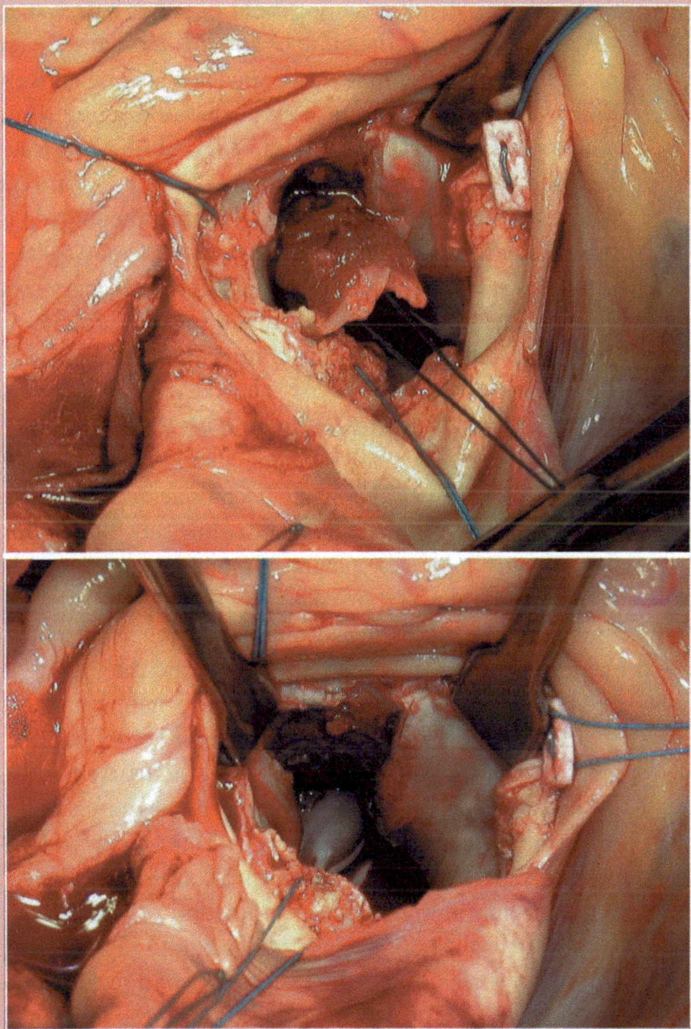

Fig. 5.25 Septal myectomy (operative view). (According to Morrow and Brockenbrough [31])

bioprosthesis. Stentless bioprosthesis does not have a stent or a sewing ring, and therefore its annulus is usually fixated into the recipient's annulus with single stitches or mattress stitches. After seating the valve inside the aortic annulus and tying the sutures, another suture line is performed to fixate the scalloped commissures (Fig. 5.26). The design of some stentless bioprostheses (see Fig. 3.20) enables the surgeon to decide individually between the technique of root replacement with subsequent reimplantation of the coronary ostia buttons or trimming the bioprosthesis for classic double-suture-line "freehand" technique of implantation (Fig. 5.27).

5.2.3.5 Aortic Valve Replacement with the Allograft

Aortic valve replacement with the allograft is performed either in subcoronary "freehand" technique or as a root replacement [32]. In the double-suture-line subcoronary implantation technique the allograft annulus is sutured into the recipient's annulus as a first step. Then the commissures of the allograft are symmetrically pulled into the recipient's root by means of transaortic mattress stitches and the second suture line is completed with a continuous stitch (Fig. 5.27). The first (annular) suture line can also be completed with a continuous stitch. In such case three stitches are inserted in the nadirs of the allograft annulus. The allograft is pulled inside the recipient's annulus, inverted into the left ventricle, and subsequently sutured with a continuous stitch to the recipient's annulus. After completion of this first suture line, the allograft is reinverted back into the aorta, the commissures are resuspended, and the second suture line is completed as described previously. This subcoronary double-suture-line technique cannot be used if unsuitable morphology is present (asymmetric or dilated sinuses of Valsalva,

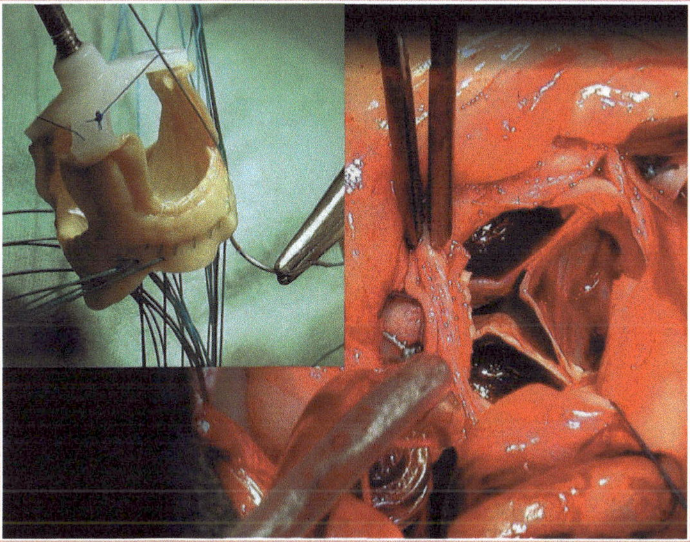

Fig. 5.26 Implantation of stentless bioprosthesis. *Inset* shows placement of sutures into the annulus of bioprosthesis

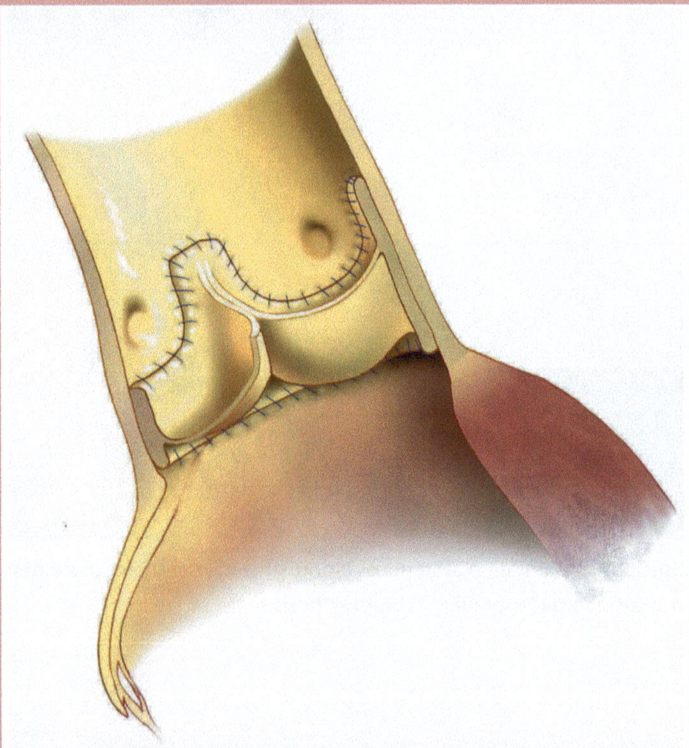

Fig. 5.27 Subcoronary freehand implantation of allograft into aortic position

dilated sinotubular junction, annulo-aortic ectasia, etc.). In these cases the technique of allograft implantation as a root replacement has to be chosen. The annulus implantation is identical to the previously described technique (isolated single sutures). Some authors recommend incorporation of a Teflon (DuPont, Wilmington, Del.) felt stripe into the suture to prevent further annular dilation and to achieve better hemostasis. Subsequently, the buttons with coronary ostia are implanted into the allograft with a continuous monofilamentous stitch. The final step is the distal anastomosis of the allograft to the distal part of the ascending aorta (Fig. 5.28). The root replacement technique has generally been preferred in recent years, and not only in cases where its choice is forced by unsuitable morphology of the patient's aortic root [33].

5.2.3.6 Aortic Valve Replacement with Concomitant Surgery of the Ascending Aorta

Optimal decision making in mild to moderate poststenotic dilation of the ascending aorta (4.0–5.5 cm) with absent dilation of the sinuses of Valsalva and of the sinotubular junction remains controversial. Recommended strategies vary from isolated aortic valve replacement with subsequent echocardiography follow-up of the ascending aorta dimensions to a radical solution: supracoronary replacement of the ascending aorta with a prosthetic graft. In between these treatment modalities there is the option to wrap up (girdle) the ascending aorta with the prosthetic-graft fabric or to perform reducing aortoplasty with concomitant girdling [34]. If the surgeon decides for the reducing aortoplasty, the approach to the aortic valve replacement is performed via a long longitudinal aortotomy that later enables the accomplishment of the aortoplasty.

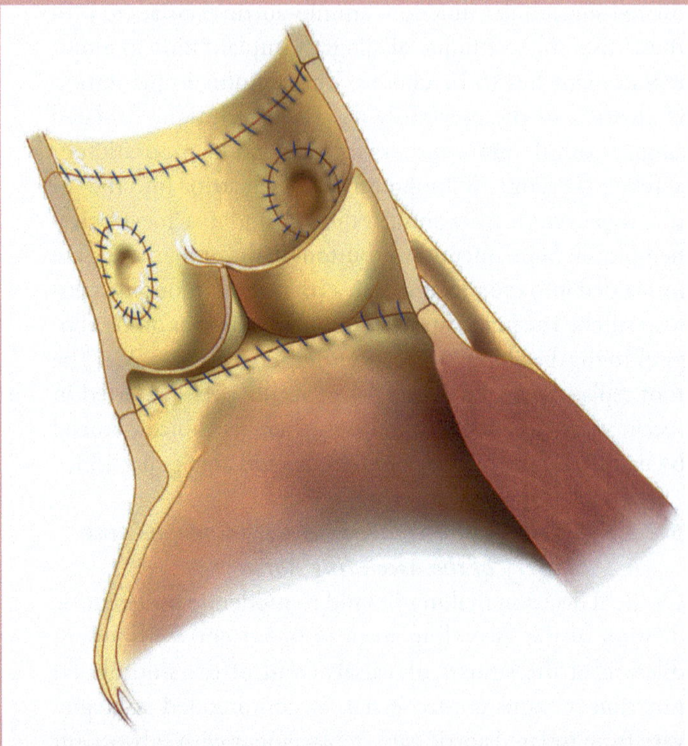

Fig. 5.28 Allograft implantation by technique of root replacement

The isolated aortic valve replacement may be considered a proper treatment in patients with a large body-surface area and an aortic diameter of approximately 4 cm. The reducing aortoplasty and external girdling (Fig. 5.29) aim to reduce the aortic diameter to at least 4 cm [35–39]. The girdling prevents further progression of aortic dilation. The girdling itself is an acceptable solution in elderly and polymorbid patients as well as in patients with smaller aortic dilation. In case of a greater extent of aortic dilation, in younger patients and in the presence of local pathologies of the ascending aorta the supracoronary aortic replacement is a more proper therapeutic option (Figs. 5.30, 5.31).

Dilation of the sinuses of Valsalva and the sinotubular junction together with ascending aortic dilation is an indication for the Bentall procedure. This operation is originally indicated for aortic incompetence at the annulo-aortic ectasia (Fig. 5.53; see Sect. 5.3.1), but in the case of aortic stenosis with dilated sinotubular junction and dilated ascending aorta, it also is a treatment of choice [40].

The principle of the Bentall procedure is simultaneous aortic valve replacement together with replacement of the dilated ascending aorta. This is accomplished by the implantation of a composite graft (conduit) that has a built-in valve prosthesis at its proximal end (Fig. 5.32). After aortic cross-clamping close to the origin of the brachiocephalic trunk, the aneurysmatic sac is open. The native aortic valve is excised and the composite graft is implanted with use of mattress pledgeted stitches (Fig. 5.33) or a continuous stitch. Then the reimplantation of the coronary ostia in the graft follows, with use of a continuous stitch. The final anastomosis is the suture of the distal end of the graft with the end of the ascending aorta. The aneurysmatic sac is partially

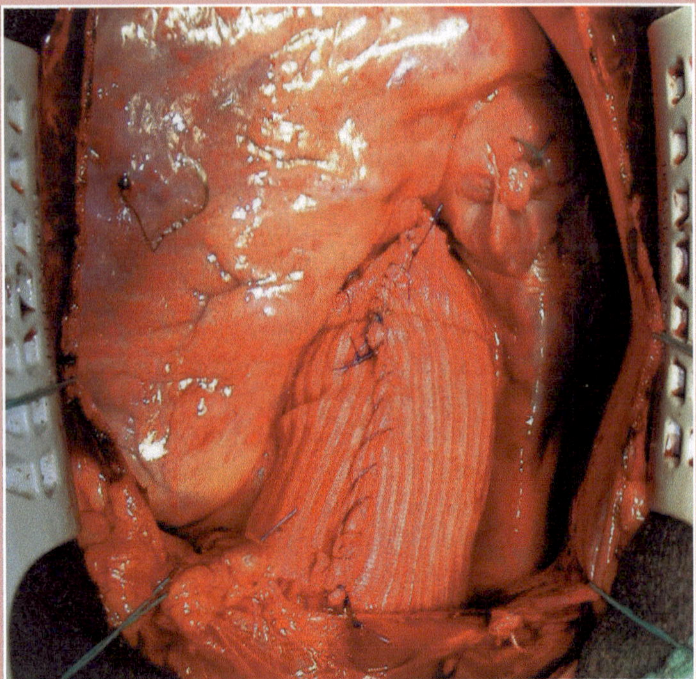

Fig. 5.29 Girdling of dilated ascending aorta

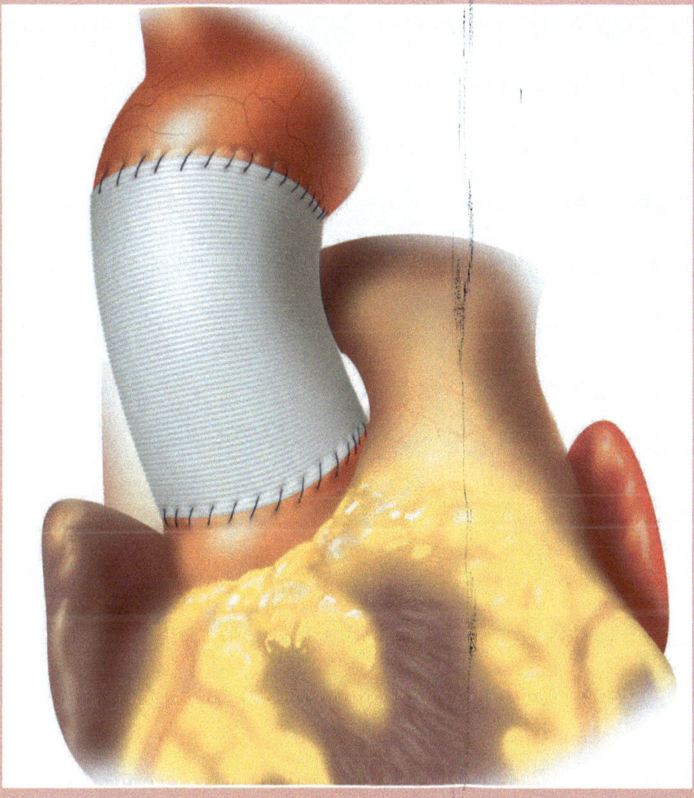

Fig. 5.30 Supracoronary replacement of dilated ascending aorta

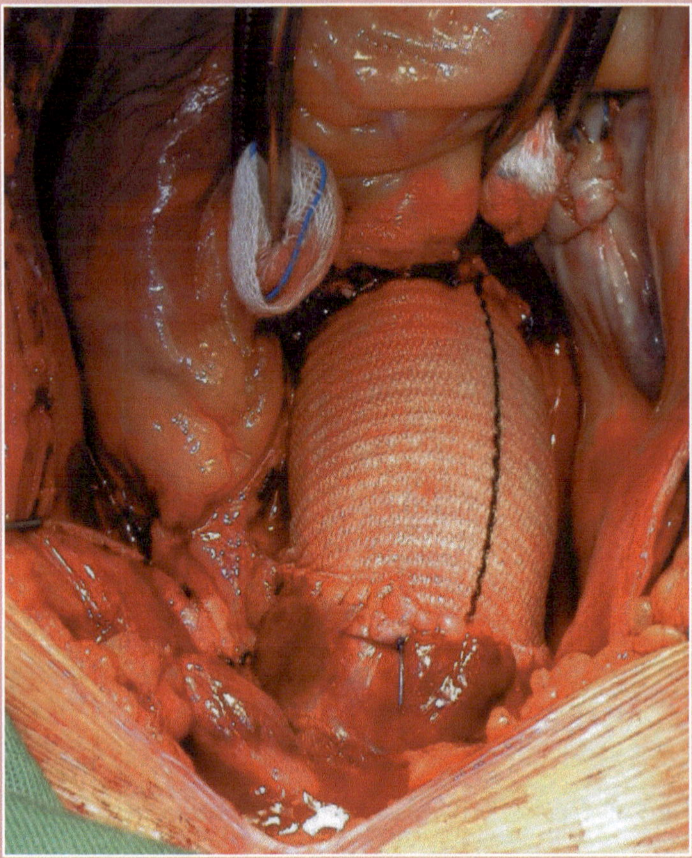

Fig. 5.31 Supracoronary aortic replacement for poststenotic aortic dilation

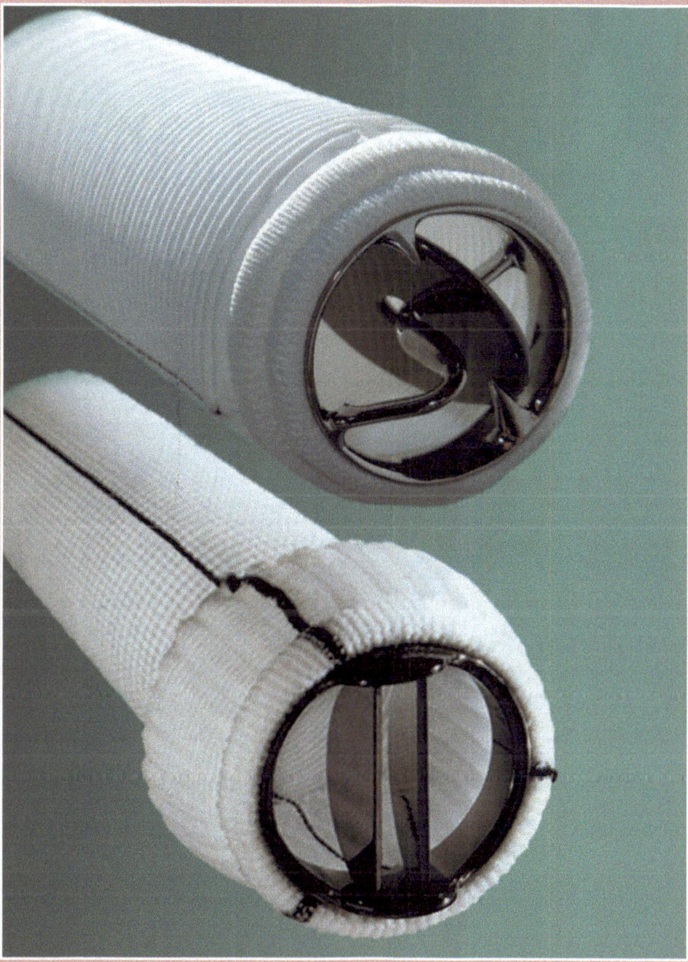

Fig. 5.32 Valved composite graft. Modern types reproduce the geometry of sinuses of Valsalva *(bottom)*

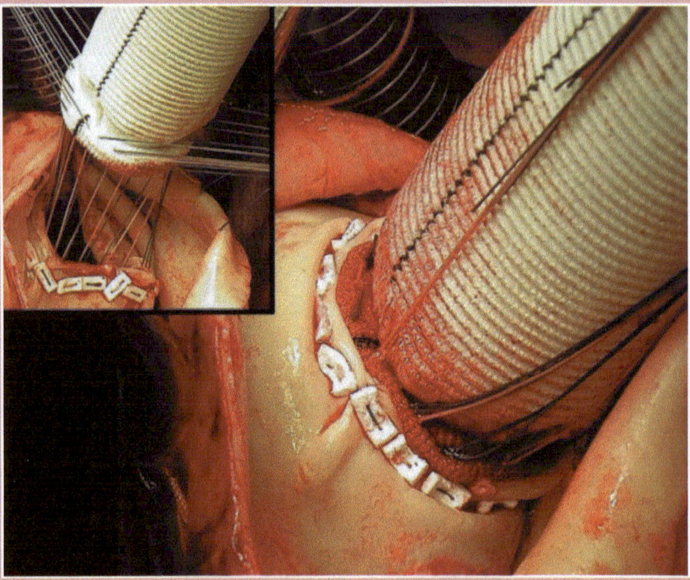

Fig. 5.33 Implantation of valved composite graft into aortic orifice with pledgeted mattress sutures

resected to a proper size and then used for wrapping up the prosthetic graft ("original Bentall technique"; Fig. 5.34) [41]. This maneuver (wrapping up) may be considered as a kind of protection against graft infection but formerly played an important role in achieving hemostasis in circumstances of diffuse bleeding through the graft fabric or some minor inaccessible leaks. In case of persistent bleeding the accumulation of blood inside the closed sac may lead to increased pressure around the graft and coronary ostia. This situation can be resolved by creation of a Cabrol shunt, which is a surgically instituted shunt between the aneurysmatic sac and the right atrium. The shunt can be accomplished either by direct suturing of the right atrial appendage to the aneurysmatic sac or by interposition of the Gore-Tex (W.L. Gore and Associates, Elkton, Md.) or saphenous vein graft. This left-to-right shunt is only temporary, because after normalization of coagulation, the prosthetic blood leakage stops and the shunt thromboses within several hours.

In recent years the implantation technique of the coronary ostia as isolated buttons into the prosthetic graft, without wrapping up with the remnants of the aneurysmatic sac, has been preferred (button technique; Fig. 5.35). The aneurysmatic sac is resected. This modern surgical technique was facilitated by the development of zero-porosity vascular grafts (impregnated with collagen or gelatin) and also employment of tissue glues.

Technical difficulties may arise during the Bentall procedure if the coronary ostia cannot be mobilized to reach the prosthetic graft (the ostia encased in firm adhesions at reoperation). In these situations connection can be accomplished by means of a vascular graft interposition. Cabrol et al. [42] described the use of an arch-like connection of

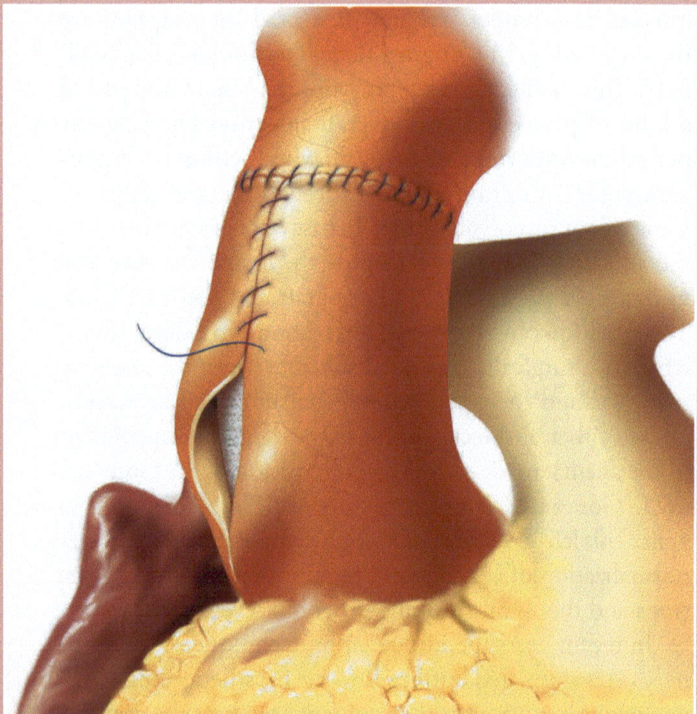

Fig. 5.34 The Bentall procedure. Original technique with wrapping of the valved graft by the remnants of the aneurysmatic sac

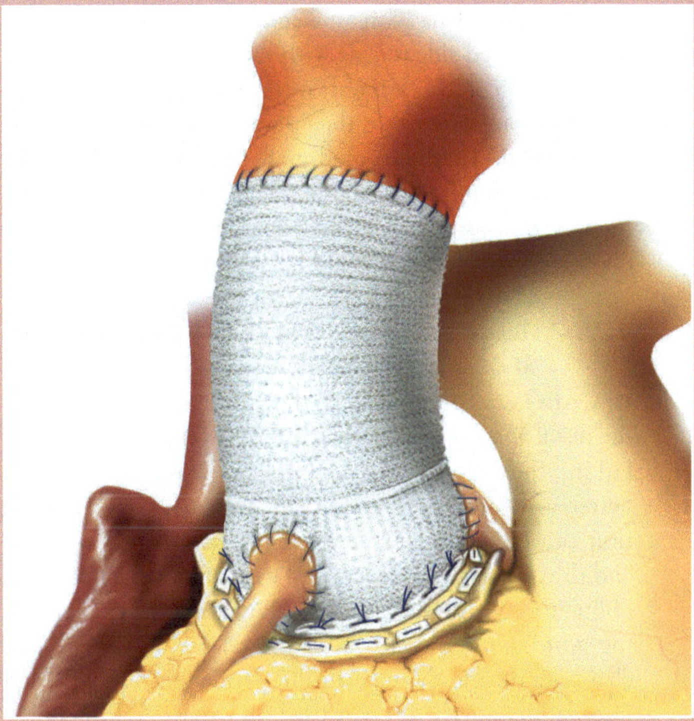

Fig. 5.35 Modification of Bentall procedure: the "button technique"

both coronary ostia with an 8-mm vascular graft, which is then connected side to side with the aortic prosthetic graft (Figs. 5.36, 5.37) [42]. If only one coronary ostium is too far from the composite graft, then the Svensson [43] technique can be used. The interposed graft from the left coronary ostium has to follow a circumferential course before entering the composite graft; otherwise, there is the risk of graft cranking (Figs. 5.38, 5.39) [43].

5.2.3.7 Aortic Valve Replacement with a Concomitant Myocardial Revascularization

In CABG concomitant with the aortic valve replacement the distal anastomoses are performed prior to valve implantation. The rationale for such practice is the advantage of better myocardial protection since the cardioplegic solution can be administered via the newly created bypasses and thus reach the areas beyond the coronary stenoses and obliterations. The proximal anastomoses with the ascending aorta are performed after the release of aortic cross-clamping during the reperfusion period. As a rule the left internal mammary artery is used for bypass grafting of the left anterior descending artery. Great care has to be taken in de-airing of the left heart cavities to avoid air embolization into newly created bypasses. The vein grafts that originate from the highest point of the ascending aorta are prone to trap the bubbles, which may result in myocardial ischemia of variable severity.

5.2.3.8 Aortic Valve Replacement with Concomitant Mitral Valve Surgery

In cases of simultaneous mitral surgery and aortic valve replacement, the mitral procedure is performed first followed

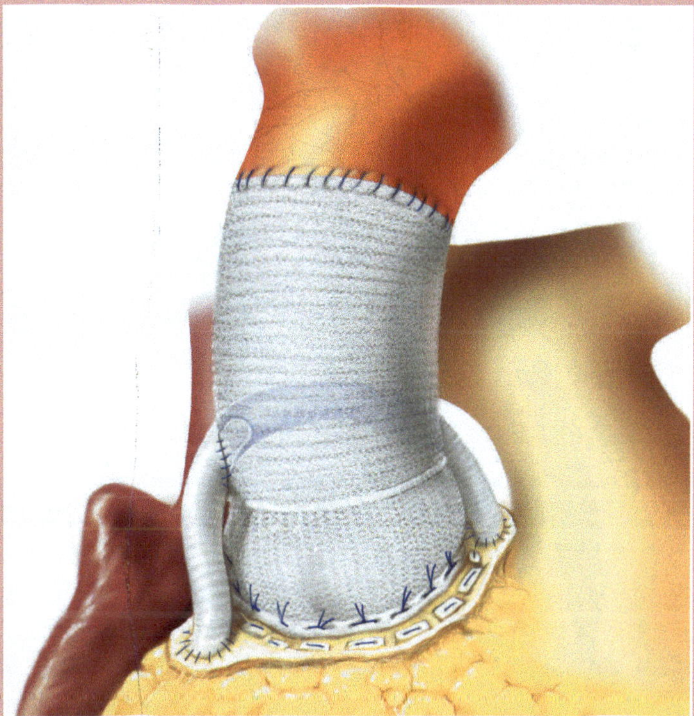

Fig. 5.36 Modification of Bentall procedure with anastomosing the coronary ostia. (According to Cabrol et al. [42])

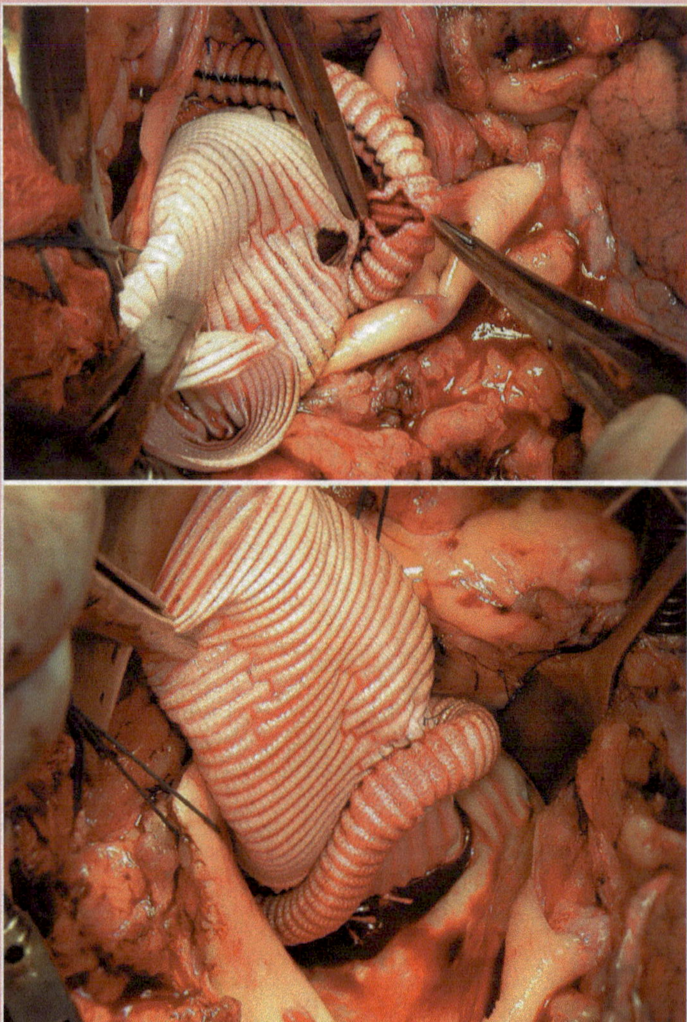

Fig. 5.37 Cabrol technique for anastomosing coronary ostia with the vascular graft (operative view). (According to Cabrol et al. [42])

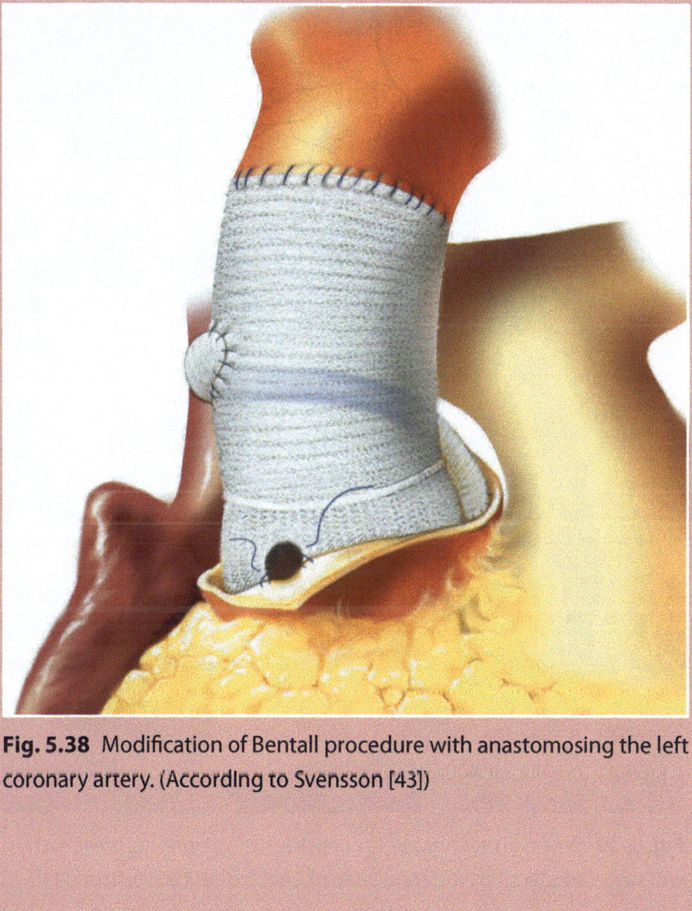

Fig. 5.38 Modification of Bentall procedure with anastomosing the left coronary artery. (According to Svensson [43])

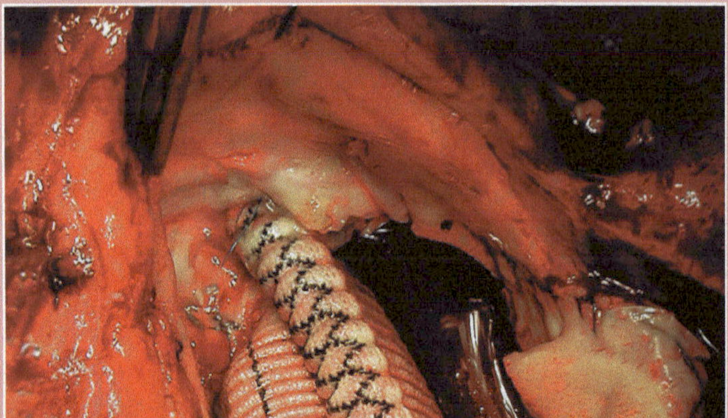

Fig. 5.39 Svensson technique for anastomosing right coronary ostium with the vascular graft (operative view). (According to Svensson [43])

by the aortic valve replacement. If mitral valve morphology is suitable for repair, excellent exposure of the anterior mitral leaflet and its chordae may be obtained through the aortic annulus after excision of the aortic valve; therefore, should the resection of the restrictive secondary chord be part of the planned mitral repair, it is advantageous to perform it easily and safely through the aortic annulus.

If the stenotic mitral valve is indicated for replacement, a good option is to cut the anterior mitral leaflet chordae at the junction with the papillary muscles again through the aortic annulus after excision of the aortic valve. The excellent exposure makes this step comfortable and safe, and the rest of the anterior leaflet excision can then be accomplished from the left atrium far more easily. After mitral valve replacement, it is advisable to repeat sizing of the aortic annulus since its size may be affected by the mitral surgery.

5.2.3.9 Aortic Valve Replacement with a Pulmonary Autograft

Aortic valve replacement with a pulmonary autograft (the Ross procedure) is a highly demanding operation, not only surgically but also due to the long duration of cardiopulmonary bypass and aortic cross-clamping. The principle of the Ross procedure is replacement of the diseased aortic valve with a pulmonary autograft. Surgically the technique of root replacement has been preferred in recent years. Continuity of the right ventricle with the pulmonary trunk is reinstituted by means of a pulmonary allograft (Figs. 5.40, 5.41). Indications and related controversies are discussed in Chap. 3.

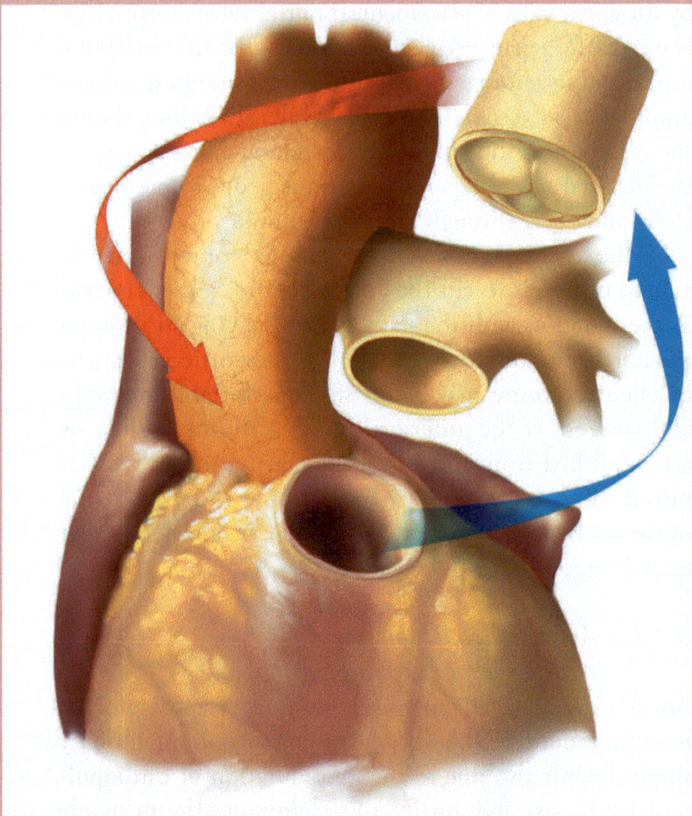

Fig. 5.40 Ross procedure: pulmonary autograft was dissected for implantation into aortic position

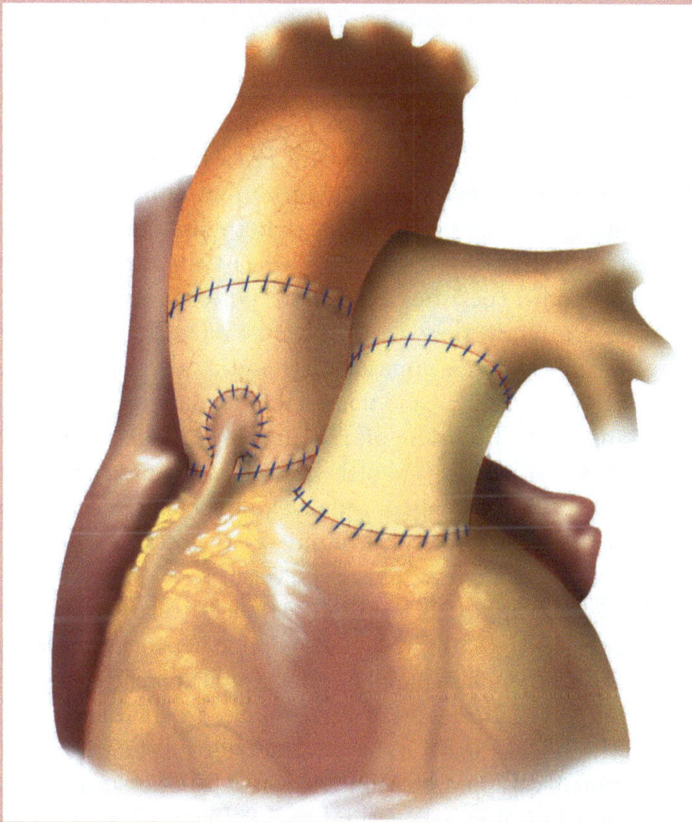

Fig. 5.41 Result of Ross procedure. Aortic root was replaced by pulmonary autograft and continuity of the right ventricular outflow tract was restored by a pulmonary allograft

5.2.3.10 Transapical Aortic Valve Implantation (J. Harrer, J. Vojacek)

There exists a population of patients who suffer from severe symptomatic aortic stenosis but their estimated operative risk is too high for a standard procedure of aortic valve replacement. Ranking of high risk is most often based on old age together with serious comorbidities (EuroSCORE higher than 20), reoperation with patent coronary grafts with other coexisting risk factors, porcelain aorta, etc.

Currently, these patients can be offered an alternative treatment option, transcatheter aortic valve implantation (TAVI), via either the transfemoral or surgical transapical approach. The transapical approach is being chosen for those patients in whom the transfemoral approach is not amenable or perhaps uncertain and risky (e.g., small lumen of the femoral artery, tortuosity or atherosclerotic aortico-iliaco-femoral vessel disease, porcelain aorta). A novel endo-vascular approach for TAVI via a left axillary artery was published recently. It may be an option in patients in whom neither the transfemoral nor transapical approaches are optimal [44]. The results of all techniques are almost identical, with slightly higher in-hospital mortality (8–17%) with the transapical approach counterbalanced by lower incidence of neurological embolic events [45–50]. Bioprosthesis Edwards Sapien is currently the only transcatheter valve on the market developed for the transapical approach. It is a balloon-expandable biological valve constructed from bovine pericardium and mounted on a steel stent (Fig. 5.42). Currently, only sizes 23 mm (designed for aortic annulus 18–21 mm) and 26 mm (for annulus 22–24.5 mm) are available. An aortic annulus with a diameter larger than 25 mm is therefore at present a contraindication of the procedure. Other

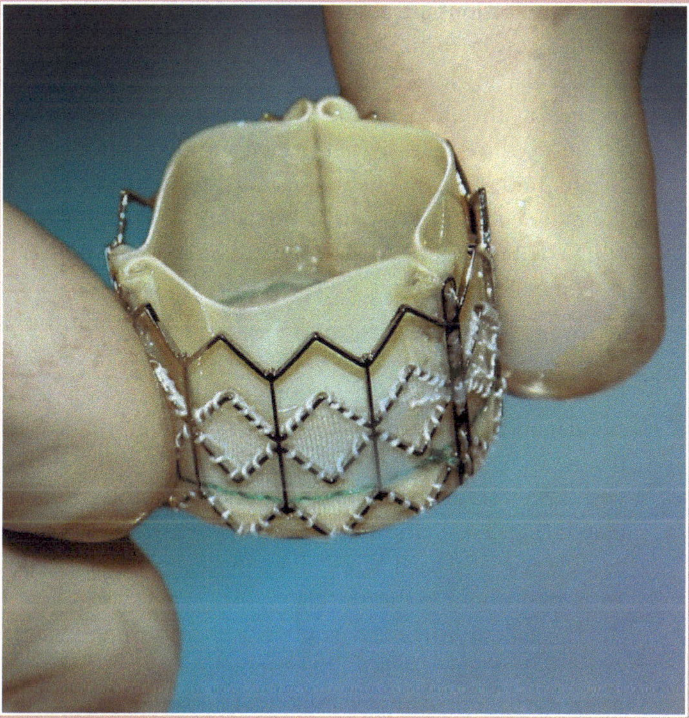

Fig. 5.42 Bioprosthesis Edwards–Sapien designed for transapical aortic valve implantation

contraindications are absence of calcifications in the aortic valve, bicuspid aortic valve, asymmetric gross calcifications, subvalvular aortic stenosis, hypertrophic obstructive cardiomyopathy, thrombus in the left ventricle, and vegetations. The procedure is being performed in a hybrid operation theater under general anesthesia. Percutaneous insertion of femoral venous and arterial guide wires is advisable to facilitate femoral cannulation for cardiopulmonary bypass in case of emergency.

The surgical approach is the anterolateral minithoracotomy (6–10 cm) in the fifth or sixth intercostal space (after echocardiography detection of position of the left ventricular apex). The pericardium is opened and the epicardial pacing leads are implanted. Two apical purse-string sutures with Teflon (DuPont, Wilmington, Del.) reinforcement are placed (Fig. 5.43). The left ventricular apex is punctured and a guide wire is passed across the stenotic aortic valve along with an introducer sheath (Fig. 5.44).

The balloon aortic valvuloplasty is then performed under rapid ventricular pacing. The biological valve is crimped upon the balloon catheter and under fluoroscopic guidance is positioned within the aortic annulus. Precise placement of the valve is extremely important and is guided by valvular calcifications and the position of the pig-tail catheter introduced retrogradely into the sinus of Valsalva. Implantation (deployment of the stent with biological valve) is performed by balloon inflation during rapid ventricular stimulation. After balloon deflation and discontinuation of the rapid pacing, the compressed valve cusps unfold. Good valve performance is confirmed by angiography and echocardiography. The wires and sheath are then removed and purse-string sutures are tied.

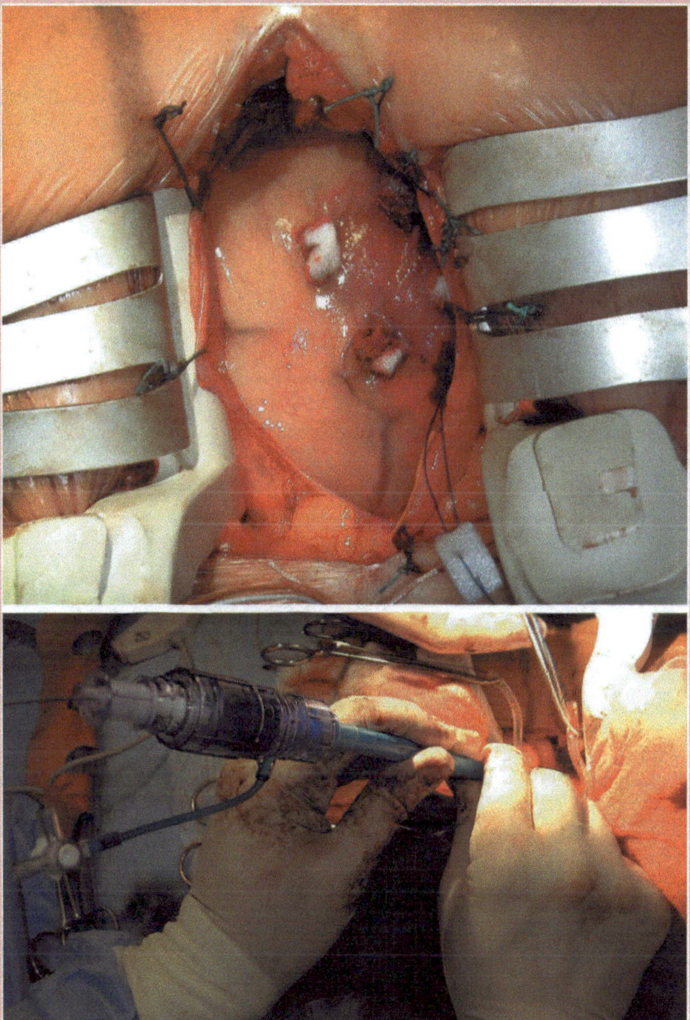

Fig. 5.43 Surgical approach to the left ventricular apex via minithoracotomy. Operative view of transapical valve implantation

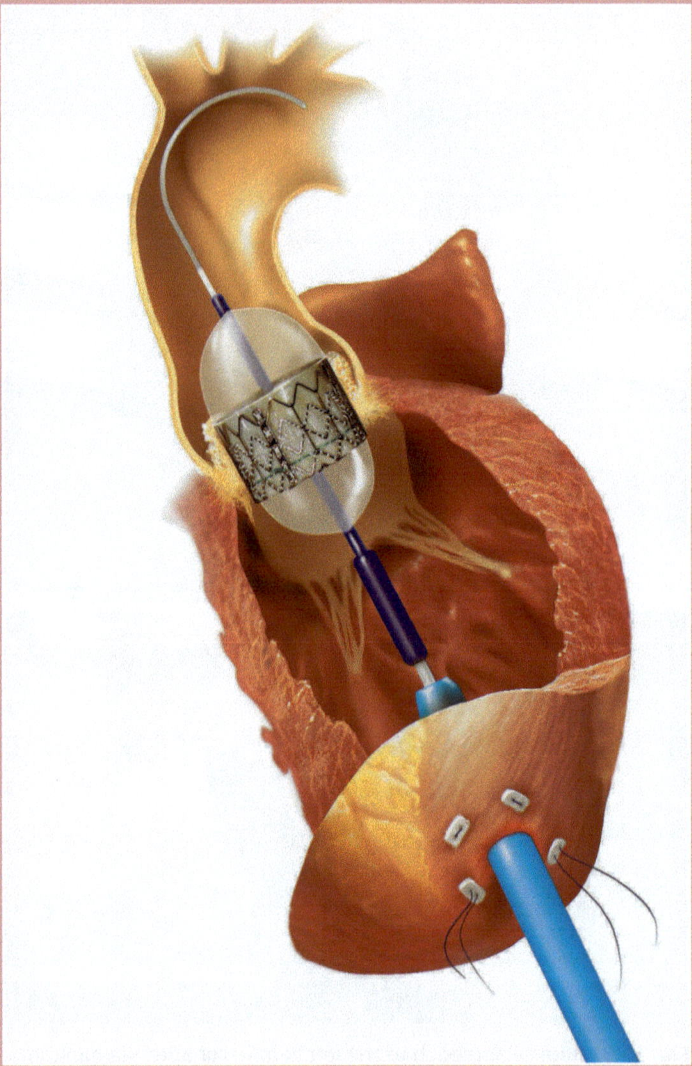

 Fig. 5.44 Transapical aortic valve implantation

Occasional complications after transapical aortic valve implantation are calcium embolization, obstruction of coronary ostia by calcifications, or even valve displacement. The occurrence of hemodynamically insignificant leaks is more frequent. Significant leaks can be minimized by valve redilation. In case of rare malfunction of the bioprosthetic cusp, a new valve can be implanted into the former one (valve in valve).

5.3 Aortic Regurgitation

Aortic regurgitation is characterized by reverse flow from the aorta to the left ventricle during diastole. In pure or predominant regurgitation disease of the aortic valve, the left ventricle complies for a long time with the volume and pressure overload due to compensatory mechanisms. The pathological condition results in eccentric left ventricular dilation and hypertrophy with corresponding increase in dimensions and volume (both end-diastolic and end-systolic). Further progression of the valve disease, however, leads to the failure of compensatory mechanisms. The left ventricular end-systolic volume continues to increase without accordant changes of the already high end-diastolic volume. As a result, the left ventricular EF decreases, whereas the left ventricular end-diastolic pressure, left atrial pressure, and pulmonary pressure increase. Clinical manifestations are fatigue, inefficiency, and dyspnea. Angina may also be present, caused by high demands of the hypertrophic myocardium in combination with coronary hypoperfusion from low aortic diastolic pressure and high left ventricular end-diastolic pressure. The symptoms (shortness of breath, fatigue, angina, palpitations) often appear very late and sometimes when the systolic dysfunction is already irreversible; thus, aortic regurgitation is not called an insidious disease for no reason, because many patients stay asymptomatic with already severe left ventricular impairment. If only the onset of advanced clinical symptoms triggers the diagnostic process, confirming poor EF and large left ventricular dimensions, the indication for surgery is a late one with high operative risk and dubious long-term results.

Operations for aortic regurgitation are less frequent than those for aortic stenosis, accounting for about 20% of all aortic valve operations.

5.3.1 Etiology of Aortic Regurgitation

Aortic regurgitation may be caused by isolated cusp involvement, dilation of the aortic annulus, the sinuses of Valsalva, the sinotubular junction, or a combination of two or more coinciding pathological factors.

Pathological changes of the aortic cusps causing valve regurgitation may be congenital (a unicuspid or more frequently a bicuspid aortic valve) or acquired. Infective endocarditis is the frequent cause of acquired valve regurgitation, either in its active phase (Figs. 5.45–5.47) or after healing of the infection (Fig. 5.48). Other etiological causes are rheumatic or degenerative sclerotic calcified (Fig. 5.49) involvement of the cusps leading predominantly to their retraction. A prolapse of one or more cusps may occur (Fig. 5.50) as well as damage to the cusps from turbulent blood flow in subvalvular aortic stenosis (see Fig. 5.9). Aortic regurgitation occurs occasionally in rheumatoid arthritis, ankylosing spondylitis, systemic lupus erythematosus, and Takayasu's disease (Fig. 5.51). In childhood aortic regurgitation may also result from an isolated right-cusp prolapse caused by

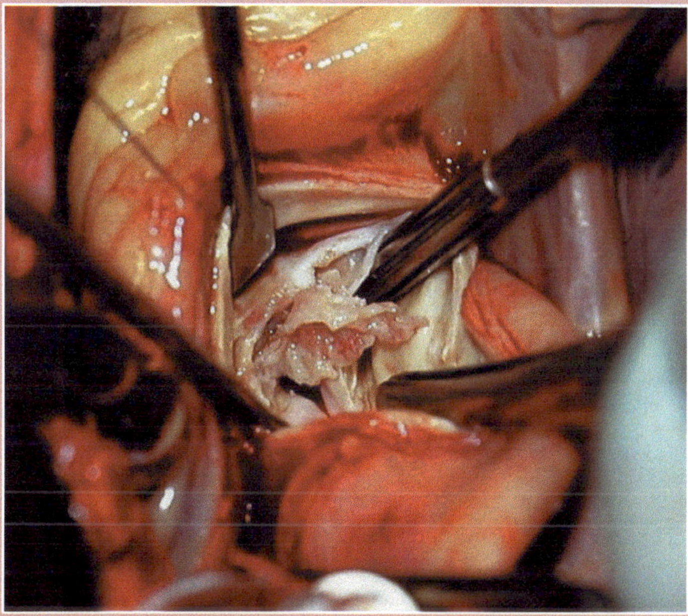

Fig. 5.45 Infective endocarditis of aortic valve with vegetations

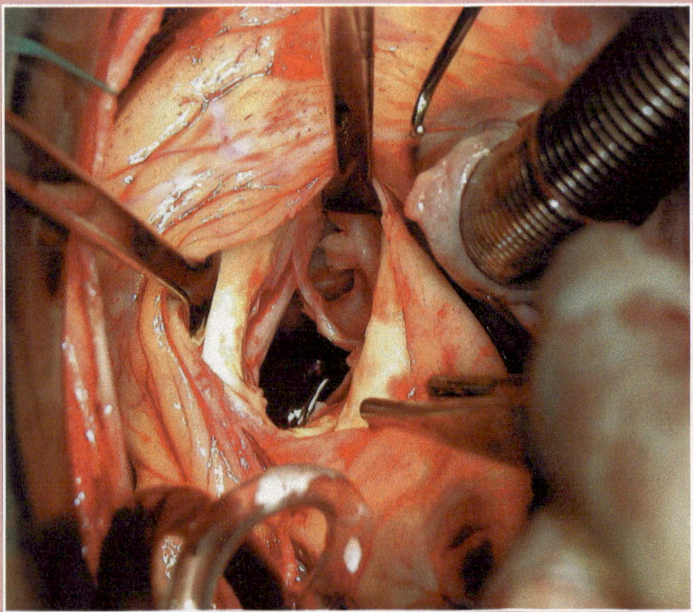

Fig. 5.46 Infective endocarditis of aortic valve with the defect in the non-coronary cusp

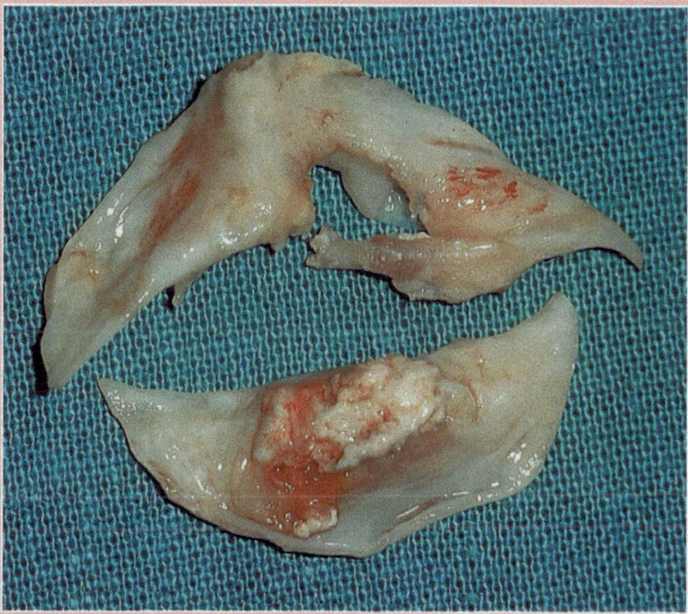

Fig. 5.47 Explanted bicuspid aortic valve with active endocarditis

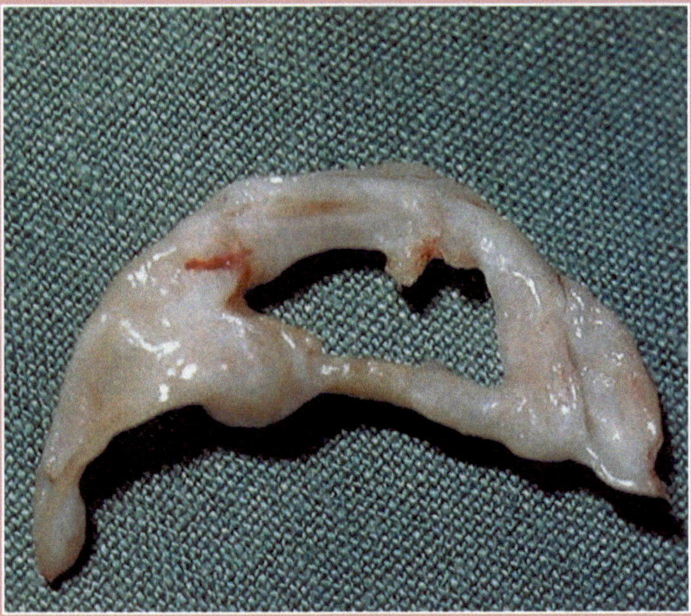

Fig. 5.48 Aortic cusp with a large defect after healing of infective endocarditis

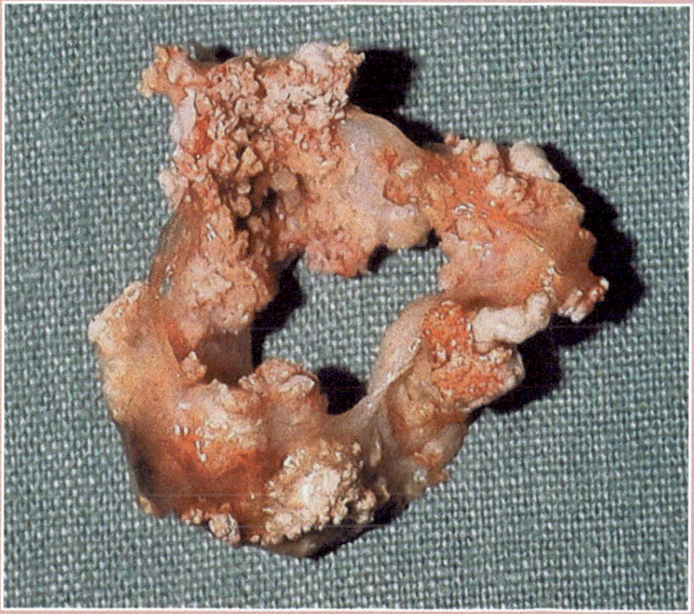

Fig. 5.49 Aortic valve turned into a ring of calcifications. Combined aortic valve disease with severe regurgitation

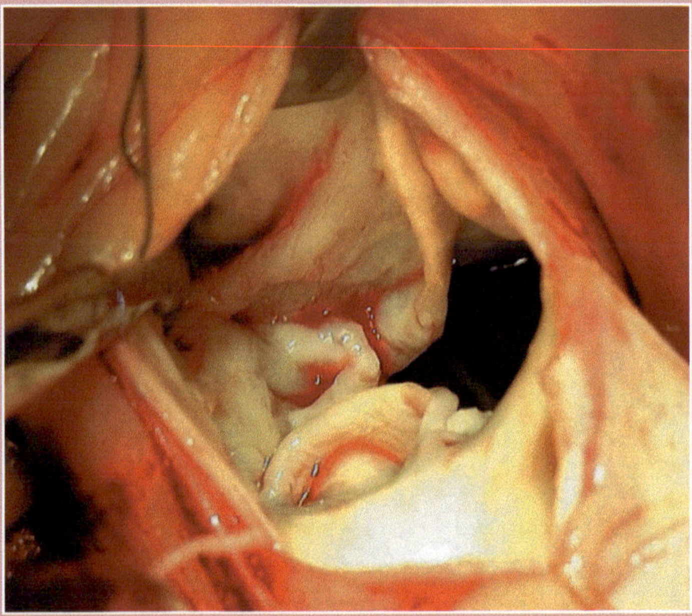

Fig. 5.50 Prolapse of thickened aortic cusps

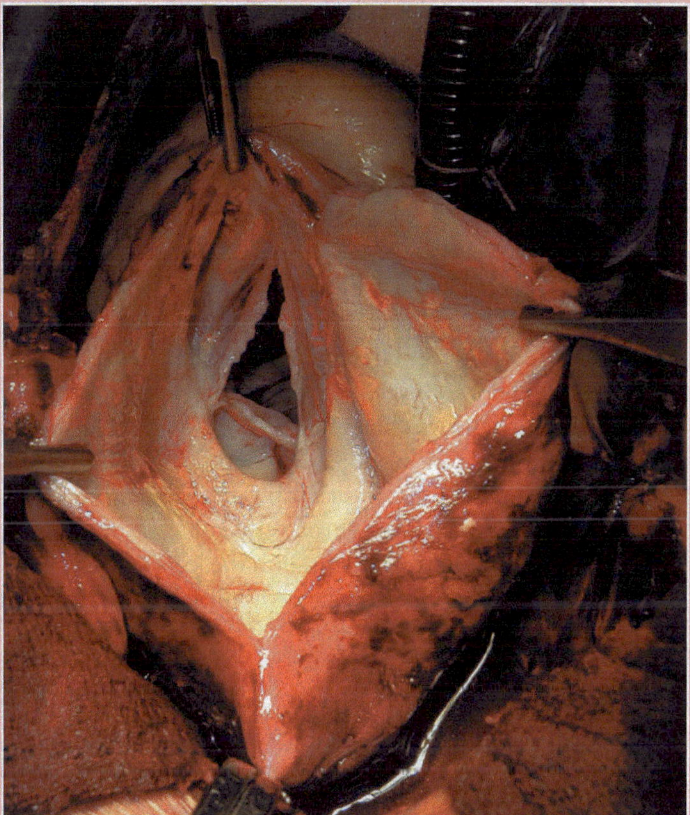

Fig. 5.51 Takayasu disease of aortic valve and ascending aorta

the loss of morphological support due to the subaortic ventricular septal defect (Fig. 5.52).

Dilation of the aortic annulus leading to the central regurgitation is often accompanied by dilation of the sinuses of Valsalva and of the sinotubular junction, thus forming the clinical entity of annulo-aortic ectasia (Figs. 5.53, 5.54). This global involvement of the aortic root may result from long-term hypertension and aortic-wall atherosclerosis, and is a typical cardiovascular manifestation of Marfan and Ehlers-Danlos syndromes.

Acute aortic regurgitation is most frequently caused by infective endocarditis during the course of which a cusp perforation or destruction develops (Figs. 5.45–5.47). Another cause of acute aortic regurgitation is aortic dissection type A. In this pathological condition the retrogradely spreading false lumen tears off the aortic valve commissure that prolapses with the adjacent cusps into the left ventricle. Acute aortic regurgitation may occur occasionally due to traumatic tearing off of the valve cusp.

5.3.2 Indications for Surgery

Aortic regurgitation is an insidious valve disease because even asymptomatic patients may already have severe aortic regurgitation and advanced left ventricular dysfunction. Indication therefore has to differentiate between symptomatic and asymptomatic patients. Symptomatic patients with severe aortic regurgitation are definitely indicated for surgery [3, 4].

The criteria for severe aortic regurgitation are as follows:

1. Regurgitation volume >60 ml/contraction
2. Regurgitation fraction >50%

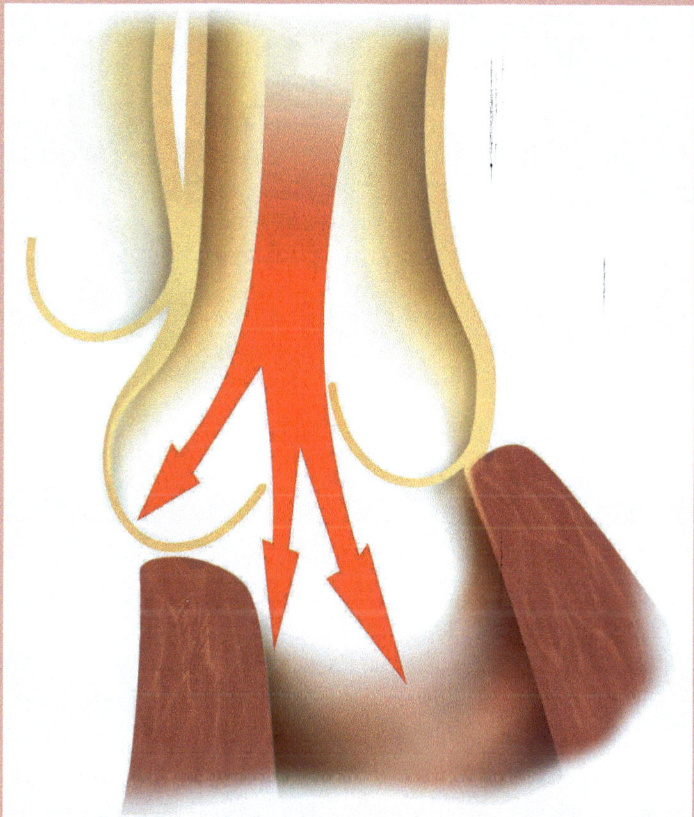

Fig. 5.52 Prolapse of the right aortic cusp in subaortic ventricular septal defect

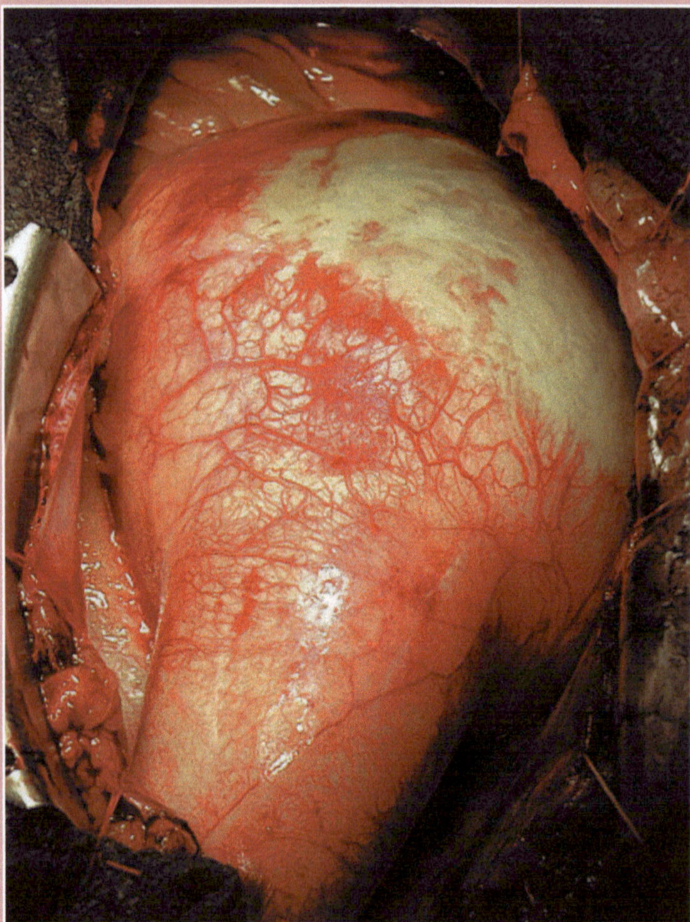

Fig. 5.53 Annulo-aortic ectasia

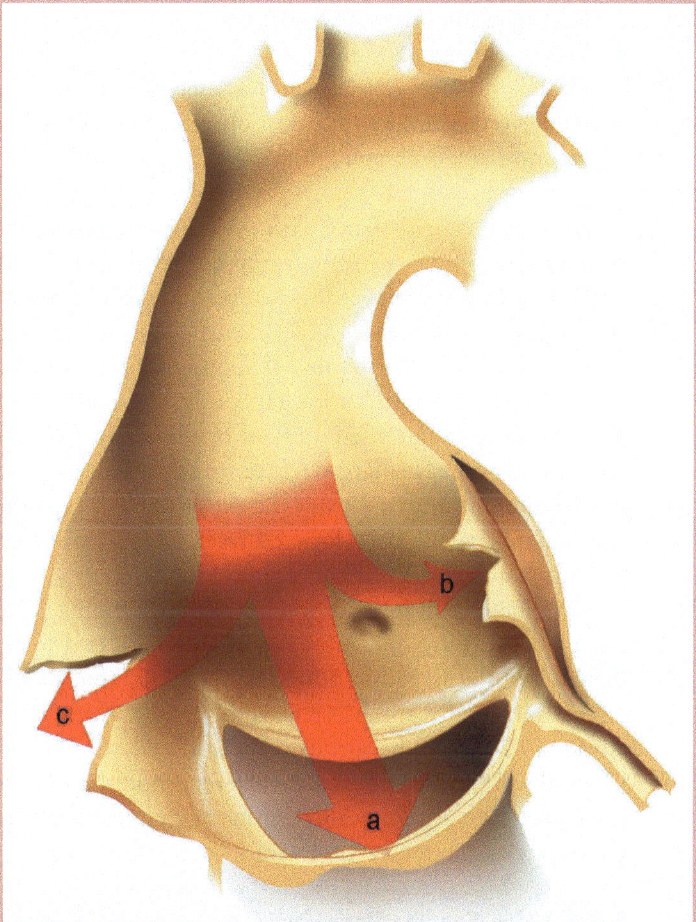

Fig. 5.54 Pathophysiological impacts of annulo-aortic ectasia. *a* Aortic regurgitation, *b* acute dissection type A, *c* aortic rupture

3. Regurgitation orifice area >0.3 cm^2
4. Vena contracta >6 mm
5. Holodiastolic reverse flow in the descending aorta
6. Undelayed equivalent contrast opacification of the left ventricle at aortography [3, 4]

Asymptomatic patients with severe aortic regurgitation are also indicated for surgery provided their EF is <50% and/or at the left ventricular end-diastolic dimension (LVEDD) >75 mm and the left ventricular end-systolic dimension (LVESD) >55 mm [3]. Constant improvement of operative results and, simultaneously, the evidence of unsatisfactory long-term results of operation in patients with already grossly enlarged left ventricle have influenced the decision making in the way the cut-off value for indication for surgery has been lowered recently to an LVEDD of 70 mm and an LVESD of 50 mm [4].

Simultaneous surgical procedure at the ascending aorta during aortic valve operation is generally indicated if the diameter of the ascending aorta reaches 50–55 mm. In bicuspid aortic valve and Marfan syndrome the operation is already indicated if the aortic diameter exceeds 45–50 mm [3, 4, 51, 52]. The indexed parameters should again be used, preferably with the cut-off value of 25 mm/m^2 for the patients with Marfan syndrome or bicuspid aortic valve.

5.3.3 Valve-Sparing Procedures in Aortic Regurgitation

Aortic valve replacement was formerly the treatment of choice for aortic regurgitation, except for acute aortic regurgitation in aortic dissection. In such cases of acute dissection the detached commissure can be sutured back to the aortic wall, and thus the competence of the valve can be restored without having to replace it (Fig. 5.55). In recent years, however, a growing body of knowledge has been accumulated concerning successful aortic valve repair in some types of aortic regurgitation. Aortic valve-sparing operations have become a challenging field for cardiac surgeons. Aortic valve repairs are offered preferably to younger patients in whom they enable avoidance of risks related to mechanical valve and long-term anticoagulation therapy. Choice of optimal surgical strategy in aortic regurgitation may sometimes be difficult. A decision has to be made between established and elaborate procedures with low operative risk and known good long-term results, and, if the operative findings allow it, a valve repair with rather uncertain early and long-term results.

Valve-sparing procedures are appropriate not only in patients with aortic regurgitation caused by isolated involvement of one or more cusps (prolapse, retraction, perforation), but also in regurgitation from annular dilation or whole aortic-root dilation provided there is little or no morphological damage evident at the cusps.

Some types of functional classifications of aortic regurgitations have already been suggested based on mechanism and pathophysiology of regurgitation. Lansac et al. [53] differentiate between two types: Type I has typical central regurgitation due to annular dilation, dilation of the sinotubular junction or of the whole aortic root, and annulo-aortic ectasia. Type II is characterized by eccentric regurgitation caused by cusp pathology (prolapse, retraction, tear, or perforation) [53]. El Khoury et al. [54] divide aortic regurgitation into three types: (a) type I (normal aortic cusps), in which the regurgitation is caused by dilation of functional aortic annulus (resembles type I according to Lansac et al.

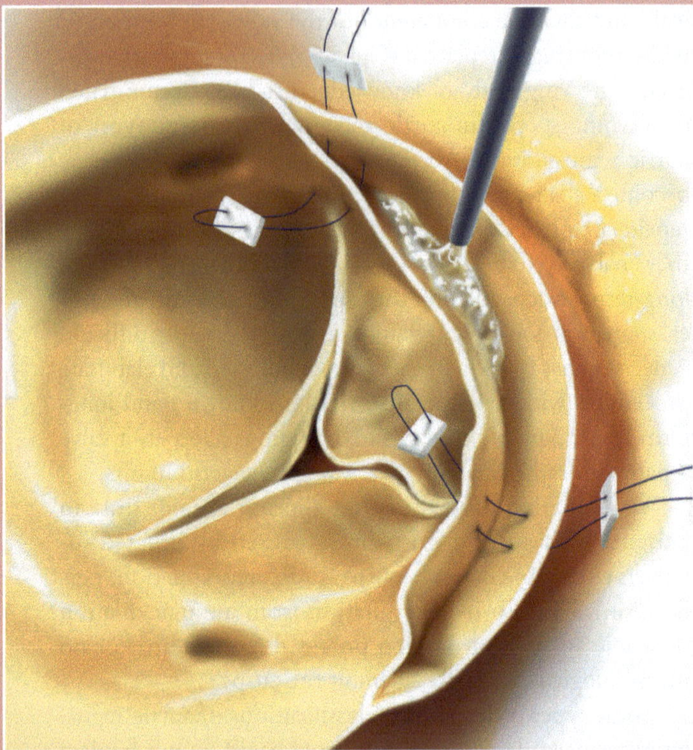

Fig. 5.55 Valve-sparing management of acute aortic regurgitation in acute dissection type A: fixation of commissures and gluing together of the dissected aortic wall layers by a tissue glue

[53]); (b) type II, featured by cusp prolapse due to tissue redundancy or a rare cusp tear-off in the commissure; and (c) type III, characterized by thickening and retraction of the cusps leading to the aortic regurgitation [54].

In cases of pure annular dilation, the surgical techniques are focused on its shortening. Circular aortic annuloplasty (Fig. 5.56) may be employed or, alternatively, only triangular subcommissural areas may be shortened by application of horizontal pledgeted mattress sutures (subcommissural annuloplasty; Fig. 5.57) [55–58].

If one cusp prolapses into the ventricle, the valve may also be spared and its good coaptation achieved with Trusler repair (Fig. 5.58) or with central plication (Fig. 5.59). Another option is triangular resection of the prolapsing aortic cusp (Figs. 5.60, 5.61) [55, 56]. A simple maneuver with Frater's stitch (Fig. 5.62) helps to assess which cusp is redundant and prolapsing. This stitch is passed through the midpoints of all three cusps (areas of noduli of Arantzius), and when it is pulled, the cusp portion that is redundant becomes clearly visible.

In prolapse of the anterior cusp of a bicuspid aortic valve, either triangular resection or central cusp plication may be performed with, in cases of wider aortic annulus, the adjunct of commissural annuloplasty. Should the raphe already be calcified, its excision is necessary (as a part of triangular resection) [56]. Cusp prolapse can also be repaired (shortened) by free margin reinforcement with "over-and--over" 7/0 polytetrafluoroethylene stitch, tied outside of the aorta (Figs. 5.63, 5.64) [57–59]. This procedure, however, is not suitable for a "paper-like" cusp due to the risk of small fenestrations. (The stitch has to be passed through the thickened edge.)

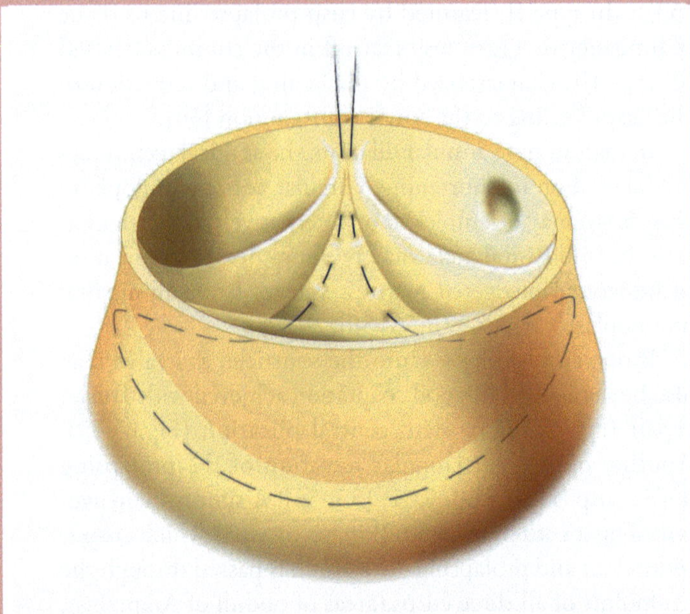

Fig. 5.56 Circular aortic annuloplasty (reduction of total circumference of dilated aortic annulus)

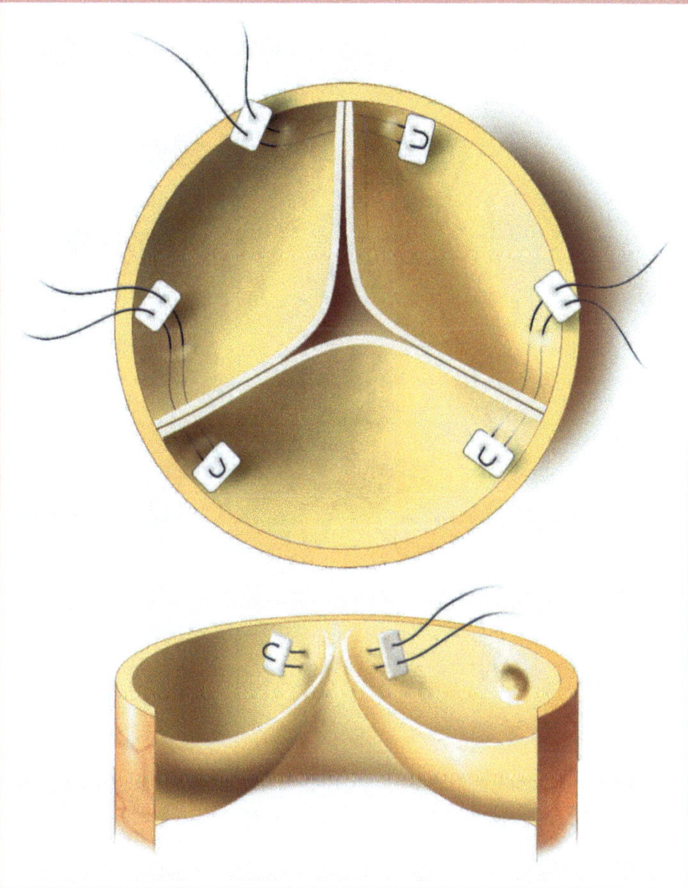

Fig. 5.57 Subcommissural annuloplasty (shortening of annulus in the areas of subcommissural triangles only)

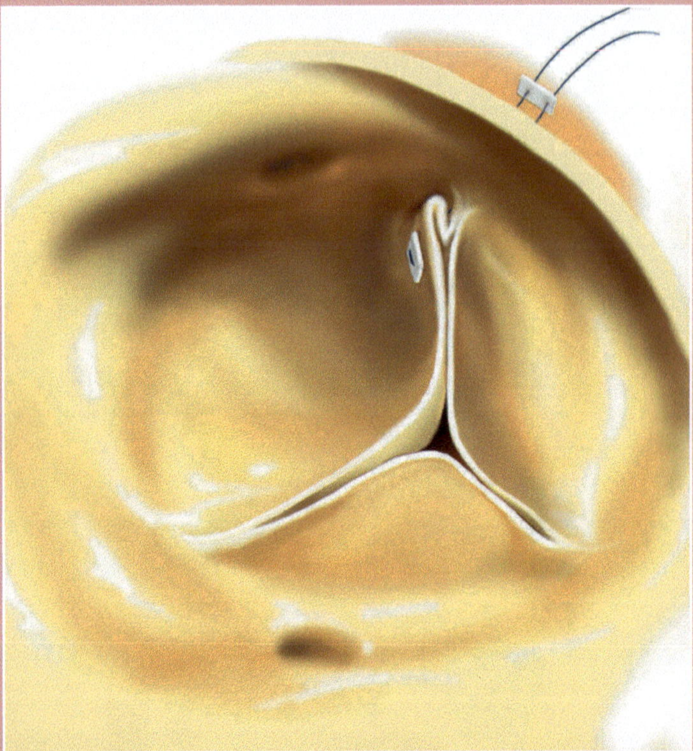

Fig. 5.58 Trusler repair (shortening of prolapsing aortic cusp by its plication at the commissure)

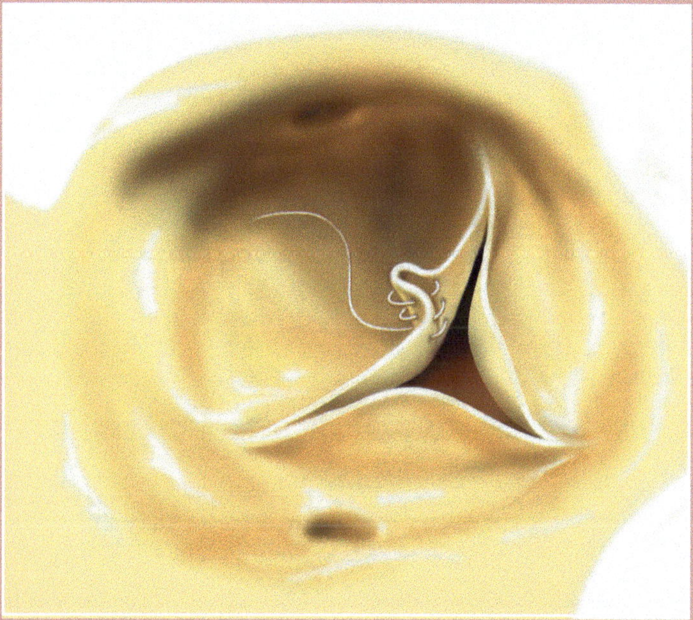

Fig. 5.59 Shortening of prolapsing aortic cusp by its central plication

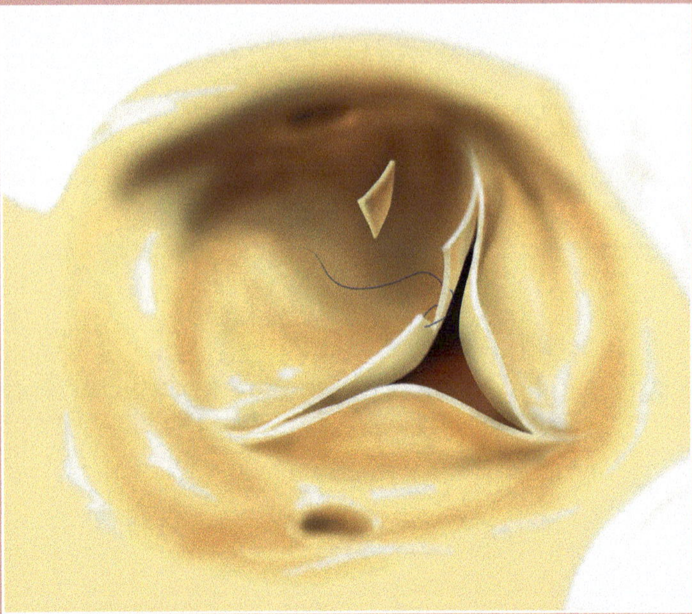

Fig. 5.60 Shortening of prolapsing aortic cusp by triangular resection

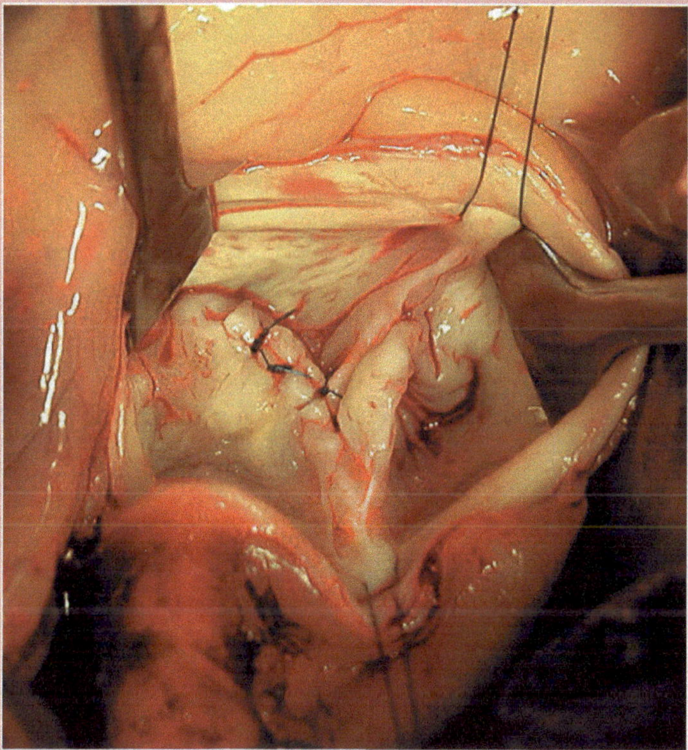

Fig. 5.61 Triangular resection of prolapsing aortic cusp (operative view)

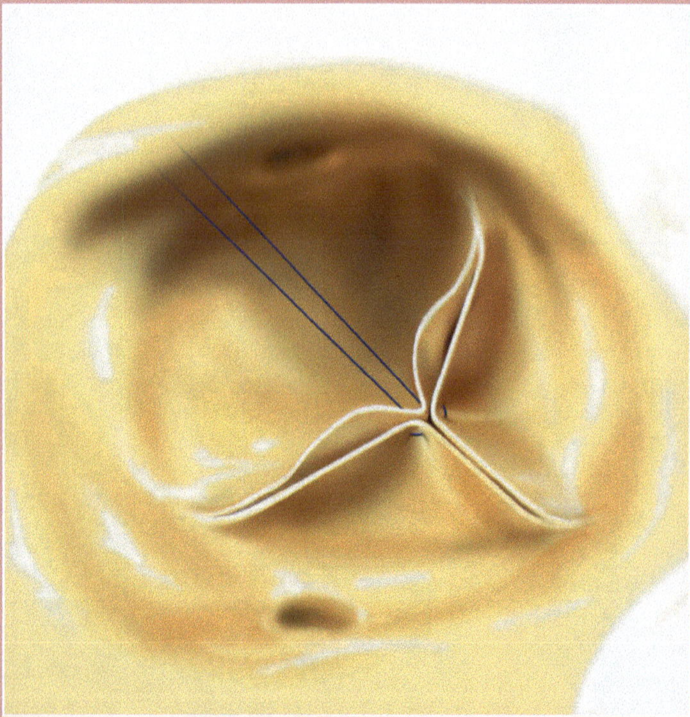

Fig. 5.62 Placement of Frater stitch facilitates analysis of prolapsing cusp and estimation of redundant length of its edge

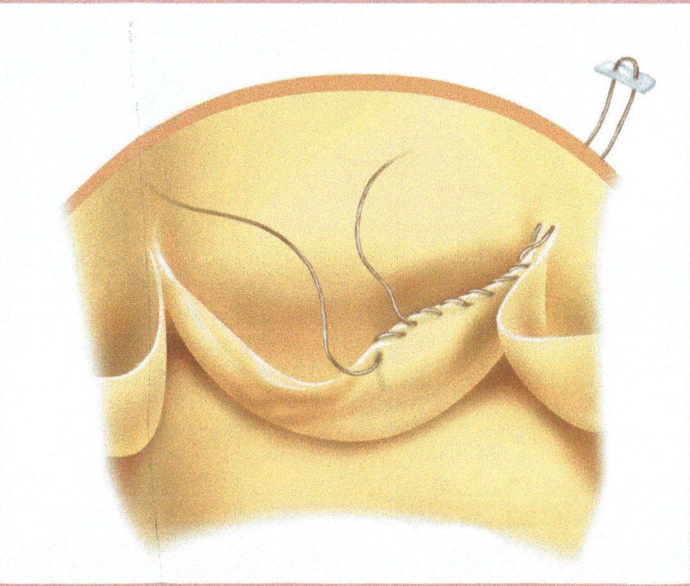

Fig. 5.63 Reduction of prolapsing aortic cusp edge by its plication with two running sutures

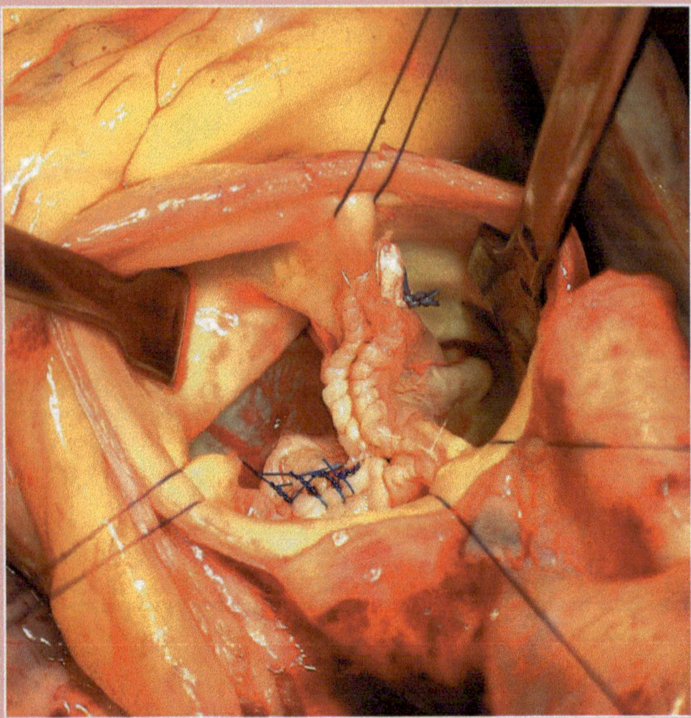

Fig. 5.64 Complex surgical restoration of aortic competence: resection of raphe; subcomissural annuloplasty; and polytetrafluoroethylene reinforcement of cusp edges

If peroperative transesophageal echocardiography confirms a residual cusp prolapse with second-degree regurgitation, a correction has to be made or the valve has to be replaced; otherwise, progression of the prolapse and worsening of regurgitation will follow, thus necessitating an early reoperation.

If the leaflets do not coapt because of lack of tissue or restricted motion, pericardial patch augmentation of the leaflets can be performed to increase coaptation surface (Fig. 5.65). The extension of aortic leaflets with glutaraldehyde-fixated autopericardium is a technically demanding procedure that is not popular among surgeons for fear of danger of patch dehiscence and late leaflet shrinkage, retraction, and calcification [60–63].

Isolated dilation of the sinotubular junction results in displacement of the commissures with loss of central cusp coaptation. Aortic valve competence can be restored by supracommissural replacement of the ascending aorta with prosthesis (see Figs. 5.30, 5.31).

If aortic regurgitation morphologically results from dilation of annulus, sinuses of Valsalva, and sinotubular junction, the clinical entity is defined as annulo-aortic ectasia. Once the aortic regurgitation and/or the dimensions of the ascending aorta meet the indicated criteria for operation, the classic treatment still remains the Bentall procedure (see Sect. 5.2.3.6). In case the aortic cusps are morphologically intact, the option of a valve-sparing procedure (aortic valve reimplantation according to David and Feindel [64]) may be considered (Figs. 5.66, 5.67) [65–69]. This procedure may also be chosen in suitable patients with acute aortic dissection type A. The aortic regurgitation caused predominantly by dilation of the sinuses of Valsalva and of the sinotubular junction with otherwise normal aortic

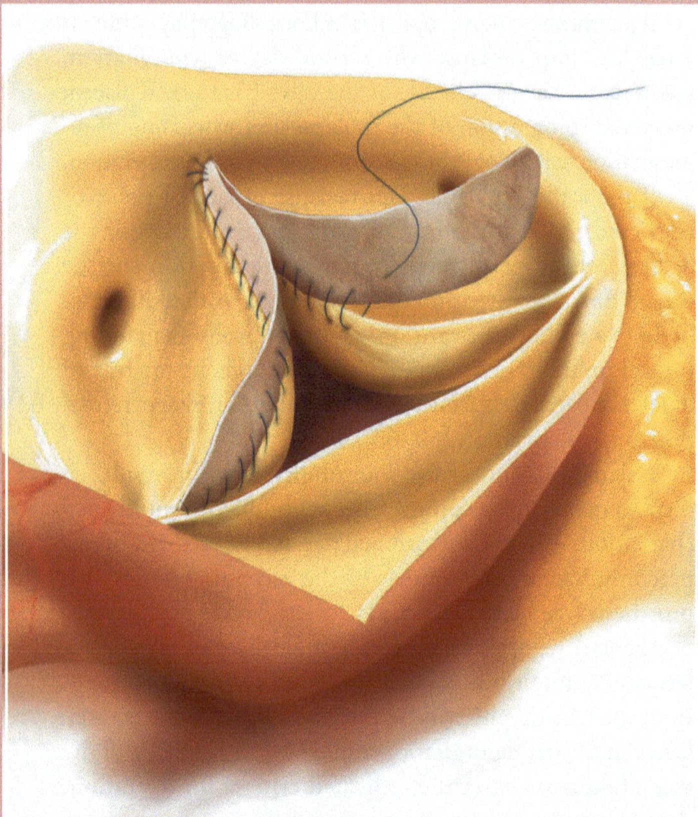

Fig. 5.65 Aortic leaflet extension by autologous pericardium fixated by glutaraldehyde

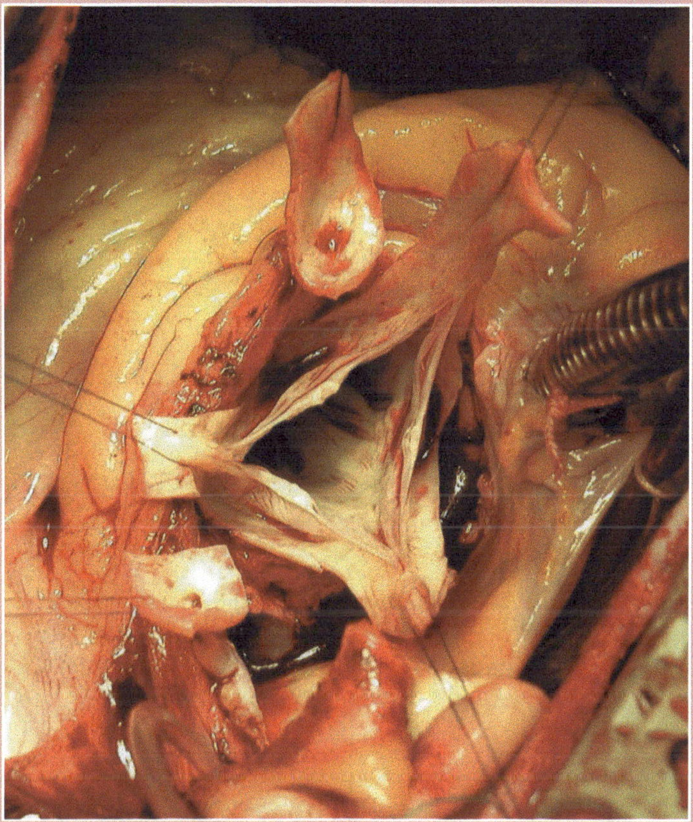

Fig. 5.66 Reimplantation of the aortic valve. (According to David and Feindel [64]). The aortic valve and both coronary ostia are dissected and prepared for reimplantation into the vascular graft

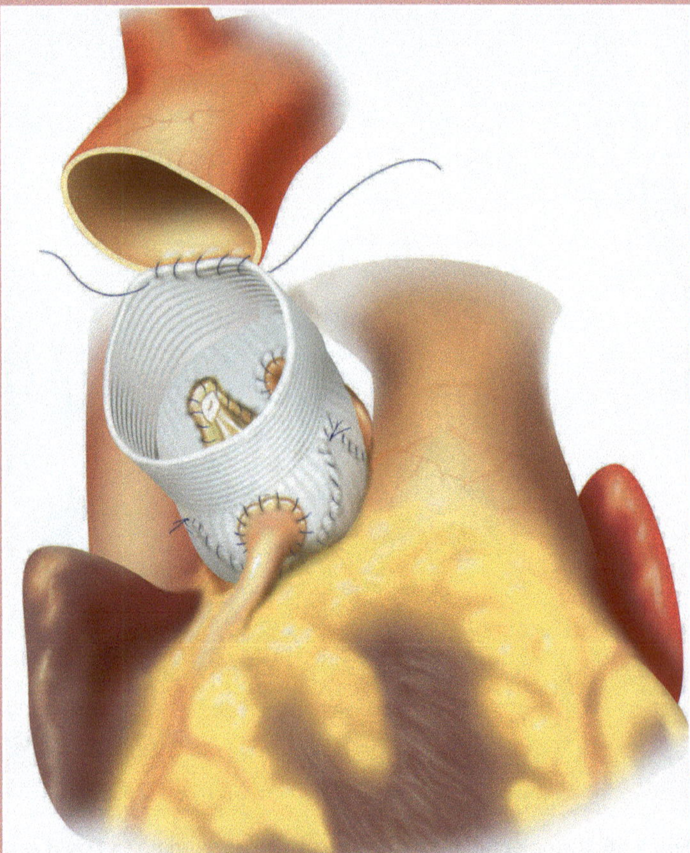

Fig. 5.67 Aortic valve reimplantation. (According to David and Feindel [64]). The aortic valve and both buttons with coronary ostia are implanted into the vascular graft

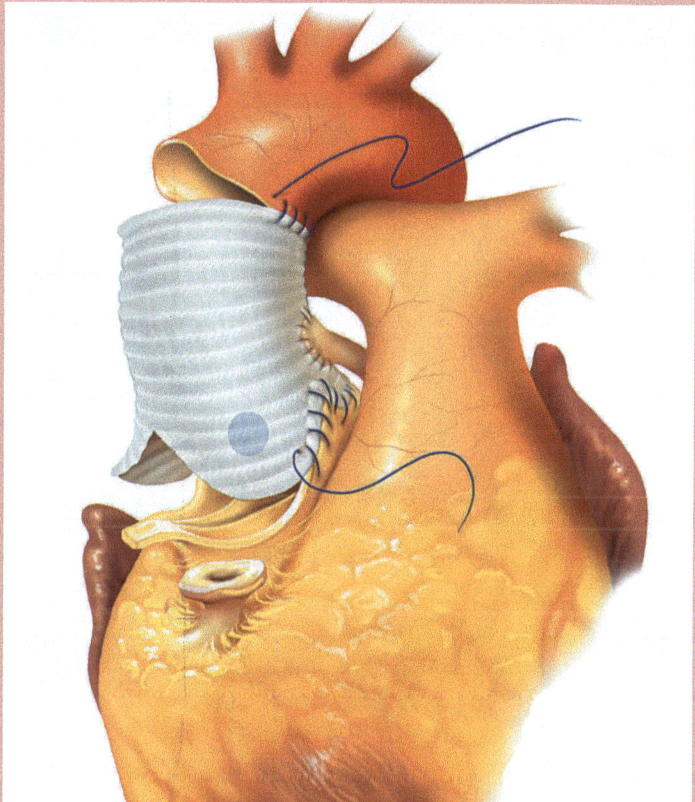

Fig. 5.68 Remodelation of the aortic root. Dilated aortic sinuses and sinotubular junction are replaced by a vascular graft. Buttons with coronary ostia are reimplanted into the vascular graft. (According to Yacoub et al. [70])

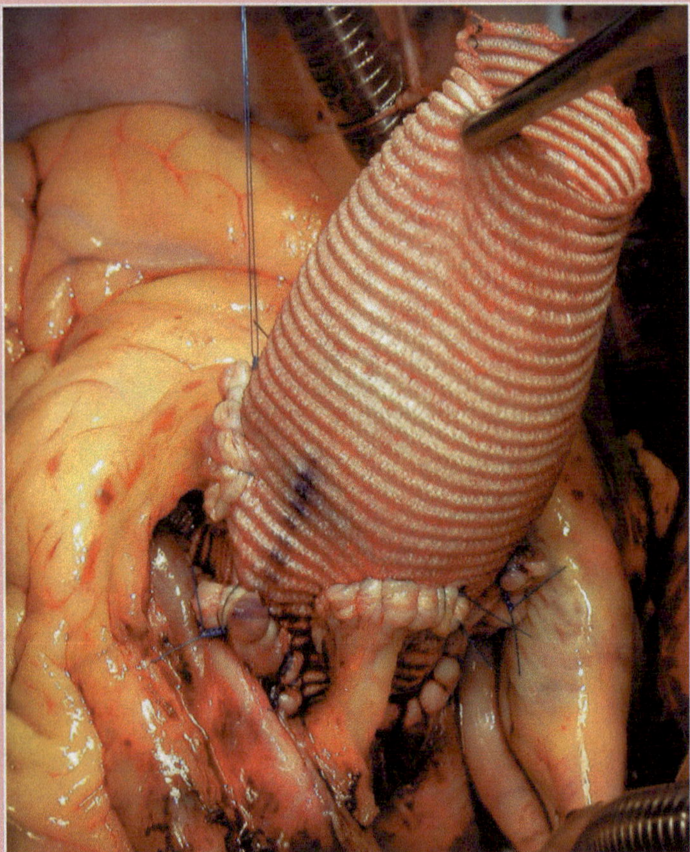

Fig. 5.69 Remodelation of the aortic root (operative view). (According to Yacoub et al. [70])

annulus may be treated by remodeling of the aortic root (according to Yacoub et al. [70]; see Figs. 5.68, 5.69) [65, 66, 71]. Despite various modifications of the aortic root remodelation technique aimed at prevention of further progression of annular dilation, the reimplantation procedure has been preferred to remodelation because of its safer long-term results. According to the multicenter analysis of 31 remodelation and reimplantation patient cohorts, the need for demanding reoperation can be expected in 9% of these patients within the first 5 years after surgery [65]. Studies over the coming years will determine whether, in the long-term, the need for reoperation will display a steep or constant increase, or a tendency to diminish.

References

1. Lewin MB, Otto CM (2005) The bicuspid aortic valve: adverse outcomes from infancy to old age. Circulation 111:832–834
2. Roberts WC, Vowels TJ, Ko JM (2009) Comparison of interpretations of valve structure between cardiac surgeon and cardiac pathologist among adults having isolated aortic valve replacement for aortic valve stenosis (±aortic regurgitation). Am J Cardiol 103:1139–1145
3. Bonow RO, Carabello BA, Kanu C et al. (2006) ACC/AHA 2006 guidelines for the management of patients with valvular heart disease. A report of the American College of Cardiology/American Heart Association Task Force on Practice Guidelines (writing committee to revise the 1998 Guidelines for the Management of Patients With Valvular Heart Disease); developed in collaboration with the Society of Cardiovascular Anesthesiologists; endorsed by the Society for Cardiovascular Angiography and Interventions and the Society of Thoracic Surgeons. Circulation 114:e84–e231

4. Vahanian A, Baumgartner H, Bax J et al. (2007) Guidelines on the management of valvular heart disease: The Task Force on the Management of Valvular Heart Disease of the European Society of Cardiology. Eur Heart J 28:230–268
5. Chambers J (2003) Low gradient, low ejection fraction aortic stenosis. Curr Treat Options Cardiovasc Med 5:469–474
6. Monin JL, Monchi M, Gest V et al. (2001) Aortic stenosis with severe left ventricular dysfunction and low transvalvular pressure gradients: risk stratification by low-dose dobutamine echocardiography. J Am Coll Cardiol 37:2101–2107
7. Subramanian H, Kunadian B, Dunning J (2008) Is it ever worth contemplating an aortic valve replacement on patients with low gradient severe aortic stenosis but poor left ventricular function with no contractile reserve? Interact Cardiovasc Thorac Surg 7:301–305
8. Piper C, Bergemann R, Schulte HD et al. (2003) Can progression of valvular aortic stenosis be predicted accurately? Ann Thorac Surg 76:676–680
9. Aris A, Camara ML, Montiel J et al. (1999) Ministernotomy versus median sternotomy for aortic valve replacement: a prospective, randomized study. Ann Thorac Surg 67:1583–1588
10. Bakir I, Casselman FP, Wellens F et al. (2006) Minimally invasive versus standard approach aortic valve replacement: a study in 506 patients. Ann Thorac Surg 81:1599–1604
11. Brown ML, McKellar SH, Sundt TM et al. (2009) Ministernotomy versus conventional sternotomy for aortic valve replacement: a systematic review and meta-analysis. J Thorac Cardiovasc Surg 137:670–679
12. Scarci M, Young C, Fallouh H (2009) Is ministernotomy superior to conventional approach for aortic valve replacement? Interact Cardiovasc Thorac Surg 9:314–317
13. Szwerc MF, Benckart DH, Wiechmann RJ et al. (1999) Partial versus full sternotomy for aortic valve replacement. Ann Thorac Surg 68:2209–2214
14. Tabata M, Umakanthan R, Cohn LH et al. (2008) Early and late outcomes of 1000 minimally invasive aortic valve operations. Eur J Cardiothorac Surg 33:537–541

15. Karimov JH, Santarelli F, Murzi M et al. (2009) A technique of an upper V-type ministernotomy in the second intercostal space. Interact Cardiovasc Thorac Surg 9:1021–1022
16. Minale C, Reifschneider HJ, Schmitz E et al. (1997) Single access for minimally invasive aortic valve replacement. Ann Thorac Surg 64:120–123
17. Nair RU, Sharpe DA (1998) Minimally invasive reversed Z sternotomy for aortic valve replacement. Ann Thorac Surg 65:1165–1166
18. Kleine P, Hasenkam MJ, Nygaard H et al. (2000) Tilting disc versus bileaflet aortic valve substitutes: intraoperative and postoperative hemodynamic performance in humans. J Heart Valve Dis 9:308–312
19. Laas J, Kleine P, Hasenkam MJ et al. (1999) Orientation of tilting disc and bileaflet aortic valve substitutes for optimal hemodynamics. Ann Thorac Surg 68:1096–1099
20. Botzenhardt F, Eichinger WB, Guenzinger R et al. (2005) Hemodynamic performance and incidence of patient–prosthesis mismatch of the complete supraannular perimount magna bioprosthesis in the aortic position. Thorac Cardiovasc Surg 53:226–230
21. Narang S, Satsangi DK, Banerjee A et al. (2008) Stentless valves versus stented bioprostheses at the aortic position: midterm results. J Thorac Cardiovasc Surg 136:943–947
22. Petracek MR (2002) Assessing options for the small aortic root. J Heart Valve Dis 11 (Suppl 1):S50–S55
23. Sintek CF, Fletcher AD, Khonsari S (1996) Small aortic root in the elderly: use of stentless bioprosthesis. J Heart Valve Dis 5 (Suppl 3):S308–S313
24. David TE, Uden DE (1983) Aortic valve replacement in adult patients with small aortic annuli. Ann Thorac Surg 36:577–583
25. Manhas DR, Stavney LS, Jones TW et al. (1980) Implantation of a larger aortic prosthetic valve in a patient with a small aortic annulus: an operative technique. Am Surg 46:597–599
26. Nicks R, Cartmill T, Bernstein L (1970) Hypoplasia of the aortic root. The problem of aortic valve replacement. Thorax 25:339–346

27. St. Rammos K, Ketikoglou DG, Koullias GJ et al. (2006) The Nicks–Nunez posterior enlargement in the small aortic annulus: immediate–intermediate results. Interact Cardiovasc Thorac Surg 5:749–753
28. Manouguian S, Seybold-Epting W (1979) Patch enlargement of the aortic valve ring by extending the aortic incision into the anterior mitral leaflet. New operative technique. J Thorac Cardiovasc Surg 78:402–412
29. Otaki M, Oku H, Nakamoto S et al. (1997) Two-directional aortic annular enlargement for aortic valve replacement in the small aortic annulus. Ann Thorac Surg 63:261–263
30. Konno S, Imai Y, Iida Y et al. (1975) A new method for prosthetic valve replacement in congenital aortic stenosis associated with hypoplasia of the aortic valve ring. J Thorac Cardiovasc Surg 70:909–917
31. Morrow AG, Brockenbrough EC (1961) Surgical treatment of idiopathic hypertrophic subaortic stenosis: technique and hemodynamic results of subaortic ventriculomyotomy. Ann Surg 154:181–189
32. Ross D (1991) Technique of aortic valve replacement with a homograft: orthotopic replacement. Ann Thorac Surg 52:154–156
33. Kilian E, Oberhoffer M, Gulbins H et al. (2004) Ten years' experience in aortic valve replacement with homografts in 389 cases. J Heart Valve Dis 13:554–559
34. Gill M, Dunning J (2009) Is reduction aortoplasty (with or without external wrap) an acceptable alternative to replacement of the dilated ascending aorta? Interact Cardiovasc Thorac Surg 9:693–697
35. Arsan S, Akgun S, Kurtoglu N et al. (2004) Reduction aortoplasty and external wrapping for moderately sized tubular ascending aortic aneurysm with concomitant operations. Ann Thorac Surg 78:858–861
36. Bauer M, Pasic M, Schaffarzyk R et al. (2002) Reduction aortoplasty for dilatation of the ascending aorta in patients with bicuspid aortic valve. Ann Thorac Surg 73:720–724

37. Cohen O, Odim J, Zerda D de la et al. (2007) Long-term experience of girdling the ascending aorta with Dacron mesh as definitive treatment for aneurysmal dilation. Ann Thorac Surg 83:S780–S790
38. Feindt P, Litmathe J, Borgens A et al. (2007) Is size-reducing ascending aortoplasty with external reinforcement an option in modern aortic surgery? Eur J Cardiothorac Surg 31:614–617
39. Maggio P, Carbone F, Lucchese G et al. (2008) Reduction aortoplasty: effective, useless or harmful? Results at 10 years. Interact Cardiovasc Thorac Surg 7:30
40. Kindo M, Billaud P, Gerelli S et al. (2007) Twenty-seven-year experience with composite valve graft replacement of the aortic root. J Heart Valve Dis 16:370–377
41. Bentall H, Bono A de (1968) A technique for complete replacement of the ascending aorta. Thorax 23:338–339
42. Cabrol C, Pavie A, Gandjbakhch I et al. (1981) Complete replacement of the ascending aorta with reimplantation of the coronary arteries: new surgical approach. J Thorac Cardiovasc Surg 81:309–315
43. Svensson LG (1992) Approach for insertion of aortic composite valve grafts. Ann Thorac Surg 54:376–378
44. De Robertis F, Asgar A, Davies S et al. (2009) The left axillary artery: a new approach for transcatheter aortic valve implantation. Eur J Cardiothorac Surg 36:807–812
45. Bleiziffer S, Ruge H, Mazzitelli D et al. (2009) Results of percutaneous and transapical transcatheter aortic valve implantation performed by a surgical team. Eur J Cardiothorac Surg 35:615–621
46. Mack MJ (2009) Transapical aortic valve implantation: Is it ready for prime time? Eur J Cardiothorac Surg 36:229–230
47. Vahanian A, Alfieri OR, Al-Attar N et al. (2008) Transcatheter valve implantation for patients with aortic stenosis: a position statement from the European Association of Cardio-Thoracic Surgery (EACTS) and the European Society of Cardiology (ESC), in collaboration with the European Association of Percutaneous Cardiovascular Interventions (EAPCI). Eur J Cardiothorac Surg 34:1–8

48. Walther T, Falk V, Borger MA et al. (2007) Minimally invasive transapical beating heart aortic valve implantation: proof of concept. Eur J Cardiothorac Surg 31:9–15
49. Walther T, Falk V, Borger MA et al. (2009) Transapical aortic valve implantation in patients requiring redo surgery. Eur J Cardiothorac Surg 36:231–235
50. Walther T, Falk V, Kempfert J et al. (2008) Transapical minimally invasive aortic valve implantation: the initial 50 patients. Eur J Cardiothorac Surg 33:983–988
51. Borger MA, Preston M, Ivanov J et al. (2004) Should the ascending aorta be replaced more frequently in patients with bicuspid aortic valve disease? J Thorac Cardiovasc Surg 128:677–683
52. Parish LM, Gorman JH III, Kahn S et al. (2009) Aortic size in acute type A dissection: implications for preventive ascending aortic replacement. Eur J Cardiothorac Surg 35:941–946
53. Lansac E, Centa I di, Raoux F et al. (2008) A lesional classification to standardize surgical management of aortic insufficiency towards valve repair. Eur J Cardiothorac Surg 33:872–880
54. El Khoury G, Glineur D, Rubay J et al. (2005) Functional classification of aortic root/valve abnormalities and their correlation with etiologies and surgical procedures. Curr Opin Cardiol 20:115–121
55. Carpentier A (1983) Cardiac valve surgery: the "French correction." J Thorac Cardiovasc Surg 86:323–337
56. Cosgrove DM, Rosenkranz ER, Hendren WG et al. (1991) Valvuloplasty for aortic insufficiency. J Thorac Cardiovasc Surg 102:571–577
57. El Khoury G, Vanoverschelde JL, Glineur D et al. (2004) Repair of aortic valve prolapse: experience with 44 patients. Eur J Cardiothorac Surg 26:628–633
58. Chiappini B, Pouleur AC, Noirhomme P et al. (2007) Repair of trileaflet aortic valve prolapse: mid-term outcome in patients with normal aortic root morphology. Interact Cardiovasc Thorac Surg 6:56–59
59. David TE, Armstrong S, Ivanov J et al. (1999) Aortic valve sparing operations: an update. Ann Thorac Surg 67:1840–1856

60. Ahn H, Kim KH, Kim YJ (2002) Midterm result of leaflet extension technique in aortic regurgitation. Eur J Cardiothorac Surg 21:465–469
61. Doss M, Moid R, Wood JP et al. (2005) Pericardial patch augmentation for reconstruction of incompetent bicuspid aortic valves. Ann Thorac Surg 80:304–307
62. Haydar HS, He GW, Hovaguimian H et al. (1997) Valve repair for aortic insufficiency: surgical classification and techniques. Eur J Cardiothorac Surg 11:258–265
63. Jeong DS, Kim KH, Ahn H (2009) Long-term results of the leaflet extension technique in aortic regurgitation: thirteen years of experience in a single center. Ann Thorac Surg 88:83–89
64. David TE, Feindel CM (1992) An aortic valve-sparing operation for patients with aortic incompetence and aneurysm of the ascending aorta. J Thorac Cardiovasc Surg 103:617–622
65. Albes JM, Stock UA, Hartrumpf M (2005) Restitution of the aortic valve: What is new, what is proven, and what is obsolete? Ann Thorac Surg 80:1540–1549
66. Hopkins RA (2003) Aortic valve leaflet sparing and salvage surgery: evolution of techniques for aortic root reconstruction. Eur J Cardiothorac Surg 24:886–897
67. Kallenbach K, Karck M, Pak D et al. (2005) Decade of aortic valve sparing reimplantation: Are we pushing the limits too far? Circulation 112:I253–I259
68. Sareyyupoglu B, Suri RM, Schaff HV et al. (2009) Survival and reoperation risk following bicuspid aortic valve-sparing root replacement. J Heart Valve Dis 18:1–8
69. Settepani F, Bergonzini M, Barbone A et al. (2009) Reimplantation valve-sparing aortic root replacement with the Valsalva graft: What have we learnt after 100 cases? Interact Cardiovasc Thorac Surg 9:113–116
70. Yacoub MH, Fagan A, Stassano P et al. (1983) Results of valve conserving operations for aortic regurgitation. Circulation 68:III-321.
71. Sarsam MA, Yacoub M (1993) Remodeling of the aortic valve annulus. J Thorac Cardiovasc Surg 105:435–438

Mitral Valve Surgery

6 Mitral Valve Surgery

6.1 Introduction

Closed-heart mitral commissurotomies followed later by open-heart commissurotomies and mitral valve replacements were the most frequent valve procedures from the 1950s to the 1970s. Aortic valve surgery gradually has become the more frequent procedure and the number of mitral procedures has slowly decreased. Presently, operation for a rheumatic mitral stenosis is relatively rare. The reason is that rheumatic mitral stenosis is becoming very rare in developed countries, and when it does occur, the patients who were formerly candidates for surgical commissurotomy are now treated by percutaneous balloon valvuloplasty. Only the relatively few patients who do not meet the echocardiographic criteria for percutaneous intervention, because of heavy calcifications and/or coexistent mitral incompetence, are indicated for surgical treatment. Nevertheless, mitral valve surgery has been constantly developing, due mainly to the increasing number of patients who need surgical treatment for a significant mitral regurgitation. The etiology of mitral regurgitation is predominantly degenerative or ischemic, and the majority of these valves are eligible for repair.

Mitral valve surgery is often associated with tricuspid valve repair (in cases of tricuspidalized mitral valve disease), coronary artery bypass grafting (ischemic mitral incompetence), and radiofrequency or cryosurgical maze procedure for paroxysmal, persistent, or permanent atrial fibrillation.

J. Dominik and P. Zacek, *Heart Valve Surgery: An Illustrated Guide*,
DOI 10.1007/978-3-642-12206-4_6,

6.2 Surgical Approaches to the Mitral Valve

Several surgical approaches to the mitral valve exist. After analysis of a given clinical situation, the surgeon chooses the approach that will ensure perfect exposure of the surgical field and optimal conditions for performing the planned procedure. This is even more important in complex mitral repairs.

Closed mitral commissurolyses and commissurotomies were accomplished via left-sided thoracotomy through the fourth intercostal space. In cases of a rare reoperation by closed-heart technique, right-sided thoracotomy was the chosen approach.

Open-heart surgery on the mitral valve (with use of cardiopulmonary bypass) is most frequently performed via median sternotomy.

The previously often-employed extensive right anterolateral thoracotomy is currently seldom performed. A short right-sided thoracotomy through the fourth intercostal space is, however, the preferred approach for minimally invasive mitral valve surgery [1–3].

Right-sided anterolateral thoracotomy can be advantageous in repeated reoperations in order to avoid the risk of right ventricle injury. Right- or left-sided thoracotomy may also be beneficial in reoperations with previously performed left internal mammary artery bypass for coronary revascularization. In such cases the procedure is best accomplished without aortic cross-clamping on a beating heart [4, 5]. The advantages are the avoidance of resternotomy and potential risk of injury to the right ventricle, avoidance of time-consuming and risky dissection of the patent mammaro-coronary graft, and maintenance of normal coronary perfusion (coronary arteries and grafts). Prior to this strategy, aortic incompetence has to be ruled out. The arterial cannula is introduced via the groin into the femoral artery and the venous return is secured with use of vacuum-assisted drainage by a long venous cannula reaching from the femoral vein up to the right atrium. If a right-sided approach was chosen, the venous drainage can be accomplished by two venous cannulae introduced through the right atrium. To avoid systemic air embolization, it is mandatory to keep the mitral valve open for the entire intracardiac surgery and to maintain continuous suction from the left ventricle. In addition to these measures a CO_2 gaseous atmosphere is replenished intrathoracically throughout the whole period of the open left atrium.

Similarly, mitral valve procedures may be carried out via a shorter right-sided thoracotomy through the fourth intercostal space on a perfused and fibrillating heart (without aortic cross-clamping). Cardiopulmonary bypass is instituted via femoral vessels. Some cardiosurgical units do employ this unusual technique, not only in reoperations but also in primary cardiac procedures, with excellent results [6, 7].

Among other less invasive surgical approaches, short right parasternal incision, limited lower sternotomy, port-access technology, or robotic surgery could be employed for mitral valve surgery, although they have not gained much popularity, except for in a few institutions [8, 9].

The exposure of the mitral valve itself (after median sternotomy in the majority of cases) is obtained most frequently by a longitudinal left atrial incision (Fig. 6.1). Deep dissection of the interatrial groove enables to carry the incision deeper and centrally, and thus to achieve a more direct view into the left atrium. Another maneuver to improve the exposure is the liberation of the superior and inferior venae cavae at the area of pericardial reflection as suggested by

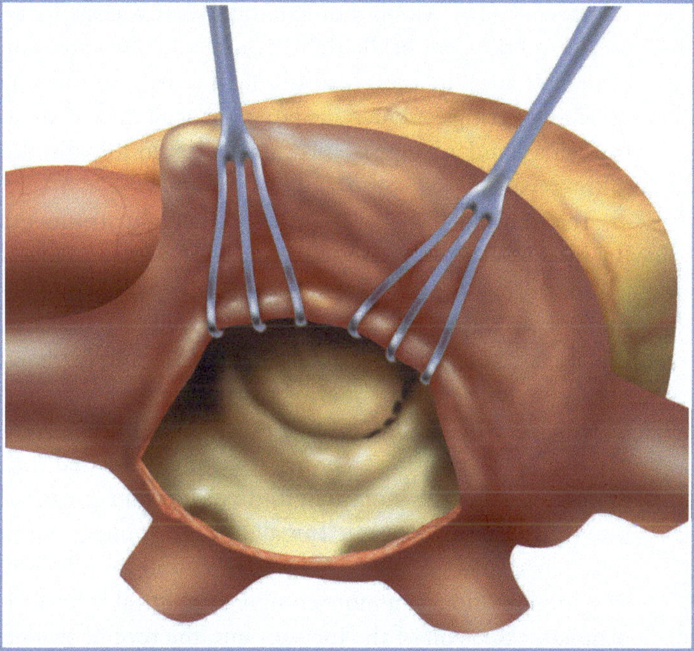

Fig. 6.1 Approach to the mitral valve via longitudinal left atriotomy (through the dissected interatrial groove in a Sondergaard's plane)

Pifarre et al. [10]. Mobilization of the venae cavae facilitates greater ventral shift of the right atrium, and also extension of the left atrial incision beneath these veins is in this way possible. Having exploited the potential of all these maneuvers, this standard approach is sufficient even for complex mitral repairs.

The transseptal approach (through the right atrium and the interatrial septum) is the second most frequently used approach (Fig. 6.2). It is preferred in patients in whom simultaneous mitral and tricuspid valve procedure is planned. It is also advantageous in mitral valve reoperations (to avoid firm adhesions after the previous left atrial approach) and in patients with small left atrium, hypertrophic left ventricle, and deep thorax. The right atrium is incised longitudinally and the same longitudinal incision is carried into the interatrial septum. This allows a convenient mitral valve replacement or an uncomplicated mitral annuloplasty ring implantation. If a more complex mitral valve repair is planned, extension of the incision into the roof of the left atrium is advisable. This extended vertical septal approach (Fig. 6.3) according to Guiraudon et al. [12] enables superior exposure of the mitral valve without harmful stress or distortion of the valve [11–14]. Sinoatrial node dysfunction is extremely rare, even in cases of transsection of the sinus node artery arising from the right coronary artery [15–17]. Safe use of this excellent approach should be preceded by coronarography analysis: a dominant blood supply of the sinus node by the left sinus node artery originating from the circumflex artery (laterally via the left atrial roof) is a favorable condition, whereas a solitary blood supply by a large right-sided sinus node artery is discouraging due to the fear of sinus node injury.

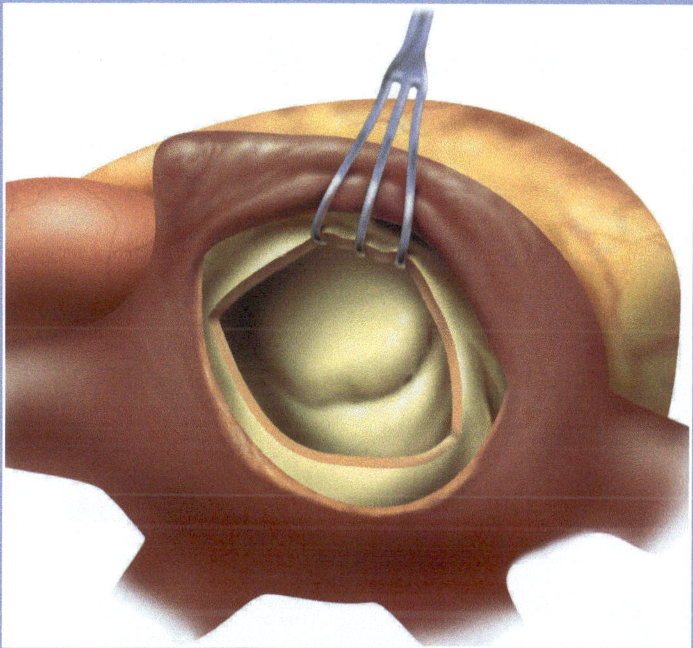

Fig. 6.2 Transseptal approach to the mitral valve (through the right atrium and the interatrial septum)

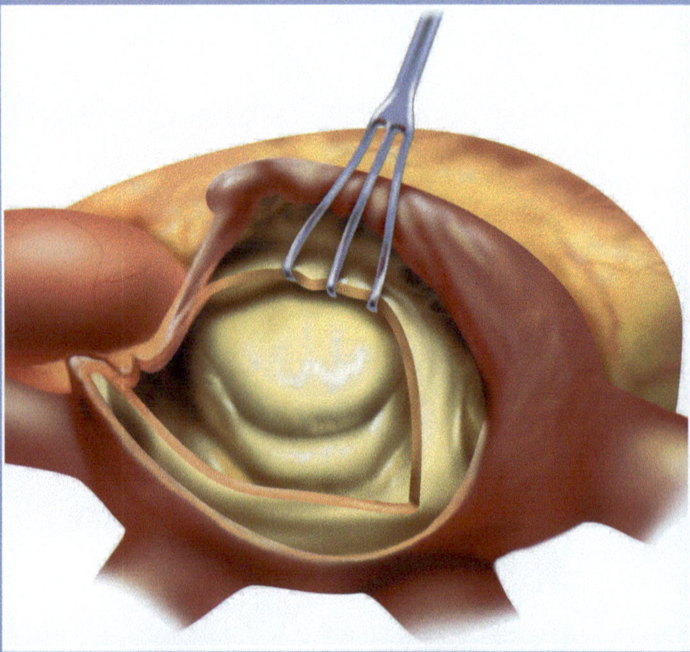

Fig. 6.3 Transseptal approach to the mitral valve (interatrial septal incision is extended into the roof of the left atrium). (According to Guiraudon [12])

Other approaches to the mitral valve have been reported but are employed less frequently. Dubost et al. described transverse incision of the right atrium and corresponding transverse incision into the interatrial septum extended far laterally between the right-sided pulmonary veins [18, 19]. We adopted a modification of this approach: instead of the lateral extension, we curve the septal incision in hockey-stick shape into the conventional upper-left atrial incision. Combination of these two principles follows the rules of surgical economy and simultaneously offers a geometrically straighter view of the mitral valve (Fig. 6.4) [20].

The superior approach reported by Meyer et al. is accomplished by a transverse incision into the left atrial roof after the ascending aorta has been pulled to the left and the superior vena cava to the right [21–24]. Carmichael et al. described mitral valve replacement via aortotomy through the aortic annulus in simultaneous aortic and mitral valve replacement [25]. In the case of the left ventricular aneurysmectomy, the mitral valve can also be replaced through the ventriculotomy.

6.3 Mitral Stenosis

Etiology of mitral stenosis is almost exclusively rheumatic. Rheumatic disease results in fibrous thickening of the mitral leaflets followed later by heavy calcification. The commissures are typically fused. The chordae are thickened and sometimes shortened to such a degree that thickened calcified mitral leaflets are attached directly to the papillary muscles (Figs. 6.5, 6.6). Development of this pathomorphology ends up in a narrow mitral orifice causing transmitral pressure gradient. Elevated left atrial pressure leads to left atrial dilation, gradually increasing pulmonary hypertension, and

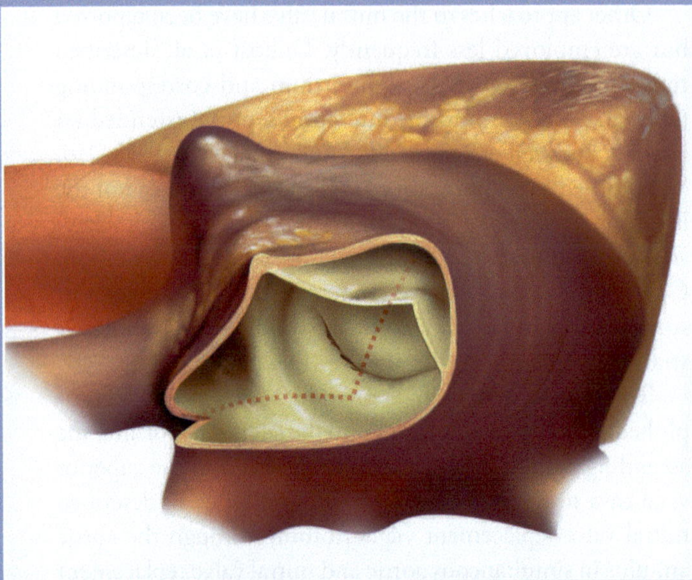

Fig. 6.4 Hockey-stick biatrial approach to the mitral valve. (According to Zacek et al. [20])

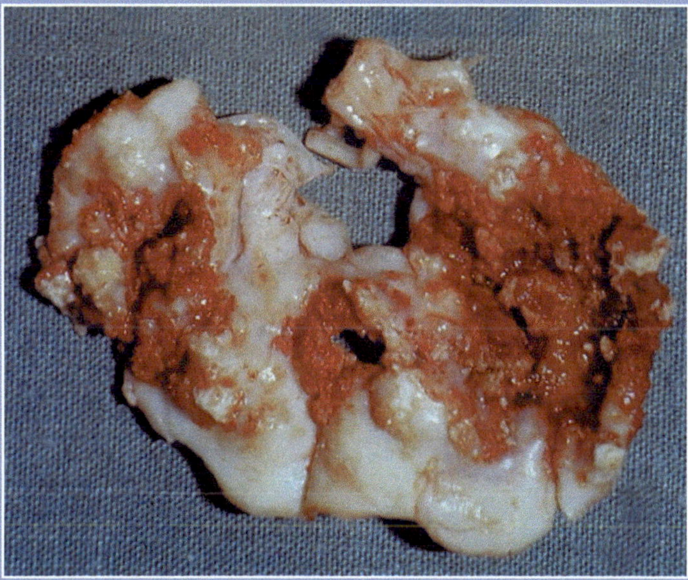

Fig. 6.5 Mitral valve is heavily calcified due to rheumatic mitral stenosis

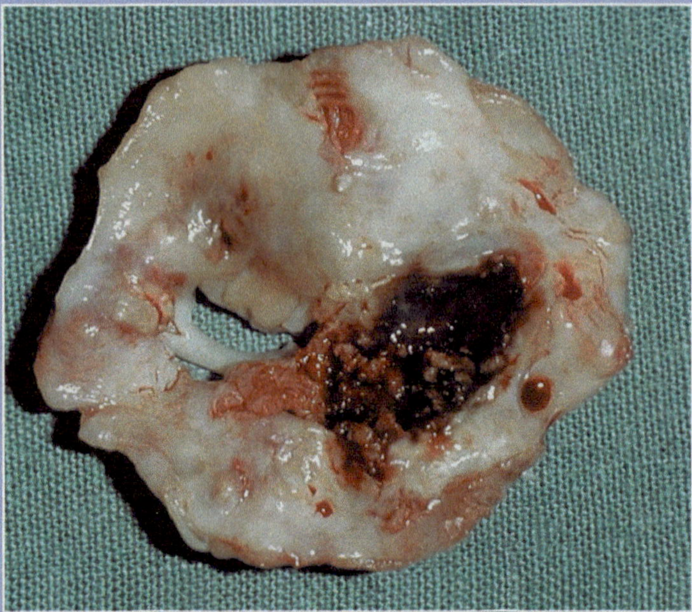

Fig. 6.6 Infective endocarditis at calcified rheumatic mitral stenosis

in the advanced stage onset of atrial fibrillation. Thrombus formation may occur in the dilated and fibrillating left atrium unless the patient is not effectively anticoagulated (Fig. 6.7). The systolic left ventricular function remains generally unaltered except for patients with history of heavy rheumatic pancarditis. Severe mitral stenosis is characterized by congestive left heart failure together with signs of low cardiac output. Clinical manifestation is worsening dyspnea and fatigue.

6.3.1 Indications for Surgery

Surgical treatment of mitral stenosis is indicated in those symptomatic patients whose mitral valve does not meet echocardiographic criteria for percutaneous transluminal balloon valvuloplasty (due to excessive calcification, commissural calcification, concomitant mitral regurgitation, or presence of thrombi in the left atrium). Severely symptomatic patients in New York Heart Association (NYHA) stage-III and stage-IV classification are indicated for surgery if their mitral valve area (MVA) is less than 1.5 cm^2 (<0.8 cm^2/m^2) and their diastolic gradient greater than 8 mmHg. Less symptomatic patients (NYHA stage II) are indicated only if their MVA is less than 1 cm^2 or if their systolic pulmonary pressure (PAP) is greater than 50 mmHg at rest or greater than 60 mmHg during exercise. Onset of atrial fibrillation and/or thrombi in the left atrium speeds up indication for operation [26, 27].

6.3.2 Closed Mitral Commissurotomy

Closed mitral commissurotomy is no longer performed in developed countries. Newly diagnosed patients with mitral valve morphology suitable for this procedure are treated

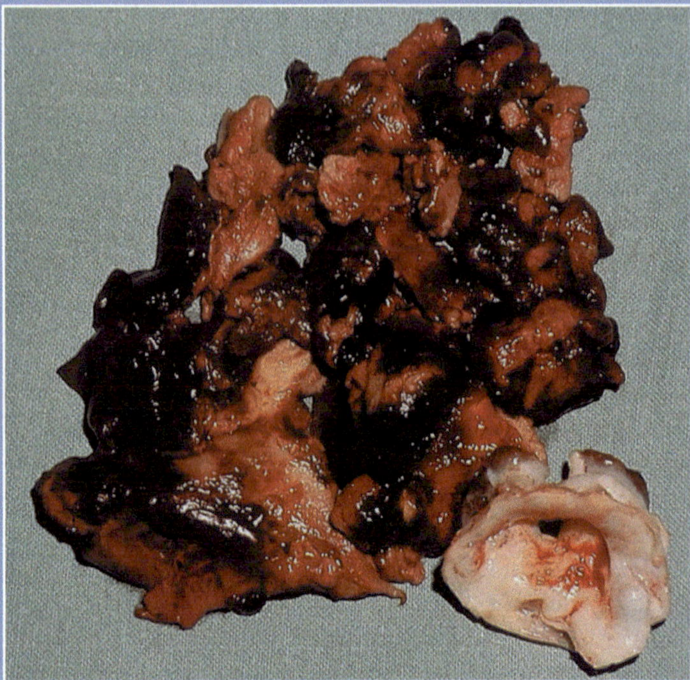

Fig. 6.7 Thrombi from the left atrium and rheumatic stenotic mitral valve (stenotic orifice, fused commissures, fibrous thickening of the leaflets with calcifications)

by percutaneous transluminal mitral balloon valvuloplasty. Those who do not meet echocardiographic criteria for percutaneous procedure are indicated for open-heart mitral surgery. Their mitral valve, however, is usually so severely diseased that replacement is the only option. For this reason open mitral commissurotomies are extremely rare.

Closed mitral commissurotomy is accomplished via left thoracotomy through the fourth intercostal space. After longitudinal pericardiotomy in front of the phrenic nerve, the left atrial appendage is encircled by a purse-string suture (in cases of narrow tubular appendage, the free left atrial wall is chosen). The surgeon then introduces his forefinger through the appendage into the left atrium and by application of pressure performs digital commissurolysis (Fig. 6.8). If the fused commissures cannot be detached by digital pressure (commissurolysis), a Dogliotti's ring on the finger has to be used for cutting the fused commissures (commissurotomy). Alternatively, some centers used the Dubost dilator introduced through the left atrial appendage into the mitral valve), or, more often, Tubbs dilator, which was introduced through the left ventricular apex into the mitral valve and its position was controlled against the surgeon's forefinger inserted through the left atrial appendage [28].

Results of the closed mitral commissurotomies were good. In-hospital mortality in large cohorts ranged between 0 and 3%. Incidence of mitral restenosis requiring reoperation within 10 years postoperatively was reported to be 20–30% [29, 30].

6.3.3 Open Mitral Commissurotomy

Only upon direct analysis of the mitral valve on opened and arrested heart does the surgeon decide whether the valve

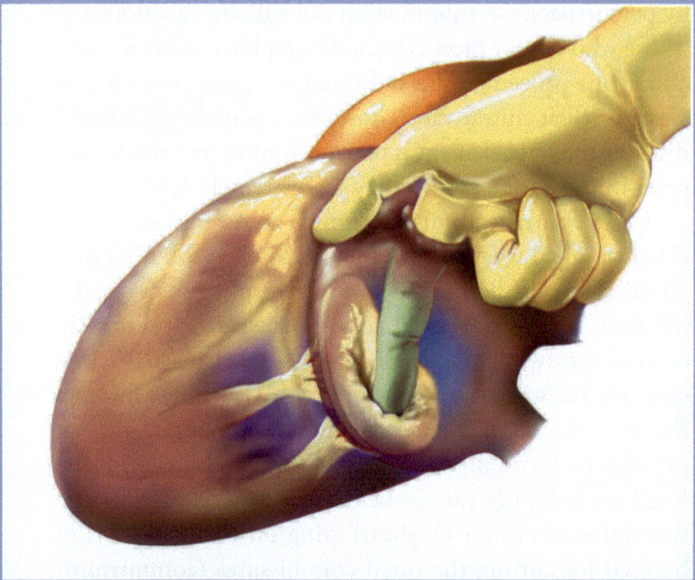

Fig. 6.8 Closed-heart digital mitral commissurolysis

can be salvaged by performing mitral commissurotomy (Fig. 6.9), or the advanced pathomorphology dictates valve replacement. When commissurotomy is attempted, the incision has to be carried across the fused commissure and stopped 2 mm before reaching the annulus. In addition, also the fused chordae usually have to be dissected down to the papillary muscles. This improves the leaflets' mobility by diminishing the degree of their retraction (Fig. 6.10) [31].

6.3.4 Mitral Valve Replacement

The approaches to the mitral valve have already been described. Mitral valve replacement is optimally started by a short incision at the base of the anterior mitral leaflet at the 12 o'clock position (from surgeon's view; Fig. 6.11). It is advisable to place immediately a pledgeted mattress stitch into the mitral annulus at the point of incision. This stitch helps to pull the annulus into the operative field. The whole anterior leaflet is then circumcised as far as the commissures (Fig. 6.12) and its chordae are divided at the tip of the papillary muscles. The posterior mitral leaflet should be left in, as recommended by Lillehei in 1964 [32]. Preservation of ventriculo-annular continuity through the retained leaflet, its chordae, and the papillary muscles is beneficial for maintenance of original left ventricular geometry. It helps to prevent acute left ventricular dilation, which may occur namely in severely impaired left ventricles after complete mitral valve excision and longer ischemic heart arrest. Decrease of left ventricular ejection fraction after mitral valve excision is also less should the posterior mitral leaflet be preserved. This strategy is recommended in mitral stenosis whenever the morphology of the valve allows it. It is, however, even more important in mitral regurgitation unsuitable for repair

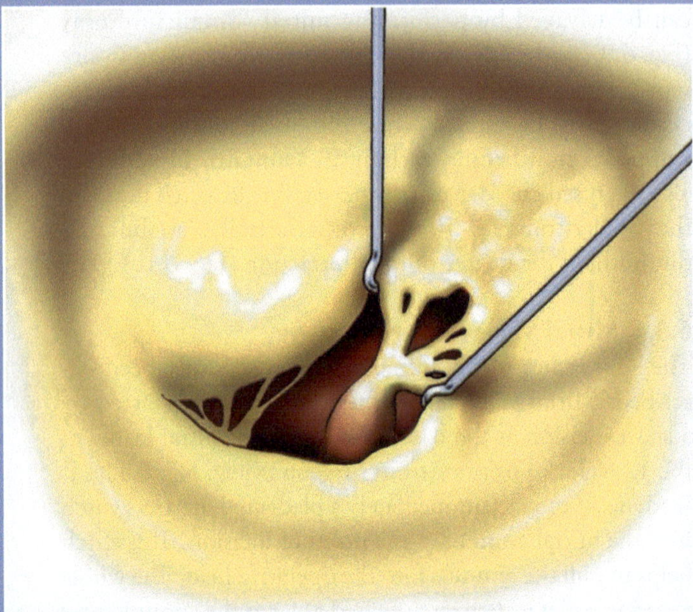

Fig. 6.9 Rheumatic mitral stenosis with fused commissures

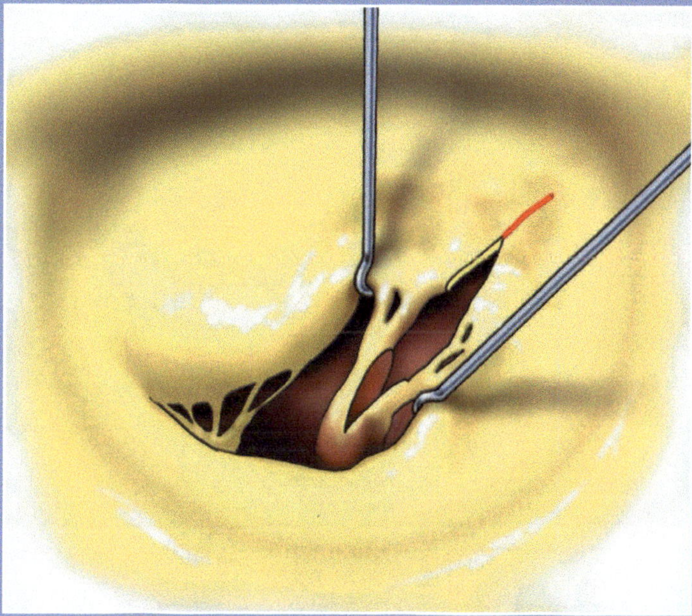

Fig. 6.10 Open-heart mitral commissurotomy

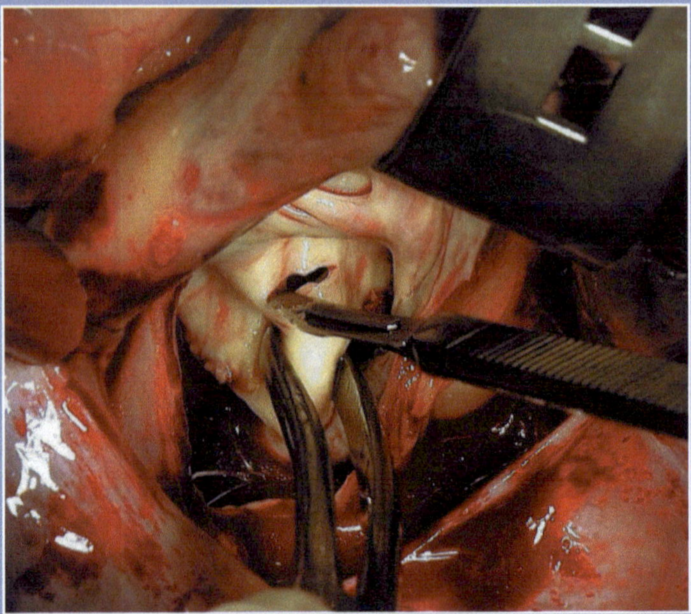

Fig. 6.11 Beginning of anterior mitral leaflet excision

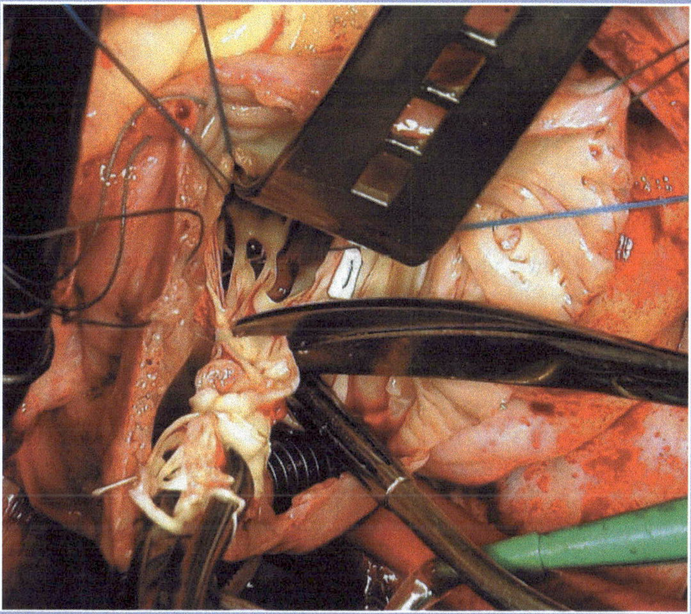

Fig. 6.12 Excision of the anterior leaflet. Chordae leading to the posterior leaflet are preserved

with a dilated, severely impaired left ventricle. Preservation of the posterior leaflet also reduces the risk of a rare but mostly fatal left ventricular rupture [33, 34]. In order to prevent left ventricular dilation and to maximize the protection of ventricular architecture, also the part of the anterior mitral leaflet with its chordae can be preserved (Fig. 6.13). A variety of other techniques and modifications have been described focused on partial anterior leaflet preservation, for example, fixation of the annulus to the papillary muscles by artificial chordae [35–40].

The mechanical valve or bioprosthesis is fixated to the mitral annulus most safely by pledgeted mattress stitches (Figs. 6.14–6.16). In cases of well-accessible firm-tissue annulus, a continuous stitch may be used for valve implantation. This technique is somewhat faster. Bileaflet heart valve should be positioned antianatomically in order to achieve optimal hemodynamics. The slit between the two leaflets should be orientated perpendicular to the original zone of coaptation of the anterior and posterior mitral leaflets (Fig. 6.15).

Patient–prosthesis mismatch may exist also in mitral valve replacement. Mild mismatch occurs if the indexed effective orifice area is within the range of 0.9 to 1.2 cm^2/m^2 and severe mismatch is defined by an effective orifice area index of less than 0.9 cm^2/m^2. Severe patient–prosthesis mismatch results in higher operative mortality, worse long-term outcome, and lesser decrease of pulmonary hypertension [41, 42]. The effort to implant a valve that is large enough is justified in small mitral annuli (rheumatic mitral stenosis with small left ventricle). On the other hand, in very large mitral annuli (mitral incompetence) the implantation of a valve bigger than 31 mm is useless. A mild undersizing

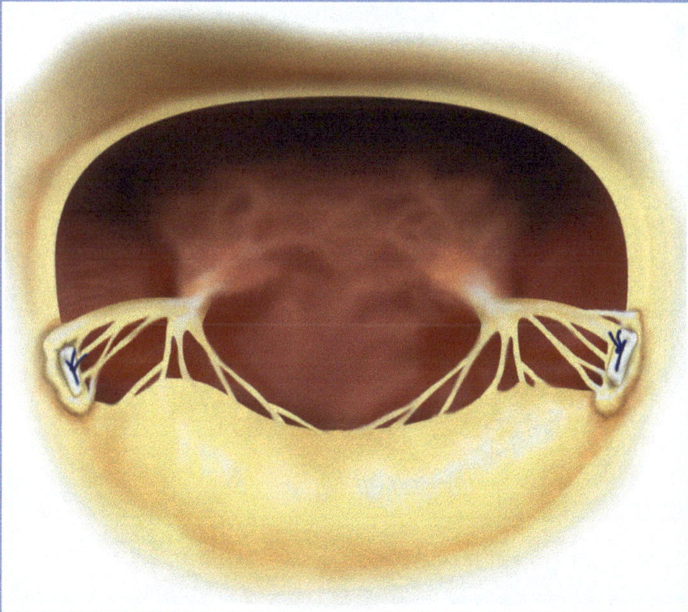

Fig. 6.13 Partial preservation of the anterior leaflet and its fixation in the area of commissures together with preservation of posterior leaflet

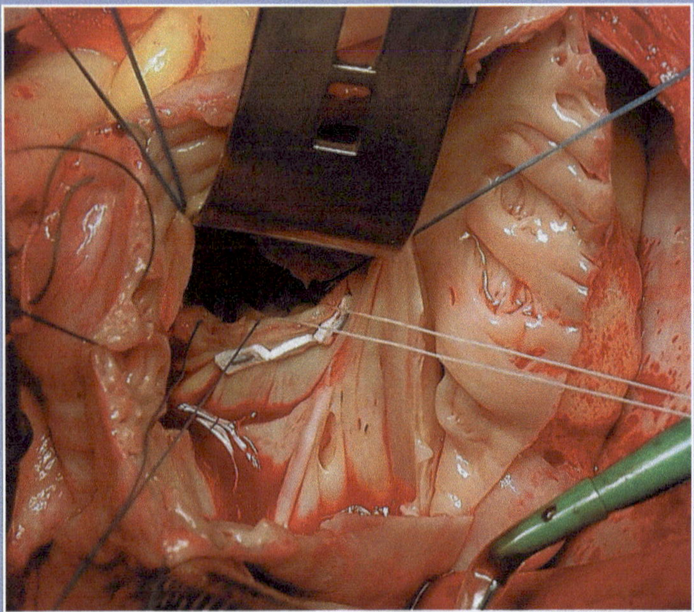

Fig. 6.14 Placement of mattress sutures into the mitral annulus with pledgets on supraannular side

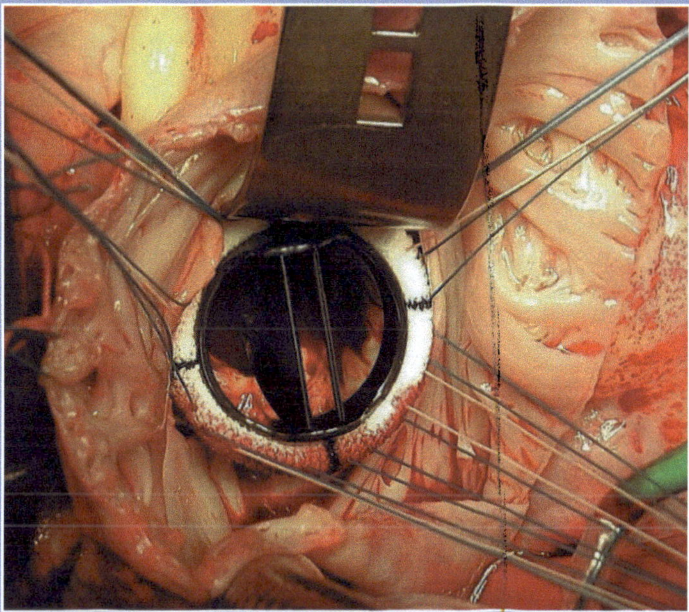

Fig. 6.15 St. Jude Medical valve seated in the mitral annulus in antianatomical orientation before tying of the sutures

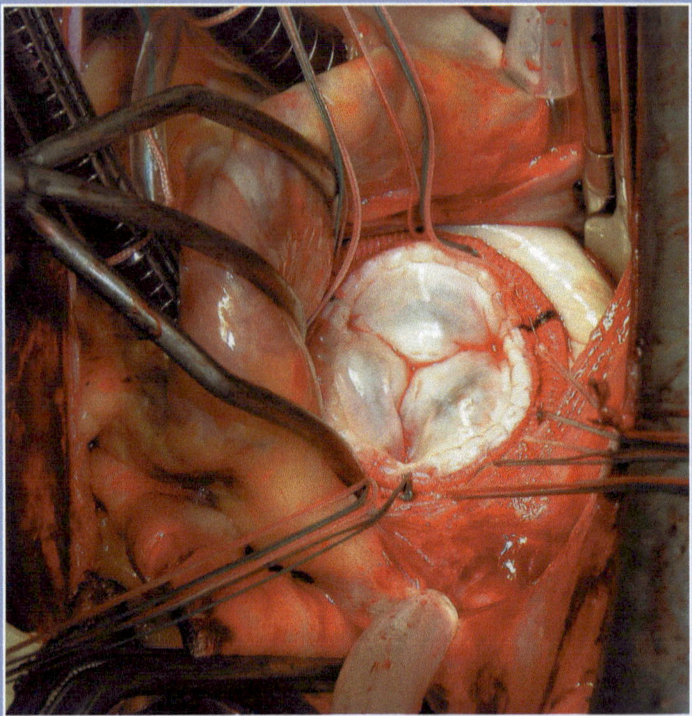

Fig. 6.16 Bioprosthesis St. Jude Medical Epic implanted into the mitral position

is reasonable and prevents the risk of disc collision with the myocardium in case of postoperative decrease of the left ventricular diameter. A proper placement of the stitches in the mitral annulus is very important at mitral valve replacement. The stitch must pass through the annulus only or through the narrow junction of the annulus and myocardium. The stitch must never pass through the myocardium. If the stitch grossly bites the myocardium, it will cut through the fragile myocardium during the tying (Fig. 6.17). Such a lesion may lead to intramyocardial hematoma or subepicardial hematoma in the atrioventricular groove, which will subsequently perforate in the course of operation or soon after operation. This is one of the causal mechanisms of the most feared complication of mitral valve replacement: left ventricular rupture [43–45]. Another cause of left ventricular rupture is an overly radical – and left untreated – excision of the calcifications that grow into the annulus and the myocardium [43, 46, 47]. Excessive annular calcifications at the base of the posterior leaflet (Fig. 6.18) can be widely excised and the area reinforced by suture with use of a pericardial patch or pledgeted stitches [48, 49]. In the opinion of the present authors, this procedure is too risky, and instead of it, a safer, faster, and easier implantation of the valve into the posterior mitral leaflet should be preferred, with leaving the calcifications in situ (Fig. 6.19). Besides these two elementary reasons for left ventricular rupture in the area of the atrioventricular groove (type-I rupture), an occurrence of this complication after forceful implantation of an overly large valve prosthesis has also been published [43, 44, 50]. Myocardial injury or even endocardial discontinuation can also happen during reoperation for dysfunction of the implanted mitral valve due to aggressive explantation of the

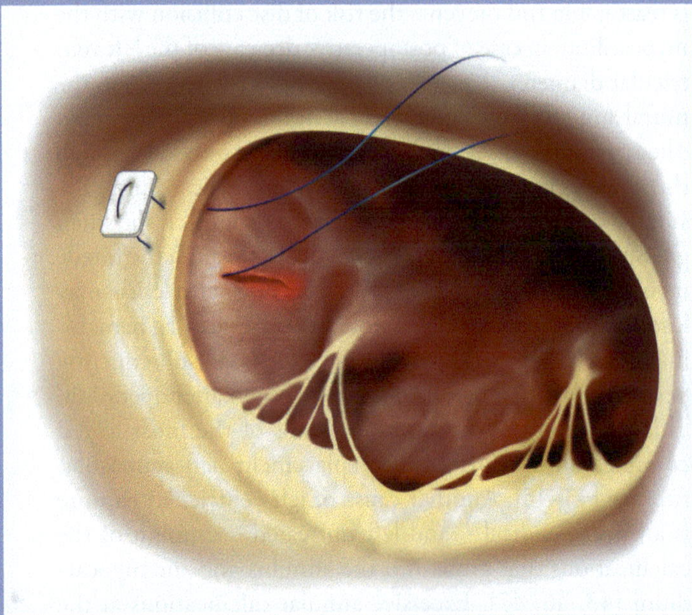

Fig. 6.17 Incorrect placement of a suture too deep in myocardium may cause left ventricular rupture

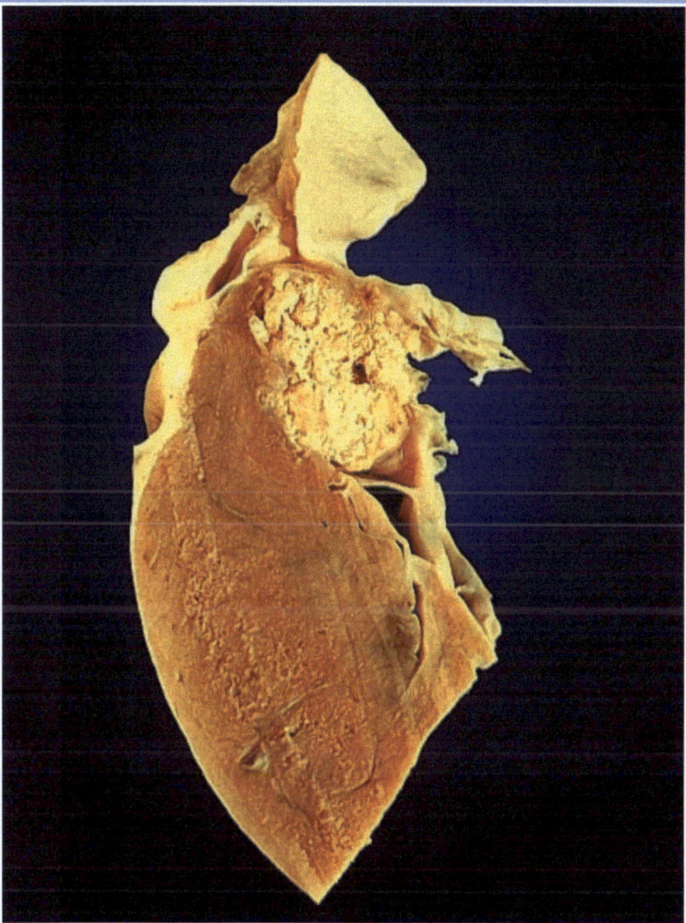

Fig. 6.18 Excessive annular calcifications in the area of posterior mitral leaflet

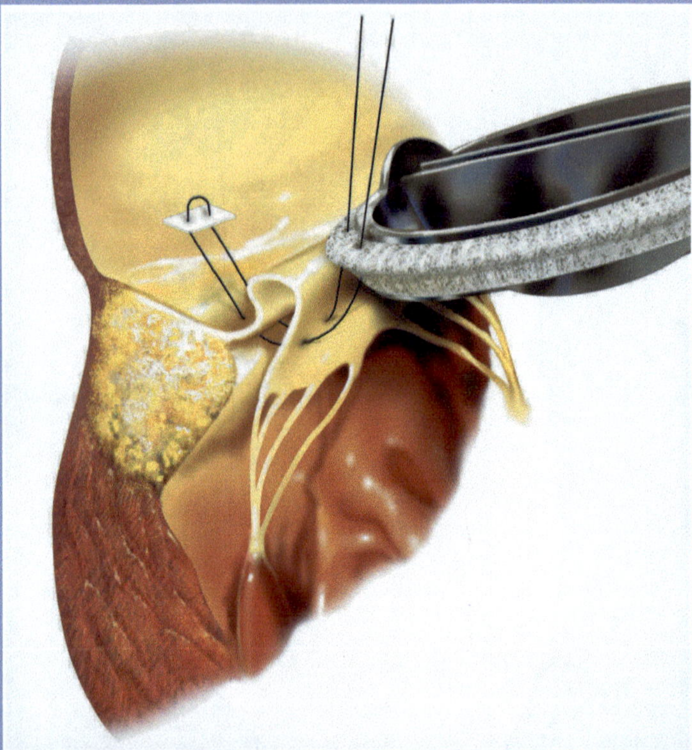

Fig. 6.19 Mitral valve replacement with preservation of annular calcifications

valve from the mitral annulus (the tips of the scissors or the lancet have to follow closely the edge of the sewing ring and point centrally below the valve and not perpendicular to the plane of its orifice) [50].

Left ventricular rupture types II and III are localized distally to the atrioventricular groove. This results from myocardial injury caused most often by a surgical tool. It may occur from the cut of the scissors tips during valve excision under poor visibility conditions (Fig. 6.20; the thickened chordae have to be cut precisely with the scissors tips under perfect visual control). Endocardial and myocardial lesions can also be caused by pressure of the sharp metallic suction device (Fig. 6.21; it is advisable to use a round-tipped glass suction device and forbid suction by the assistant, who has an obstructed view of the operative field). Similarly, the strut of the bioprosthetic stent can get buried in the myocardium and cause a deep lesion (Fig. 6.22; pushing of the stent into the ventricle during the tying has to be avoided and countertraction of the stitch has to be used instead) [43, 51]. All these mechanisms can cause either a complete tear or a partial lesion first followed by intramyocardial and later subepicardial hematoma, which can end in perforation even after several hours.

Left ventricular rupture is a rare but highly lethal complication (65–80%) [43, 47, 50]; therefore, all abovementioned risk factors for its occurrence during mitral valve replacement have to be kept in mind. Surgical management of the rupture is potentially possible but very difficult and often unsuccessful due to the inability to localize its origin and treat the precise pathway of the rupture (pledgeted stitches, pericardial patch, glue, etc.). Chance for salvage of the patient is higher if the complication manifests when

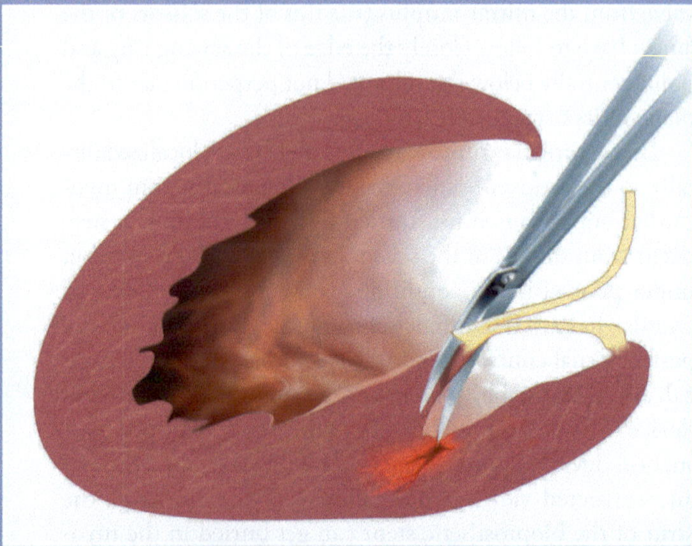

Fig. 6.20 Myocardial injury caused by scissors tips is a potential cause of left ventricular rupture

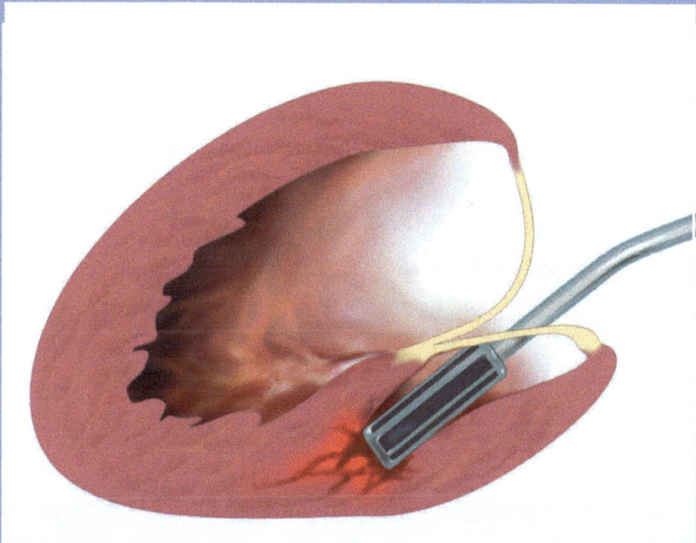

Fig. 6.21 Sharp cardiotomy sucker may injure the myocardium with subsequent left ventricular rupture

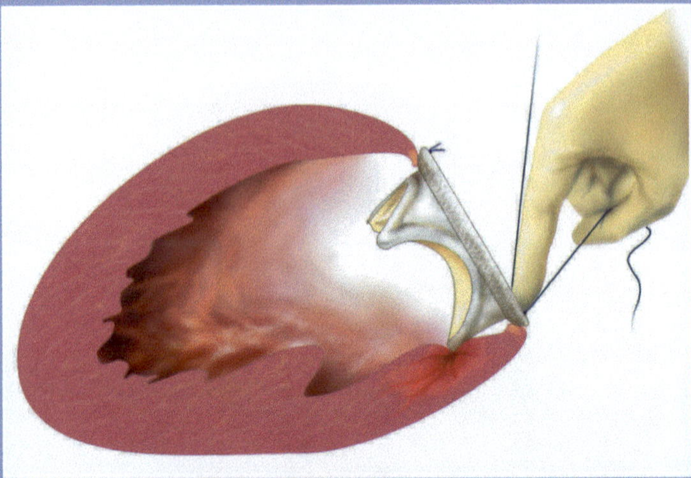

Fig. 6.22 Myocardial tear caused by the strut of bioprosthesis during tying of sutures

the cardiopulmonary bypass is still instituted than at the end of the operation or even at the intensive care unit in the moment of rupture of subpericardial hematoma. Some authors therefore recommend gentle lifting of the heart and inspection of the posterior left ventricular wall and the area of atrioventricular groove at every mitral valve replacement before disconnecting the cardiopulmonary bypass [45, 46].

6.4 Mitral Regurgitation

Surgical procedures for mitral regurgitation are the second most frequent valve operations. Regurgitant flow from the left ventricle into the left atrium causes volume overload of the left ventricle. This volume overload in the long-term course leads to left ventricular dilation and hypertrophy, dilation of the left atrium with onset of atrial fibrillation, and, without treatment, to a significant impairment of the left ventricular ejection fraction. The first clinical symptoms are weakness, fatigue, palpitation, and exertional dyspnea. The majority of mitral regurgitation cases can be treated by valve repair. In recent years a significant shift toward much earlier indications for operation, even in asymptomatic patients, has been witnessed, supported by excellent early and long-term results of mitral repairs and, on the other hand, worse early and uncertain long-term outcome in cases of delayed surgery.

6.4.1 Etiology of Mitral Regurgitation

Degenerative disease is the most common cause of mitral regurgitation. This involves myxomatous degeneration (Barlow's disease with leaflets billowing into the left atrium, floppy mitral valve), fibroelastic leaflets degeneration leading to their prolapse (Fig. 6.23), leaflets prolapse caused by rupture or elongation of the chordae, mitral regurgitation in Marfan and Ehlers-Danlos syndromes, and also annular calcifications (Fig. 6.18) and sclerotic changes of the leaflets. Mitral regurgitation caused by degenerative etiology is in most cases amenable to valve repair.

Ischemic etiology is the second most common cause of mitral regurgitation. In ischemic mitral regurgitation the valve itself is not altered morphologically, but its incompetence results from dysfunction of the ischemic left ventricular myocardium (remodelation, akinesis, dyskinesis, papillary muscles displacement; Fig. 6.24) [52]. Ischemic mitral regurgitation can be almost always resolved by annuloplasty ring implantation. Rare papillary muscle rupture (Fig. 6.25) in acute myocardial infarction leads to acute mitral regurgitation, which necessitates acute surgery, i.e., repair or replacement of the mitral valve.

Third in order of incidence is the functional (secondary, non-organic) mitral regurgitation in which the valve again is not altered but regurgitation develops from annular dilation and left ventricular remodelation with displacement of papillary muscles (dilated left ventricle due to dilated cardiomyopathy or aortic valve disease, mainly aortic regurgitation). In functional mitral regurgitation the left ventricular systolic function used to be significantly impaired. The majority of these functional regurgitations can be treated by annuloplasty ring implantation.

Infective endocarditis, either active (Fig. 6.26) or healed (Fig. 6.27), can lead to mitral regurgitation due to infective destruction of the valve (leaflet defects, periannular abscesses, chordae ruptures). Infective mitral regurgitation in acute endocarditis where fulminant and uncured infection

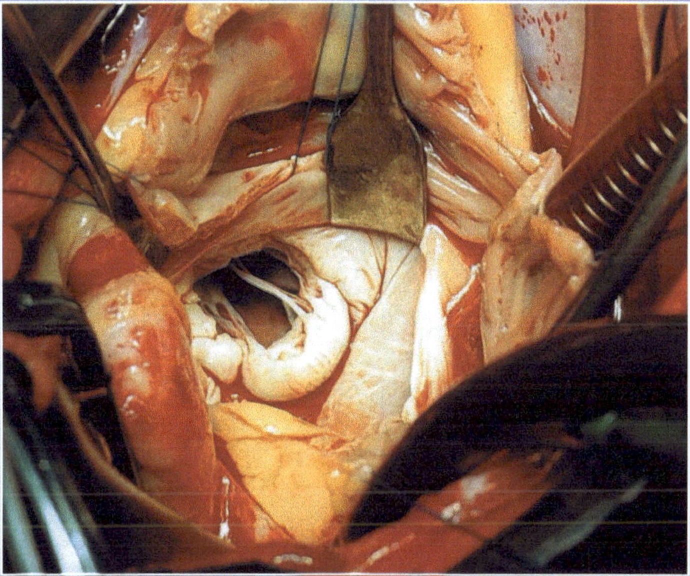

Fig. 6.23 Posterior mitral leaflet prolapse (P2)

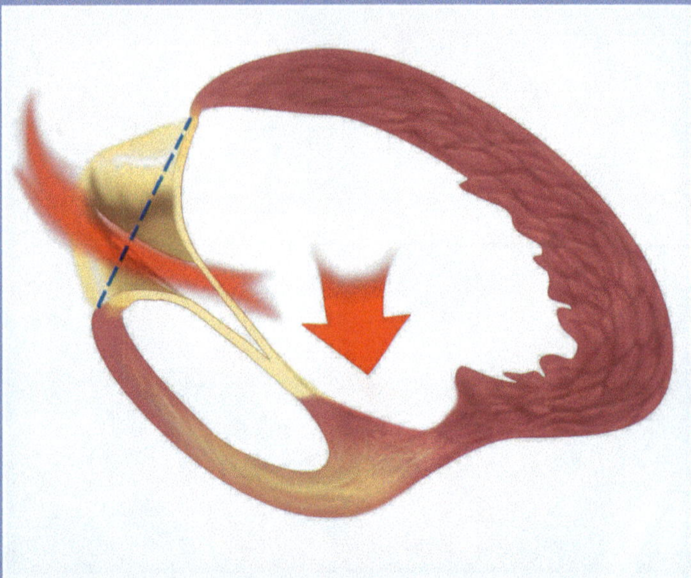

Fig. 6.24 Ischemic mitral regurgitation due to left ventricular remodelation in ischemic ventricular dysfunction. *Dashed line* represents the plane of the mitral annulus, arrow indicates posteromedial papillary muscle displacement.

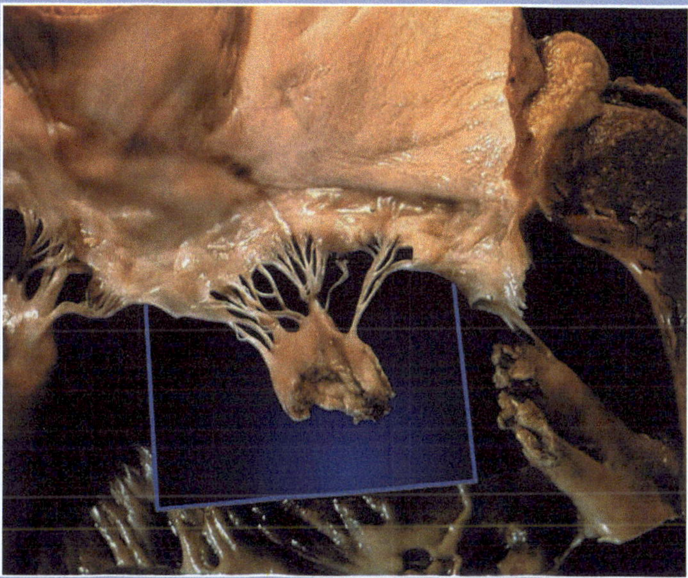

Fig. 6.25 Ischemic papillary muscle rupture

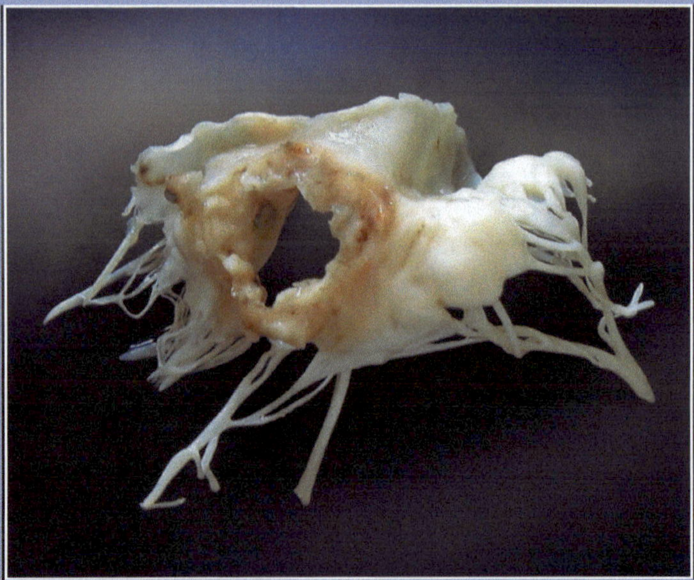

Fig. 6.26 Excised anterior mitral leaflet with large defect in acute phase of infective endocarditis

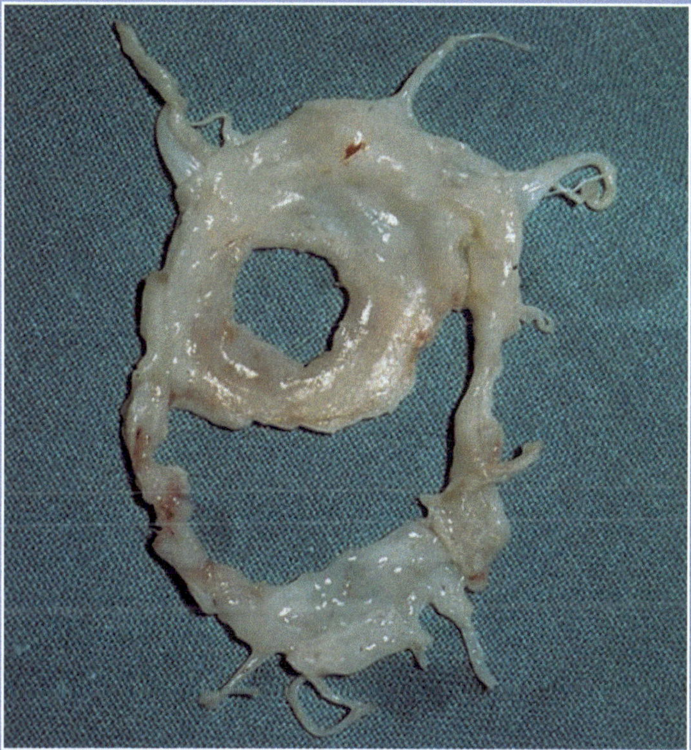

Fig. 6.27 Excised mitral valve (deteriorated from Barlow's disease) after healing of infective endocarditis (defect in the anterior leaflet)

process destroyed the valve leaflets requires valve replacement. If the infection is restricted (e.g., to a portion of the posterior leaflet only) or had caused the perforation, valve repair may be considered (partial posterior leaflet resection, closure of the leaflet perforation with a pericardial patch). Mitral regurgitation after healed endocarditis can sometimes also be treated by a valve-sparing procedure [53].

Rheumatic etiology of mitral regurgitation is rare in developed countries and may be encountered in the elderly population only. On the other hand, in developing countries it is still very common mainly in young girls and women. Rheumatic mitral regurgitation is usually not very suitable for valve repair, because it is associated mostly with valvular stenosis and advanced rheumatic dystrophy of the leaflets, their commissures, and chordae (Fig. 6.28). Moreover, the ongoing rheumatic process impacts negatively in the long term on the result of the valve repair, which is, due to the nature of rheumatic involvement, scarcely ideal even at the surgery.

The commonest type of congenital mitral regurgitation is the cleft of the anterior mitral leaflet in atrioventricular septal defect (Fig. 6.29). The easiest treatment is suture of the cleft. In adulthood the complete form of the atrioventricular septal defect is not to be met as a subject of primary operation, but sometimes reoperations for steno-incompetence of the mitral valve are required after previous surgical corrections of a complete or incomplete form in childhood. Such findings usually end up with mitral valve replacement.

An iatrogenic lesion of the mitral valve during balloon mitral valvuloplasty is one of the rare causes of acute mitral regurgitation (Fig. 6.30). It happens when the pressure of the inflated balloon does not cause the desired loosening

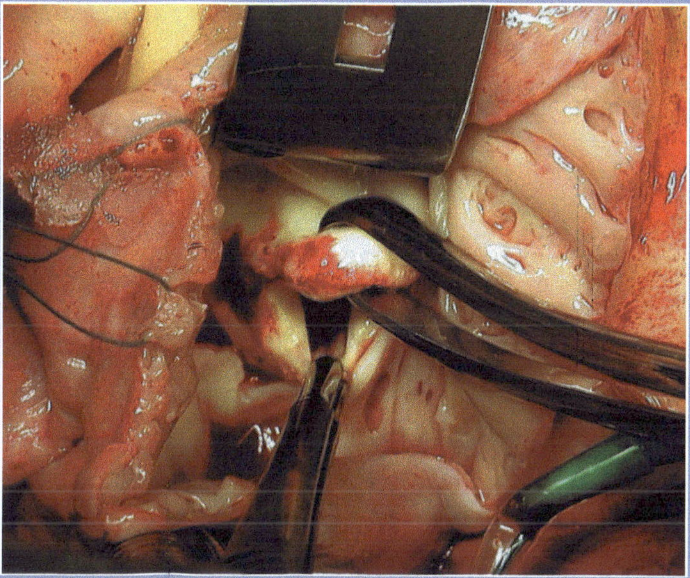

Fig. 6.28 Rheumatic mitral valve disease. Both leaflets display fibrotic thickening and commissures are fused

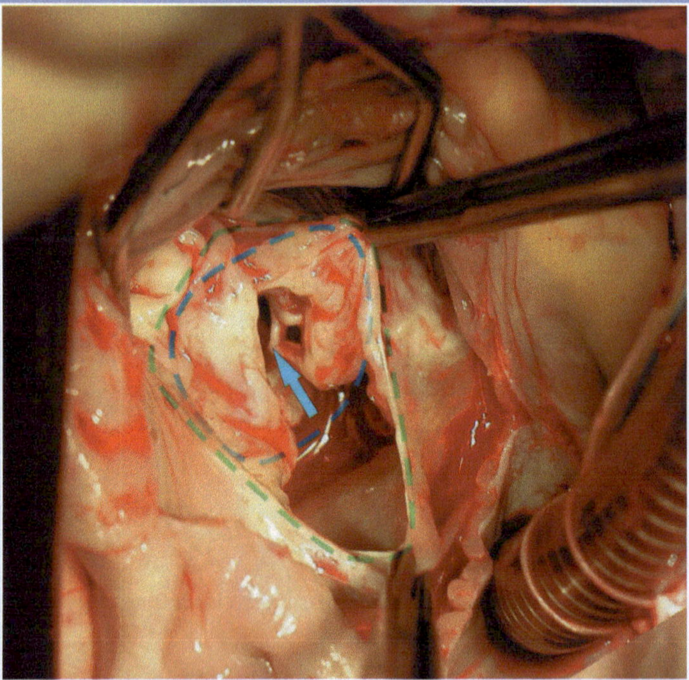

Fig. 6.29 Cleft of anterior mitral leaflet *(arrow)* in incomplete atrioventricular septal defect. *Green curve* represents margins of atrial septal defect, *blue curve* represents mitral annulus

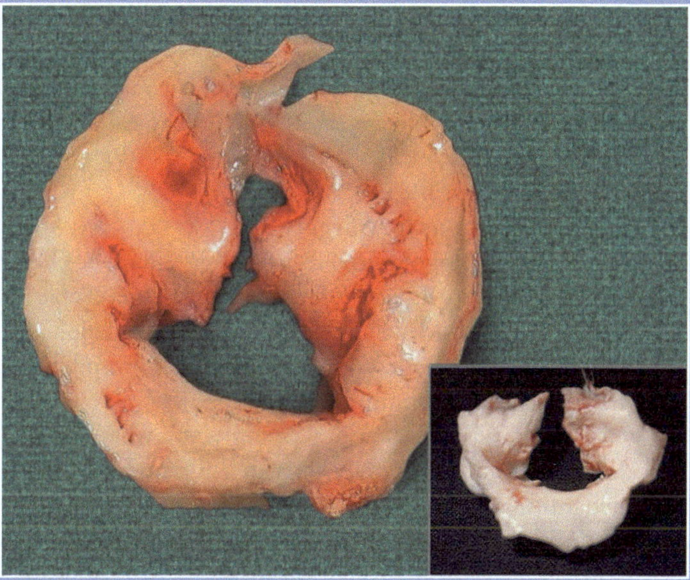

Fig. 6.30 Iatrogenic tear of anterior mitral leaflet occurred during percutaneous balloon mitral valvuloplasty. *Inset* Complete rupture of the anterior mitral leaflet

of the fused commissures but tears the valve in the place of least resistance, usually across the anterior leaflet. Acute surgery is inevitable. A rheumatic diseased valve with disrupted leaflet has to be replaced by a mechanical prosthesis or bioprosthesis.

6.4.2 Indications for Surgery

Surgical treatment of mitral regurgitation should be offered to patients early, i.e., before development of irreversible left ventricular dysfunction and dilation, left atrial dilation, pulmonary hypertension, onset of atrial fibrillation, and finally, tricuspidalization of mitral valve disease [54].

Patients with severe mitral regurgitation who are symptomatic are unequivocally indicated for surgery. Hemodynamically severe mitral regurgitation is determined by regurgitation volume (RV) >50 ml, regurgitation fraction >50 %, effective regurgitation orifice (ERO) >0.4 cm^2, vena contracta >6–7 mm, and by impaired left ventricular functional parameters (EF <60% and end-systolic left ventricular diameter, LVESD, >40–45 mm). The onset of atrial fibrillation and development of pulmonary hypertension (systolic pulmonary pressure >50 mmHg) are the signs of long-term presence of significant mitral regurgitation [26, 27].

In cases of ischemic mitral regurgitation, the indication criteria for surgery are stricter. Mitral valve repair should be performed as an adjunct to coronary bypass grafting in already mild to moderate ischemic mitral regurgitation, i.e., provided that RV is >30 ml and ERO >0.2 cm^2. These strict criteria need not be applied – and often even should not be – in patients with significant comorbidities and in those over 75 years. Except for increased operative risk, the quality of life would remain unaffected, keeping in mind that mitral regurgitation is only mild to moderate and overall life expectancy shorter [55, 56].

Indications for surgery are not easy to identify in symptomatic patients with chronic mitral regurgitation and poor left ventricular function (EF <30 %). In general, mitral valve repair should be performed if there is evidence of contractile reserve. Current progress in myocardial protection and perioperative care has influenced the indication criteria. Patients with severe mitral regurgitation and low ejection fraction who would have been formerly rejected for surgery are currently operated with acceptable outcome. If the decision remains controversial, the left ventricular end-diastolic diameter (LVEDD) also has to be taken into account. The surgery can be recommended at LVEDD below 65 mm. Operative risk rapidly increases when dimensions exceed 65 mm, and at LVEDD of 85 mm the surgery is no longer indicated. These patients with poor ejection fraction, large ventricular dimensions, and no contractile reserve are amenable to medical therapy only or could be considered candidates for heart transplantation.

Asymptomatic patients with severe mitral regurgitation are followed-up by echocardiography. Surgery is indicated when the first signs of the left ventricular impairment appear (EF <60%, LVESD >45 mm,) ERO >40 mm^2, at the onset of atrial fibrillation or pulmonary hypertension (at-rest pulmonary systolic pressure >50 mmHg) [26, 27, 54, 57, 58].

6.4.3 Mitral Valve Repair

Perfect performance of the mitral valve depends on correct function and coordination of all components of the mitral valve complex (i.e., mitral annulus, mitral leaflets, chordae, papillary muscles, and left ventricular myocardium). The mitral leaflets have to coapt along the whole line of closure in a safe coaptation zone of several millimeters in height (Fig. 6.31). A lesion of whichever mitral valve component can lead to severe regurgitation based on the loss of coaptation of the mitral leaflets.

Morphological classification of mitral regurgitation has been mentioned previously (i.e., degenerative, ischemic, functional, rheumatic, congenital, and iatrogenic types). For surgery there is important functional classification into three basic types according to Carpentier [31]. Type I is characterized by normal leaflet mobility (Fig. 6.32). Regurgitation results from loss of coaptation due to annular dilation, left ventricular dysfunction, or occasional perforation of a leaflet. In type II there is mitral leaflet prolapse caused by elongation or rupture of the chordae or papillary muscles (Fig. 6.33). Type III is characterized by restricted motion of the leaflets caused by shortening of the chordae in rheumatic disease (Fig. 6.34) or by traction of the chordae due to ischemic left ventricular remodelation.

A prerequisite of successful surgery is proper preoperative echocardiographic analysis of the regurgitation mechanisms. Selection of the repair technique is based on knowledge of the regurgitation etiology, pathomorphology findings, and functional type of the regurgitation. The effect of the repair should be durable and simultaneously the valve must not become stenotic. The main principle to be pursued in all repair techniques is achievement of safe and wide coaptation of the mitral leaflets. The effect of the accomplished repair has to be proved by peroperative echocardiography after weaning off cardiopulmonary bypass.

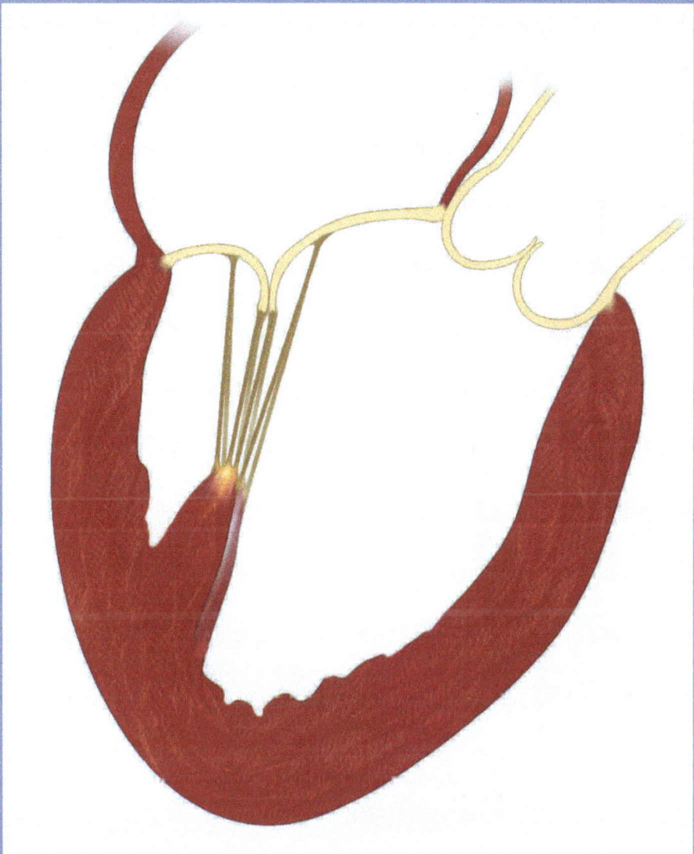

Fig. 6.31 Competent mitral valve with sufficient zone of coaptation

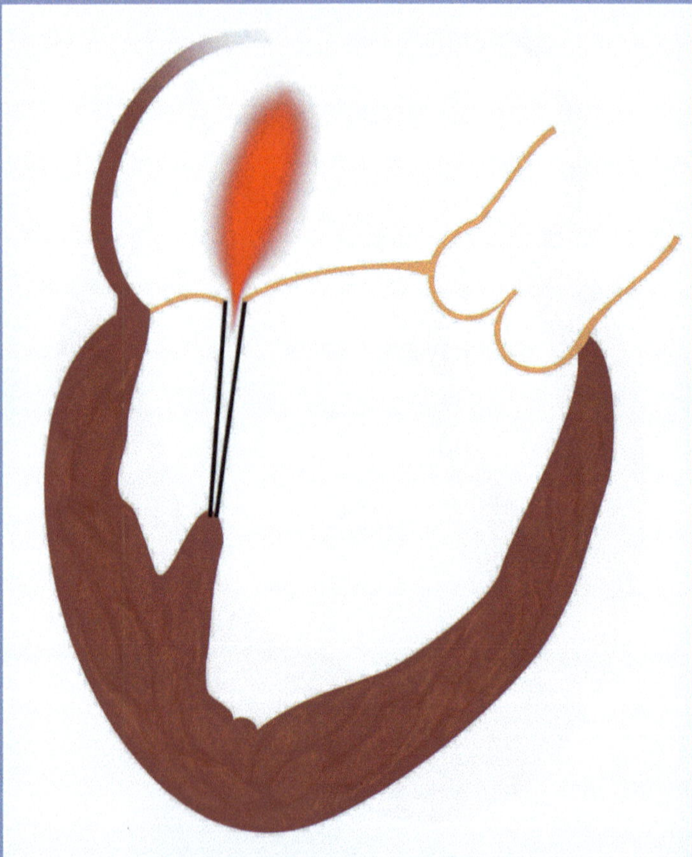

Fig. 6.32 Mitral regurgitation type I (normal leaflet mobility, annular dilation). (According to Carpentier [31])

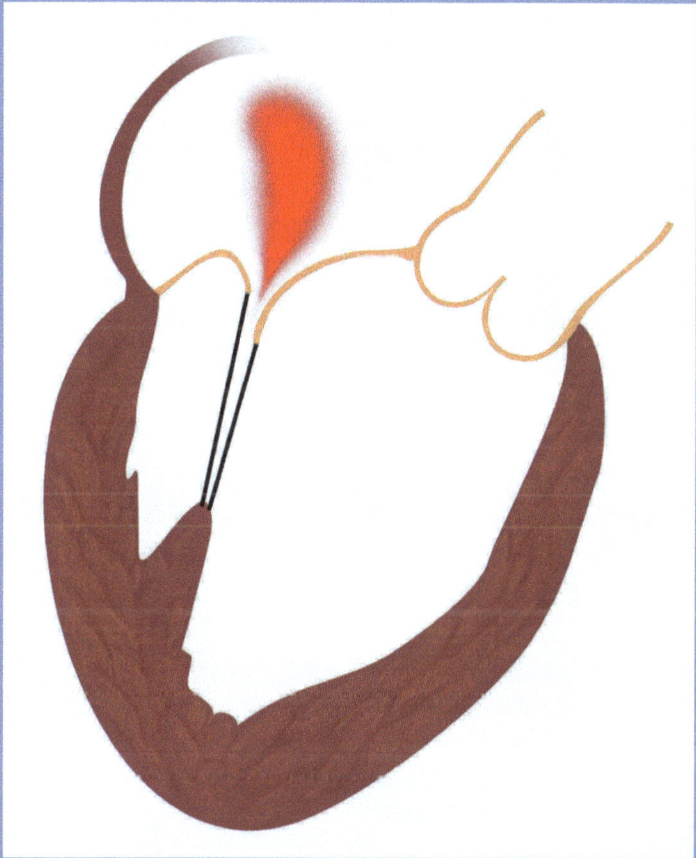

Fig. 6.33 Mitral regurgitation type II (prolapse of one or both leaflets – depicted is the posterior leaflet prolapse). (According to Carpentier [31])

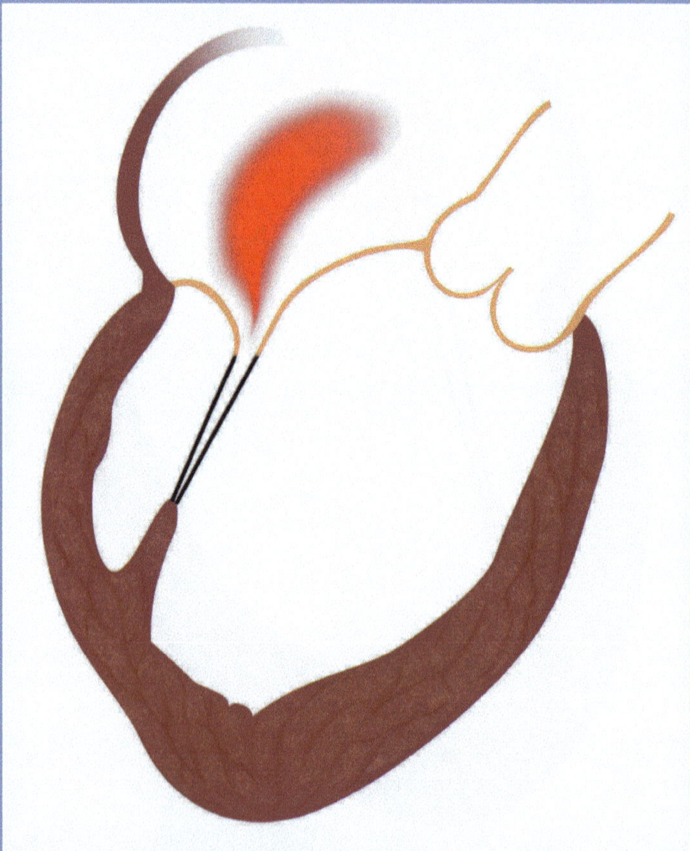

Fig. 6.34 Mitral regurgitation type III (restricted leaflet mobility due to chordal retraction). (According to Carpentier [31])

6.4.3.1 Annuloplasty Procedures

Chronic hemodynamically significant mitral regurgitations existing over a long time display one common feature: dilation of the mitral annulus. The dilation does not develop symmetrically along the whole annular circumference but only in the area of the posterior leaflet and both commissures. Annular length of the area belonging to the anterior leaflet remains unaltered (Fig. 6.35) [59]. This finding determines the philosophy of annuloplasty ring implantations as well as other repair techniques. Annuloplasty rings are being implanted in a manner to reduce the dilated portion of the annulus only. The mattress sutures in the area of the posterior leaflet and both commissures take wider bites along the annulus but are passed through the ring in narrower intervals (Fig. 6.36). In this way the annular circumference can be plicated and intentionally reduced. Annuloplasty rings are very effective in most Carpentier type-I mitral regurgitations

A variety of annuloplasty rings have been designed and marketed (Fig. 6.37). They are rigid (e.g., Carpentier–Edwards, St. Jude Medical Rigid Saddle, AnuloFlo-CarboMedics), semiflexible (e.g., Carpentier–Edwards Physio, St. Jude Medical Sequin, Sorin MEMO3D), and flexible (e.g., Medtronic–Duran, Sorin–Sovering, AnuloFlex–CarboMedics, ATS Simulus FLX-O) [60, 61].

Some rings are designed without the anterior leaflet portion (resembling horizontal figure of C, e.g., Colvin–Galloway, Cosgrove–Edwards, ATS Simulus FLX-C, or AorTech MRS) or this portion can be either used or trimmed off (St. Jude Medical Tailor, AnuloFlex–CarboMedics) [59, 62]. All rings are biocompatible, and some of them are even carbofim coated (Sorin–Sovering) or produced from polytetrafluoroethylene (PTFE; Jostra).

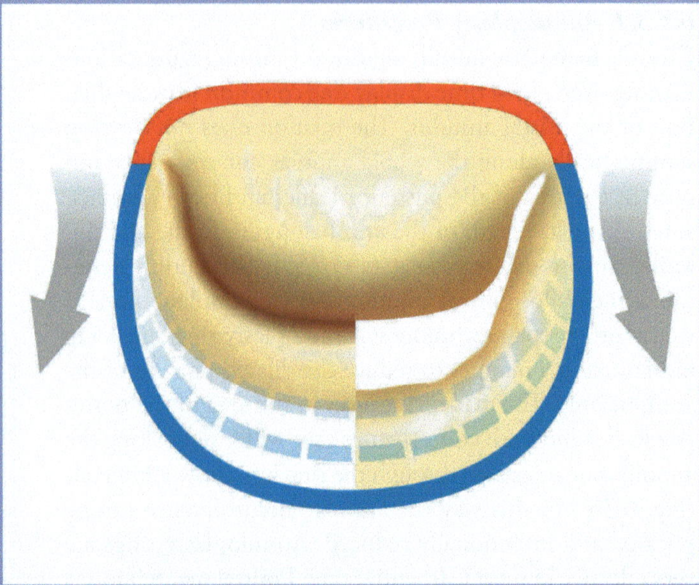

Fig. 6.35 Disproportional dilation of mitral annulus. The area of anterior leaflet does not dilate. The dilation develops at circumference belonging to posterior mitral leaflet

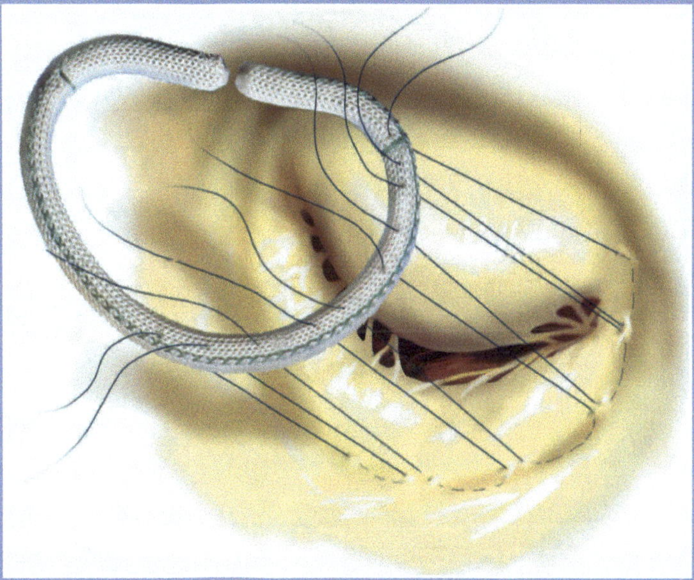

Fig. 6.36 Principle of implantation of annuloplasty ring. Mattress sutures placed in the area of posterior leaflet take wider bites than their intervals in annuloplasty ring

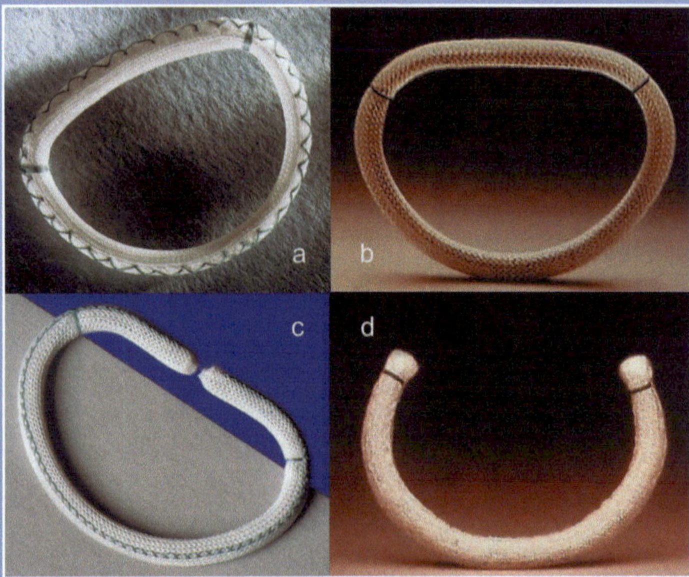

Fig. 6.37 Mitral annuloplasty rings. **a** St. Jude Medical–Seguin. **b** Carpentier–Edwards Physio. **c** Carpentier–Edwards (rigid). **d** Cosgrove–Edwards

There is a possibility to implant a new adjustable annuloplasty ring, St. Jude Medical Attune. This ring offers symmetrical adjustability by pulling both purse-string-suture ends equally or asymmetrical adjustability by pulling one purse-string-suture end more than the other (Fig. 6.38). Very similar adjustable rings, such as Puig–Massana–Shiley and St. Jude Medical BiFlex, were used in the 1980s [63].

The GeoForm ring is geometrically designed to treat mitral regurgitation caused by the enlargement of the left ventricle. Anteroposterior distance of the mitral annulus is reduced and the P2 zone is elevated in the ring.

A novel annuloplasty ring design, Myxo-ETlogix (Edwards) [64], is also aimed at prevention of systolic anterior motion (SAM) in patients with myxomatous leaflet degeneration (Barlow's disease). This ring has a significantly longer anteroposterior diameter and saddle-like elevation in the area of P2.

The proper size of the ring is decided upon by measuring the distance between the two commissures marked with the first two mattress sutures (Fig. 6.39). In ischemic and secondary mitral regurgitation, a sole annuloplasty ring implantation is an adequate procedure (Figs. 6.40, 6.41). The effect of the annuloplasty lies not only in reduction of the dilated annular portion but also in true remodelation of the almost circular dilated mitral annulus into its correct original "kidney-shaped" appearance. This brings the two leaflets closer together and thereby enables restoration of their proper coaptation. Annuloplasty rings are also being implanted after complex reconstructive repairs of the mitral valve to prevent any later redilation of the annulus and reoccurrence of mitral regurgitation. Some authors recommend securing each mitral repair by annuloplasty ring implantation [65].

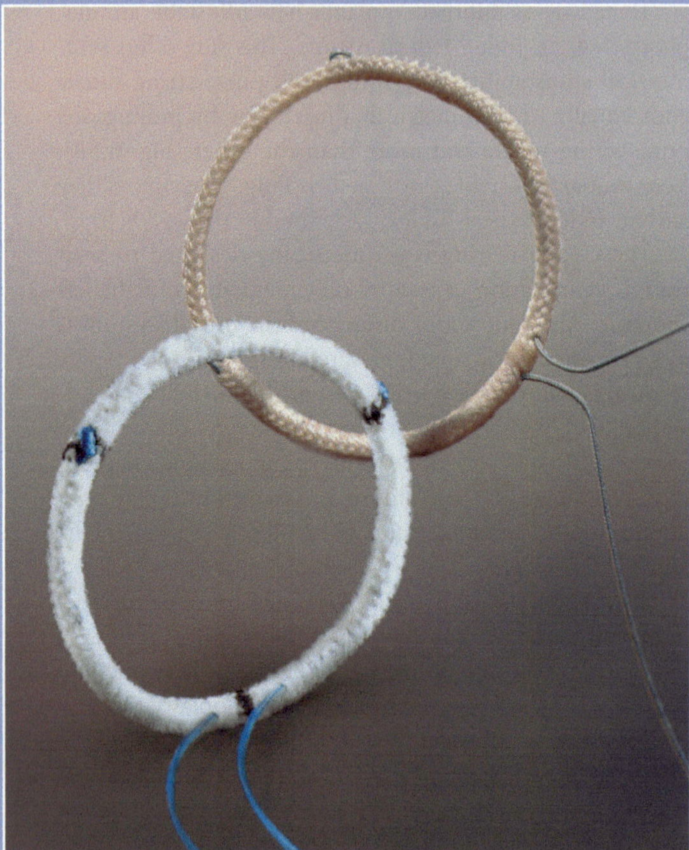

Fig. 6.38 Adjustable annuloplasty ring St. Jude Medical–Attune and Puig–Massana–Shiley *(top)*

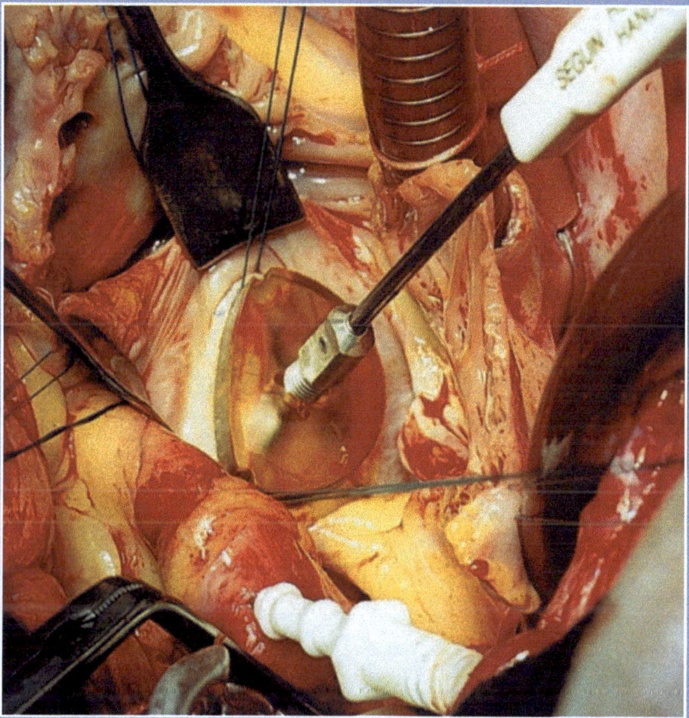

Fig. 6.39 Measuring proper size of annuloplasty ring

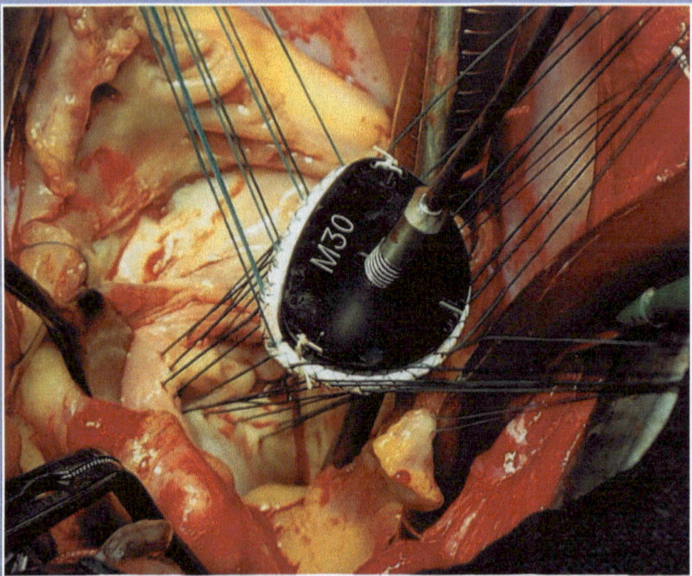

Fig. 6.40 Running down of annuloplasty ring into the mitral annulus

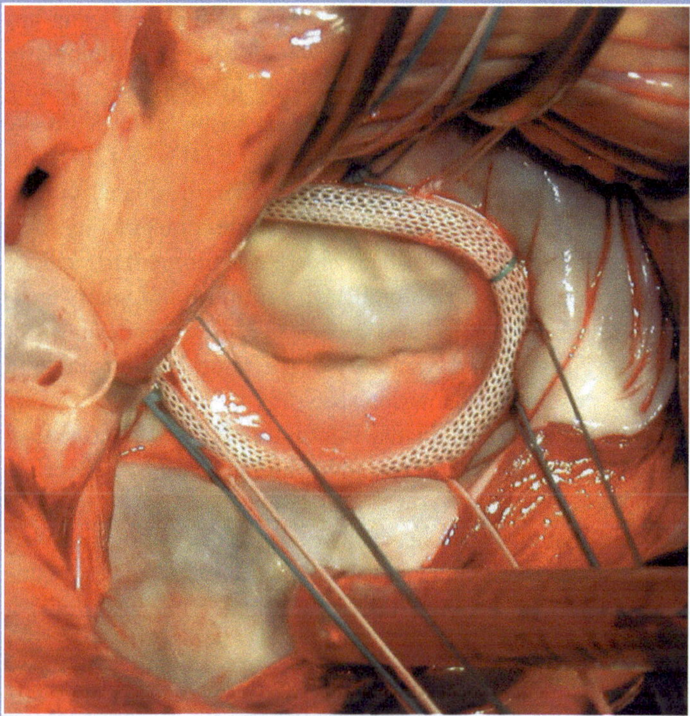

Fig. 6.41 Implanted mitral annuloplasty ring

A result similar to that achieved by flexible C-ring implantation can be obtained by a semicircular annuloplasty according to Burr et al. [66]. With this technique running sutures are passed through the posterior leaflet from the commissures toward the midpoint of P2 (Fig. 6.42). Tightening of the sutures leads to reduction of the dilated annular portion (Fig. 6.43). It is advisable to use company ring sizers (usually 26 mm for women and 28 mm for men) to facilitate proper degree of tightening. This suture annuloplasty technique is simple, fast and inexpensive, preserves flexibility of the annulus, and durability of the result is comparable to that of ring implantations [66–68].

Reduction of dilated mitral annulus as a treatment of mitral regurgitation was published in 1958 by Kay et al., who coined the term "annular plication" [69]; however, the method published by Wooler et al. [70] in 1962 has become more popular and widely used [28]. The principle of the Wooler repair involves shortening of the annulus at both commissures and adjacent portions of the posterior leaflet (Figs. 6.44, 6.45). It is a very fast and simple annuloplasty (commissuroplasty) that can resolve not only regurgitation located in the commissural area but also central regurgitation from mitral annulus dilation, because it also brings the leaflets closer together. Nonetheless, implantation of the annuloplasty ring seems currently to be a more proper way of treatment for these cases, because it guarantees postoperatively long-term prevention of redilation of the annulus; therefore, use of the Wooler repair is presently justified in occasional situations only (long duration of cardiopulmonary bypass in complex procedures, elderly patients, difficult exposure of mitral valve due to deep chest, in reoperations, etc.).

6.4.3.2 *Leaflet and Chordae Procedures*

Besides the abovementioned classic and relatively easy mitral valve repair techniques, also more demanding procedures are being performed at the mitral leaflets and chordae. Annuloplasty ring implantation is, however, usually added as a final step also in these techniques.

Prolapse of one or both mitral leaflets from degenerative etiology (Carpentier classification type II) is the commonest situation that requires such procedure. Prolapse occurs most often at the posterior leaflet, predominantly at the middle portion (P2; Figs. 6.23, 6.46). Quadrangular or triangular resection of the posterior leaflet is the treatment of choice that can be accomplished irrespective of the actual cause of prolapse (elongated or ruptured chordae, excessive leaflet tissue, or a combination of both). The prolapsing portion of the posterior leaflet is cut off, the remaining portions (P1 and P3) are sutured together, and long-term durability of the repair effect is secured by annuloplasty ring implantation (prevention of annular redilation; Fig. 6.47) [31, 65, 71]. If too much excessive tissue remains, even after quadrangular leaflet resection, and its height exceeds 1.5 cm, sliding plasty is indicated. With this method the leaflet resection is extended periannularly and cuneiform areas of the excessive leaflet tissue are excised (Fig. 6.48). Sliding plasty is considered to be prevention of occurrence of SAM, i.e., collapsing of the anterior mitral leaflet into the left ventricular outflow tract in systole. Since their publication by Carpentier in the mid-1980s, both techniques have been popular [31, 72].

In 2006 Calafiore et al. published a new concept regarding how to treat the excess of posterior leaflet tissue and named it "posterior leaflet longitudinal plication" [73]. The principle is very simple and lies in shortening of

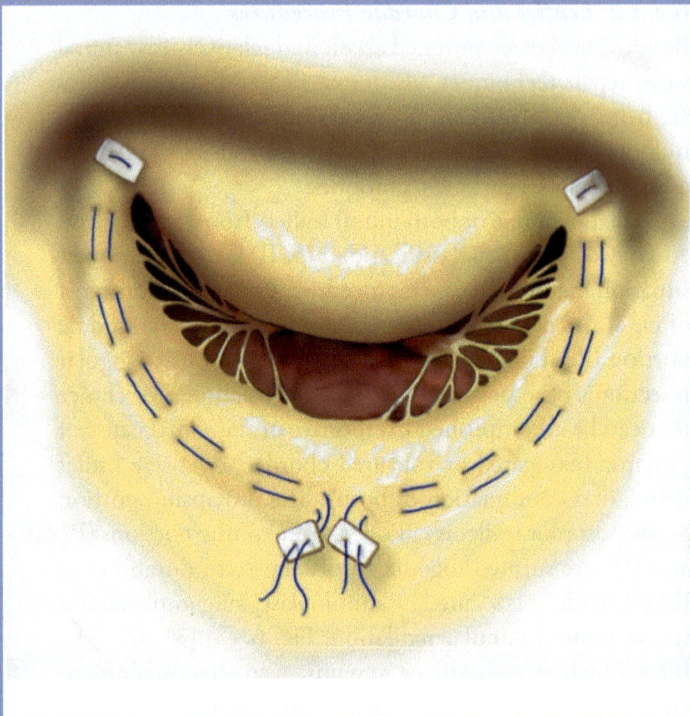

Fig. 6.42 Placement of sutures at repair. (According to Burr et al. [66])

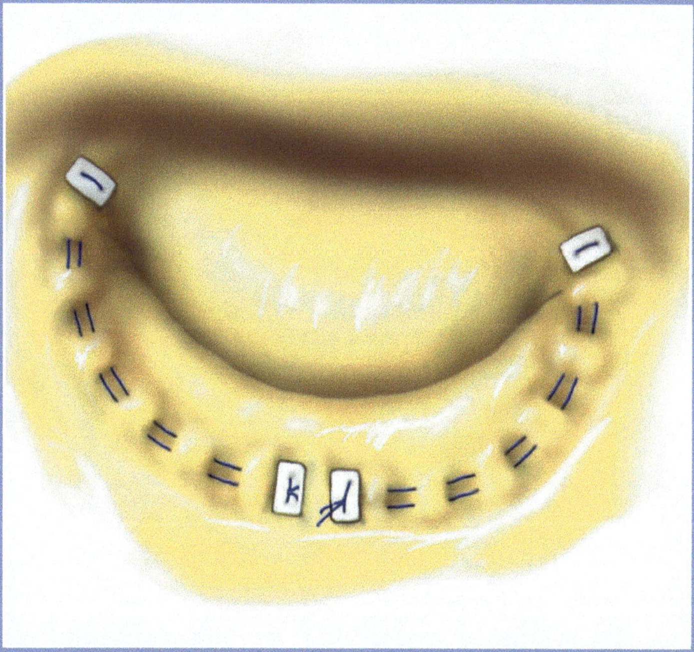

Fig. 6.43 Result of repair after tying of the sutures (reduction of posterior leaflet annulus). (According to Burr et al. [66])

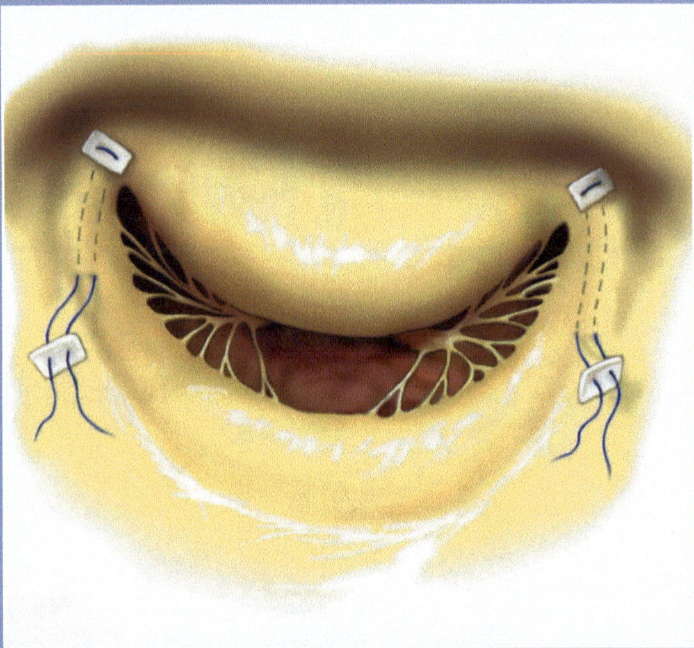

Fig. 6.44 Placement of sutures at repair. (According to Wooler et al. [70])

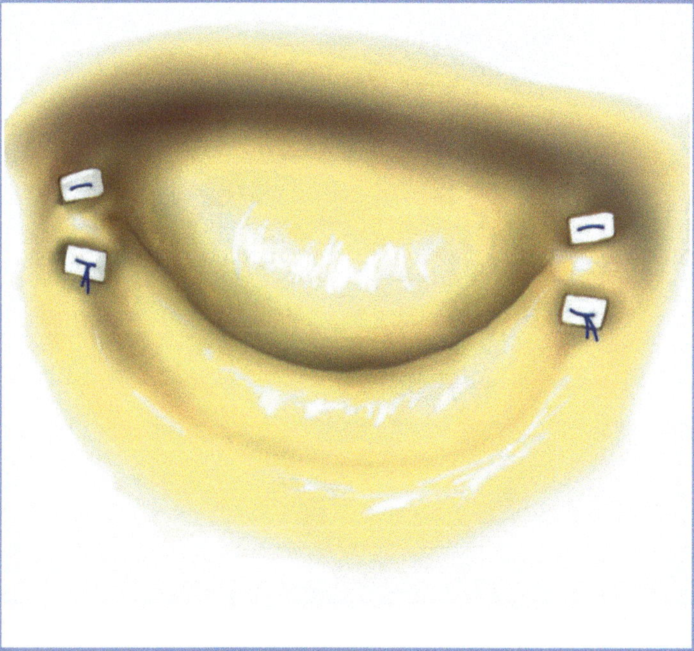

Fig. 6.45 Result of repair. (According to Wooler et al. [70])

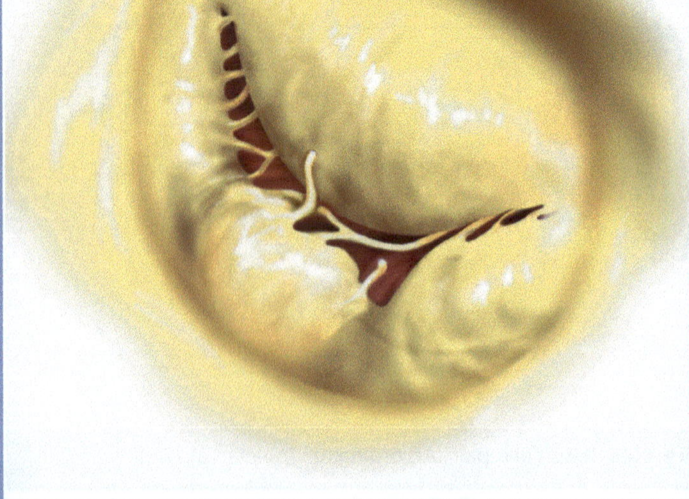

Fig. 6.46 Posterior mitral leaflet prolapse (P2) due to chordal rupture

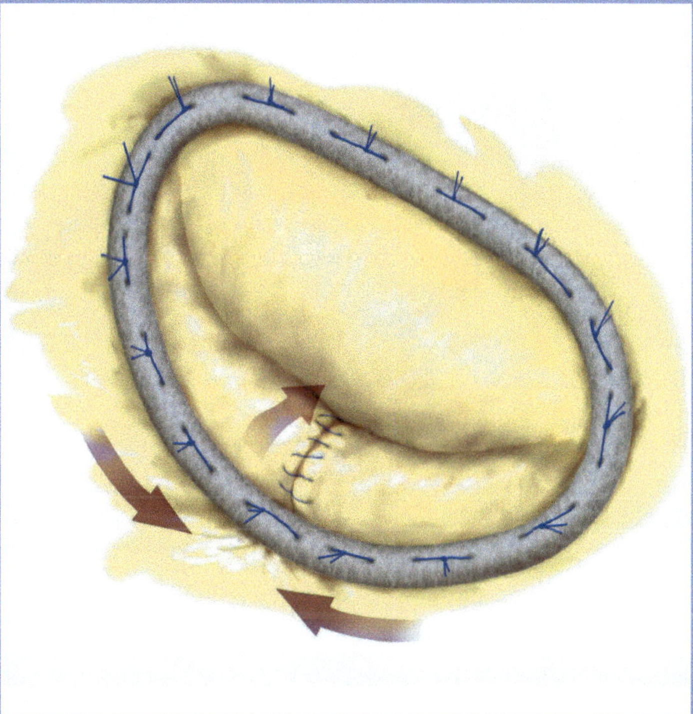

Fig. 6.47 Result of posterior leaflet resection (P2) and implantation of annuloplasty ring

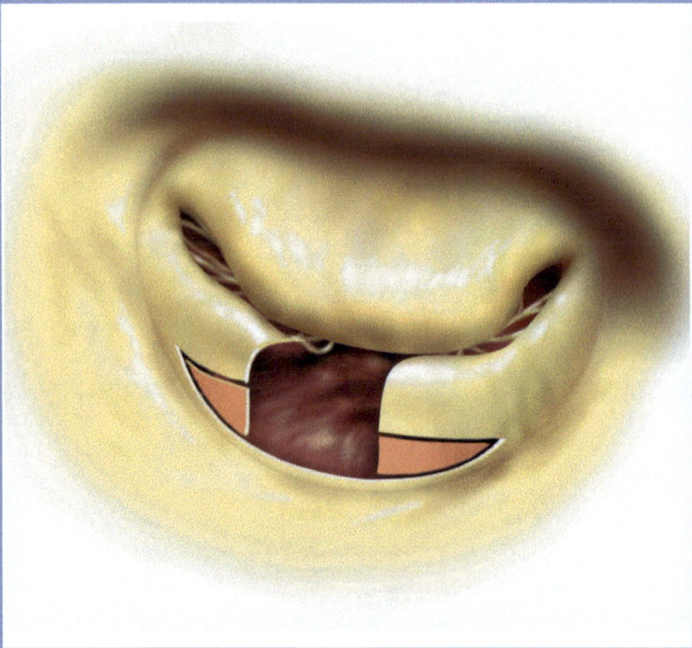

Fig. 6.48 "Sliding" plasty of the posterior leaflet (marked are the quadrangular resection of P2 and cuneiform excisions from P1 and P3)

the posterior leaflet height by several mattress sutures led through the annulus and prolapsing portion of the posterior leaflet (Fig. 6.49). Despite limited experience, the technique seems to be promising in the prevention of SAM.

While the classic concept of mitral repair is based on some reduction in the area of posterior leaflet, a different, more conservative approach has recently been advocated by Perier et al. [74]. In their strategy "respect rather than resect" they try to save the patient's prolapsing posterior leaflet tissue as much as possible and to transform it, by means of PTFE chordae, into a smooth vertical buttress. Similarly, Tabata et al. suggest remodeling of the excessive posterior leaflet tissue by one or more sutures, which would pull in the prolapsing edge beneath the body of the posterior leaflet (Figs. 6.50, 6.51) [75].

The occurrence of SAM after mitral valve repair is a serious perioperative complication that causes left ventricular outflow tract obstruction and also mitral regurgitation (Fig. 6.52). Incidence of this troublesome situation after mitral valve repair is reported usually in 5% of cases. Numerous authors claim to not have encountered this complication, although others report its incidence as up to 10% [76, 77]. Controversy exists regarding the origin of SAM, thus reflecting the diversity of potential causes. The main risk factors for SAM are: (a) excessive amount of leaflet tissue; (b) an overly large posterior leaflet left; (c) small annuloplasty ring; (d) left ventricular hypertrophy; (e) interventricular septal hypertrophy; and (f) hyperkinetic circulation [60, 77]. The danger is increased if several potential risk factors are present simultaneously. Most authors emphasize the role of an excessive amount of posterior leaflet tissue left. The height of the posterior leaflet should not

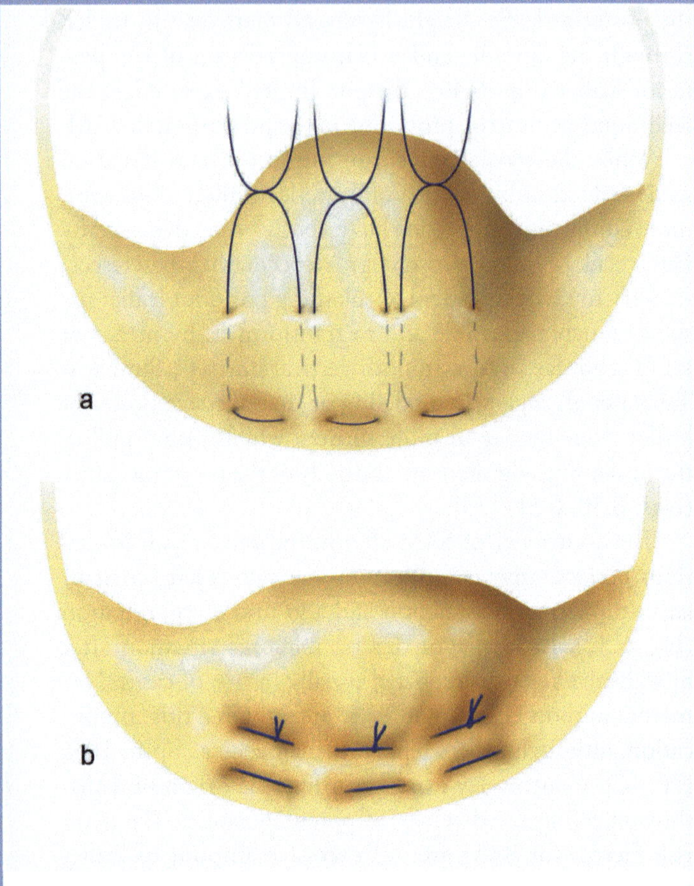

Fig. 6.49 Longitudinal plication of posterior leaflet. **a** Placement of sutures. **b** Shortening of posterior leaflet height after tying of the sutures. (According to Calafiore et al. [73])

exceed 1.5 cm; otherwise, performing a sliding plasty is recommended [78]. In small and hypertrophic left ventricle also preservation of excessive anterior leaflet tissue may increase the risk of SAM. In such situations Quigley in 2005 recommended performance of anterior leaflet reduction by a semilunar excision parallel to the annulus of the anterior leaflet [79].

Systolic anterior motion after mitral valve repair occurs predominantly as a result of the disparity between the excessive area of leaflet tissue left compared with the size of the left ventricle and width of the left ventricular outflow tract, as well as a small-size annuloplasty ring implantation (Fig. 6.52). As a rule, testing of the completed repair on an arrested heart demonstrates excellent leaflet coaptation; however, peroperative transesophageal echocardiography on a beating heart reveals SAM causing pressure gradient in the left ventricular outflow tract, and simultaneously the presence of mitral regurgitation. Management remains always problematic and individual. The principal decision concerns the necessity of mitral valve surgical reintervention. This decision can be facilitated by several tests, which may lead to cessation of SAM. The most important test is volume expansion (i.e., increase of preload). The patient's hypovolemia has to be excluded. The effect of volume expansion can be forecasted by a quick maneuver performed by partial compression of the ascending aorta by clamp or fingers. In this way, during several systoles the increased preload leads to cessation of both SAM and mitral regurgitation. If cessation of SAM is achieved, the volume expansion is continued together with administration of small doses of beta--blockers to suppress the left ventricular hypercontractility. In this case surgical reintervention on the mitral valve is not

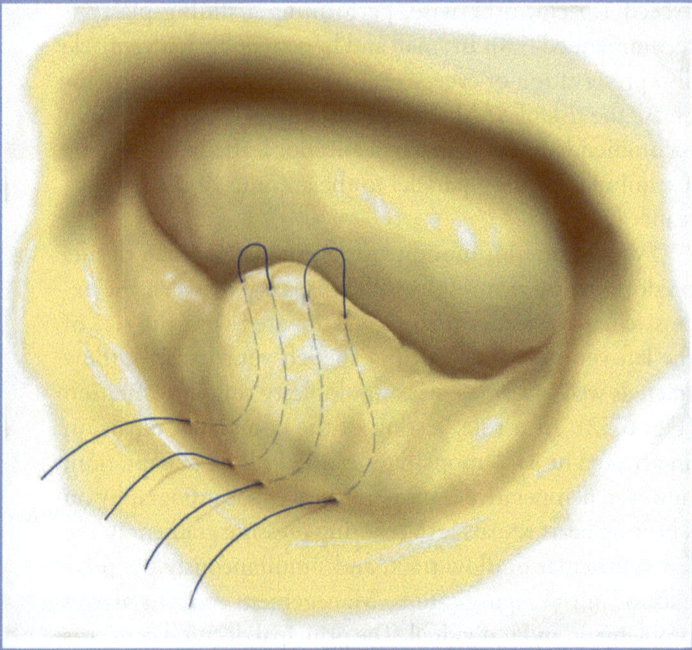

Fig. 6.50 Remodeling of the excessive posterior leaflet tissue. (According to Tabata et al. [75])

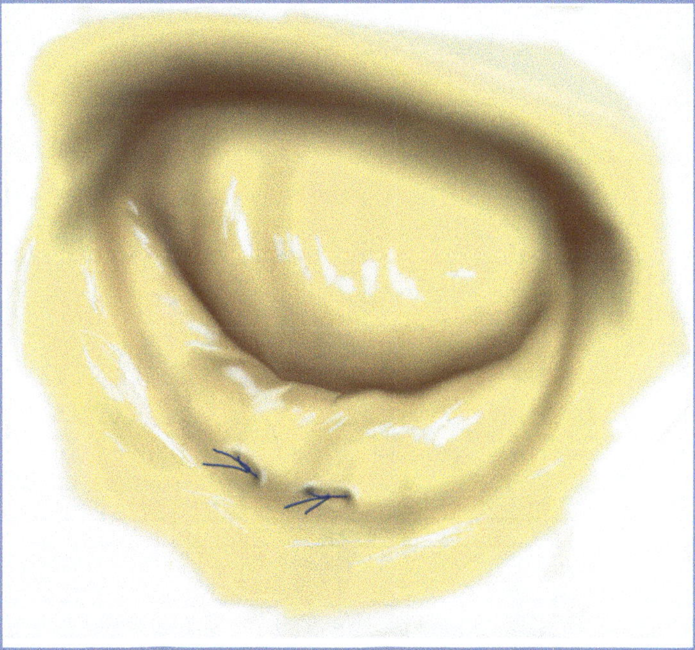

Fig. 6.51 Result of folding valvuloplasty of posterior leaflet. (According to Tabata et al. [75])

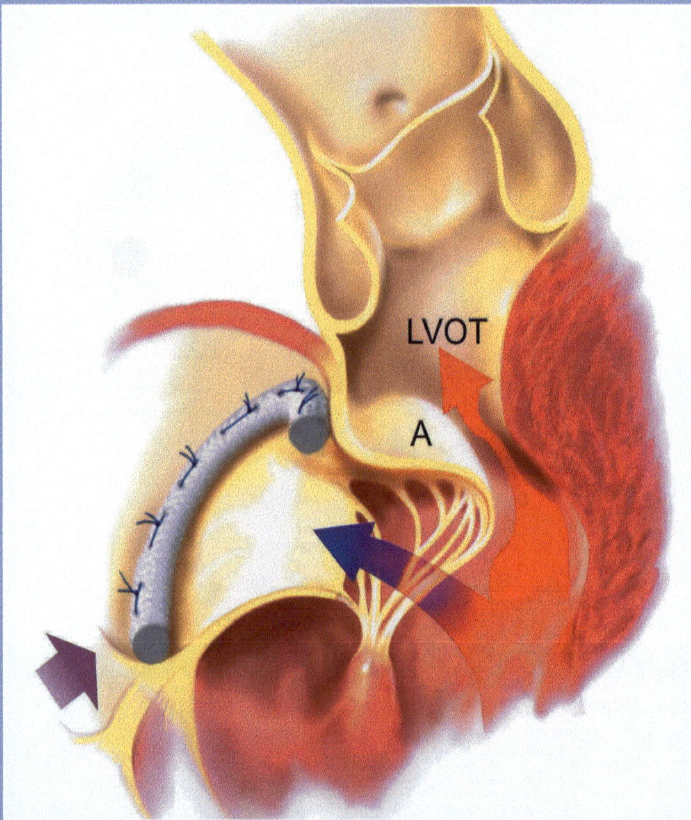

Fig. 6.52 Systolic anterior motion after implantation of mitral annuloplasty ring causes both left ventricular outflow tract obstruction and mitral regurgitation. *A* anterior mitral leaflet, *LVOT* left ventricular outflow tract

deemed necessary. Postoperatively, volume expansion and beta-blocker administration are continued, hypovolemia has to be strictly avoided, and repeated echocardiography controls are performed [76, 80, 81]. If, however, SAM persists in the operating room despite the testing maneuvers, surgical intervention has to be undertaken. The easiest solution is Alfieri edge-to-edge repair (see below), provided, however, the initial mitral procedure did not already result in a significant mitral annulus "undersizing" (borderline mitral orifice area) [82]. If the cause of SAM is clearly detected, its correction may be attempted at the reintervention; otherwise, namely after a time-consuming primary complex mitral valve repair, fast mitral valve replacement is the safest alternative compared with an uncertain and long repair correction. Failure in attempting repair correction will result in further reintervention (valve replacement), and the total of three cardiopulmonary bypass periods may have a deleterious impact.

Procedures for anterior leaflet prolapse are more difficult than for posterior leaflet prolapse. Isolated anterior leaflet prolapse occurs rarely compared with isolated posterior leaflet prolapse. Anterior leaflet prolapse is usually part of bilateral leaflet prolapse. In bilateral leaflet prolapse a relatively new Alfieri repair can be performed [83, 84]. With this technique the incompetent mitral orifice is transformed into two competent orifices by suturing the midpoints of the anterior and posterior leaflets together ("double-orifice" or "edge-to-edge" repair). It is important to place the sutures at some distance from the edge of the leaflets to shorten their length and to secure a sufficient zone of coaptation of newly created orifices (Fig. 6.53). Suturing is performed with over-and-over sutures or, in the case of thin leaflets,

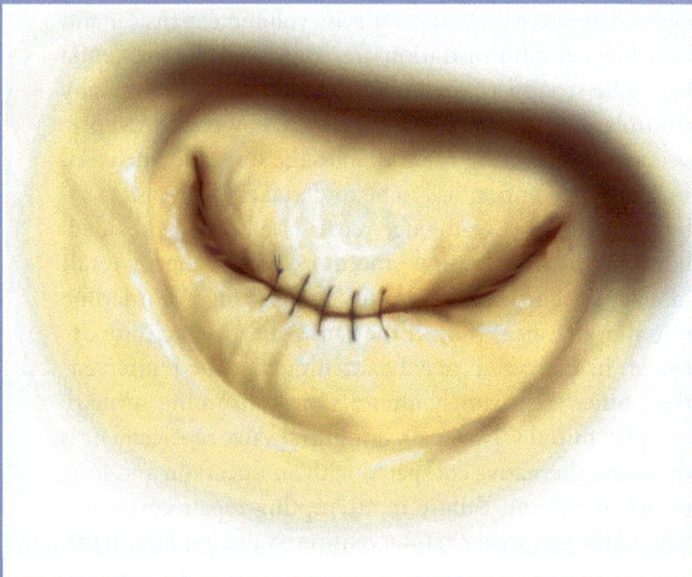

Fig. 6.53 Alfieri repair ("edge to edge," "double orifice")

with pledgeted mattress sutures. It is an extremely simple and fast technique, but it is still controversial, having both supporters and opponents.

A classic and still used method in anterior leaflet prolapse is triangular resection, which is performed by cutting off a narrow triangle from the most prolapsing portion of the anterior leaflet (Fig. 6.54). Occasionally, the excessive area of the anterior leaflet can be reduced by suture plication of the anterior leaflet edge as described by Fundaro et al. (Fig. 6.55) [85, 86].

Elongated chordae of the anterior and posterior leaflets can be shortened by their insertion into the papillary muscles (Fig. 6.56) [31]. Ruptured and recently also the elongated chordae are being replaced by artificial chordae from PTFE sutures (Figs. 6.57, 6.58) [87–89]. They can also be excised and replaced by transposition of the nearest thick secondary chord. Sometimes the secondary chordae retract the midportion of the anterior leaflet ("seagull-sign" deformation of the anterior leaflet on echocardiography examination) and thereby worsen the degree of mitral regurgitation. Their resection, as a part of mitral valve repair, improves the anterior leaflet mobility toward the coaptation zone (Fig. 6.59).

In some cases of mitral regurgitation caused by ischemic left ventricular remodelation, it has been recommended to suture together both heads of papillary muscles by a pledgeted mattress stitch (sandwich plasty) [90]. Reapproximation of the anterior and posterior papillary muscles reduces tethering and improves the leaflet coaptation [91].

Rheumatic mitral valve disease results in Carpentier type-III mitral regurgitation characterized by shortening and retraction of chordae and papillary muscles. Should

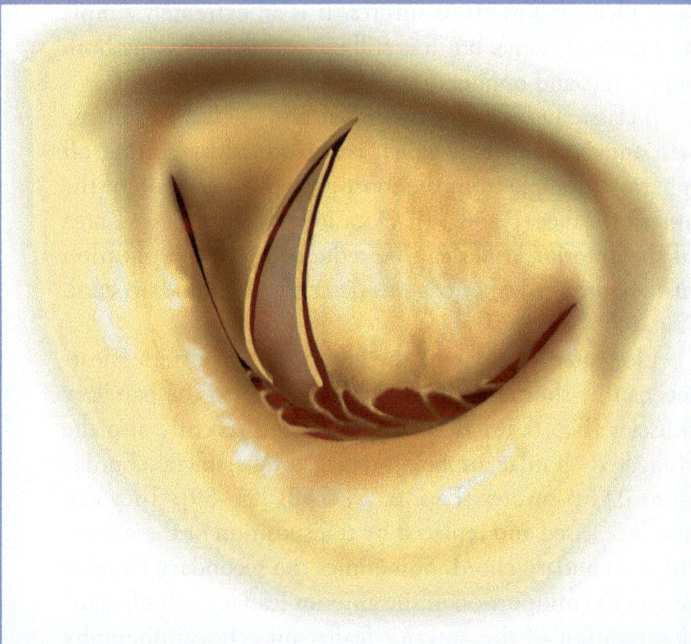

Fig. 6.54 Triangular resection of the anterior mitral leaflet for its prolapse. Marked is the extent of resection

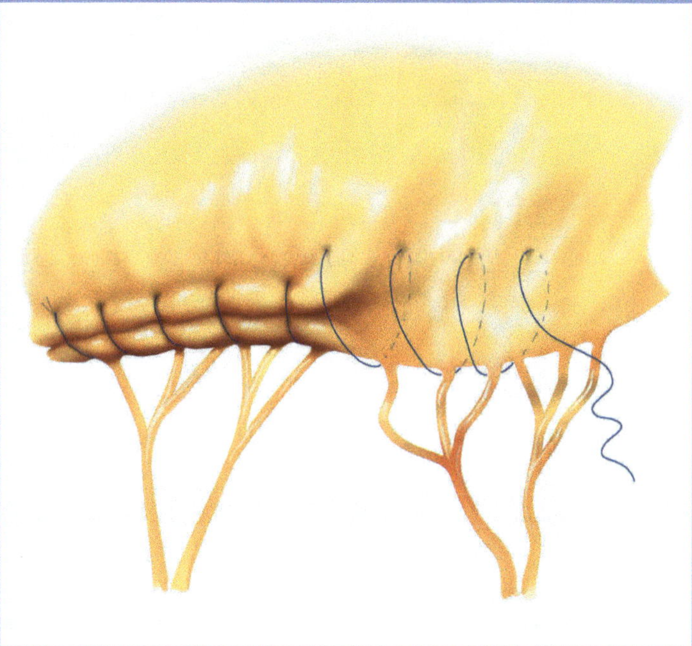

Fig. 6.55 Anterior leaflet plication. (According to Fundaro et al. [85, 86])

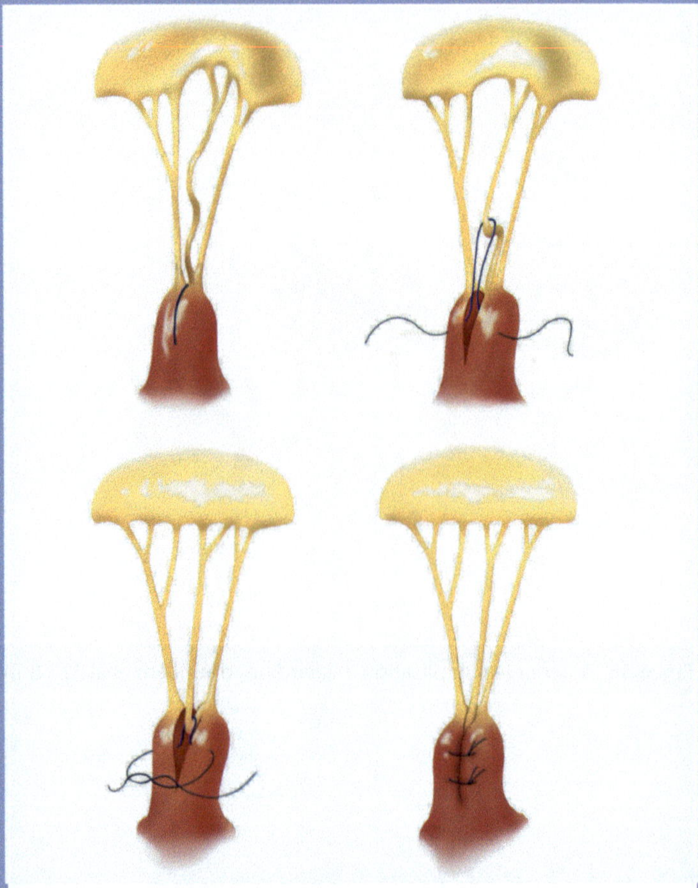

Fig. 6.56 Shortening of the chordae achieved by its plunging into a papillary muscle

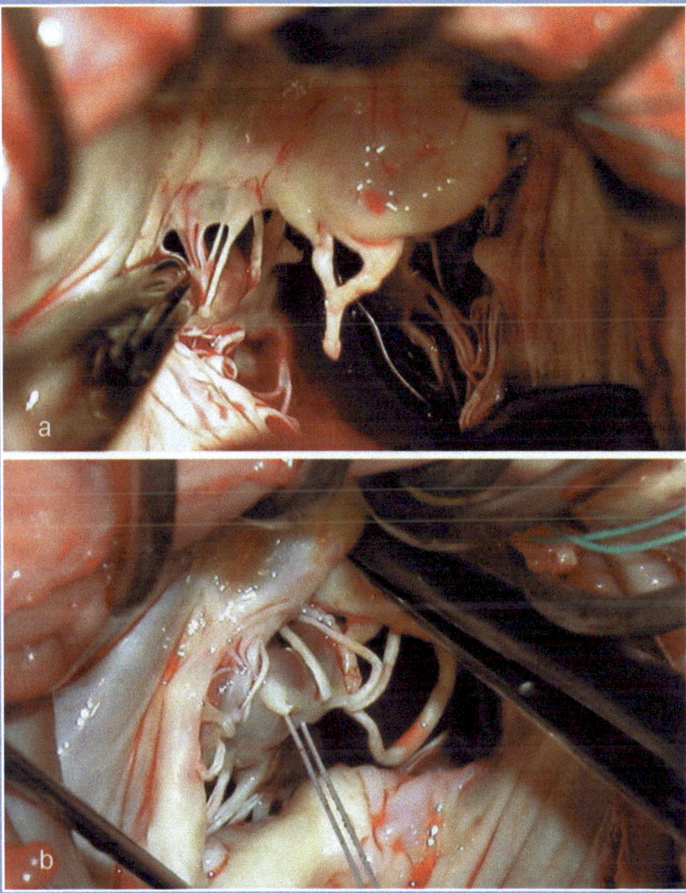

Fig. 6.57 **a** Rupture of primary chord of anterior mitral leaflet. **b** Placement of polytetrafluoroethylene (PTFE) suture into the papillary muscle (artificial chord)

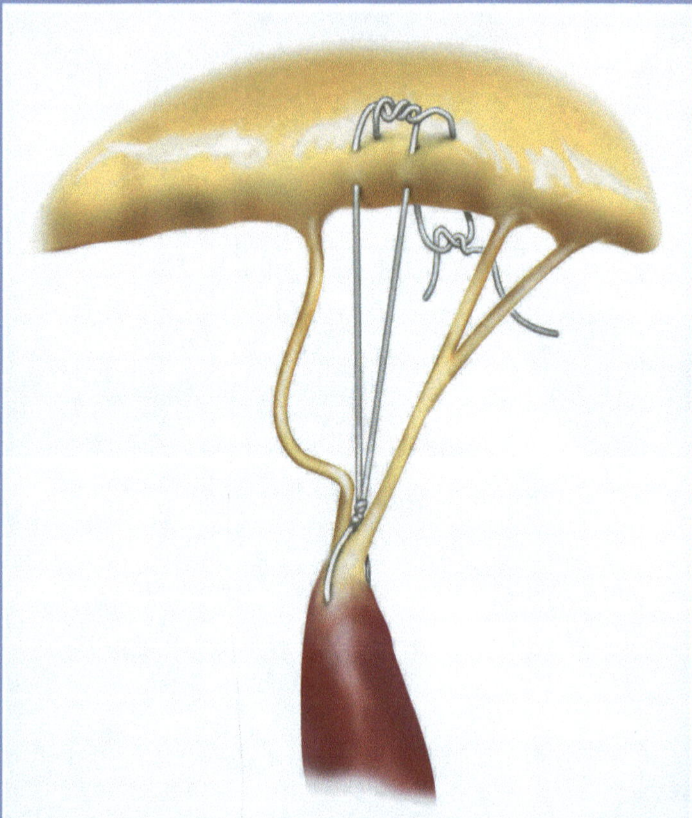

Fig. 6.58 Anchoring and securing PTFE suture at the edge of the anterior mitral leaflet. (According to Perrier [74])

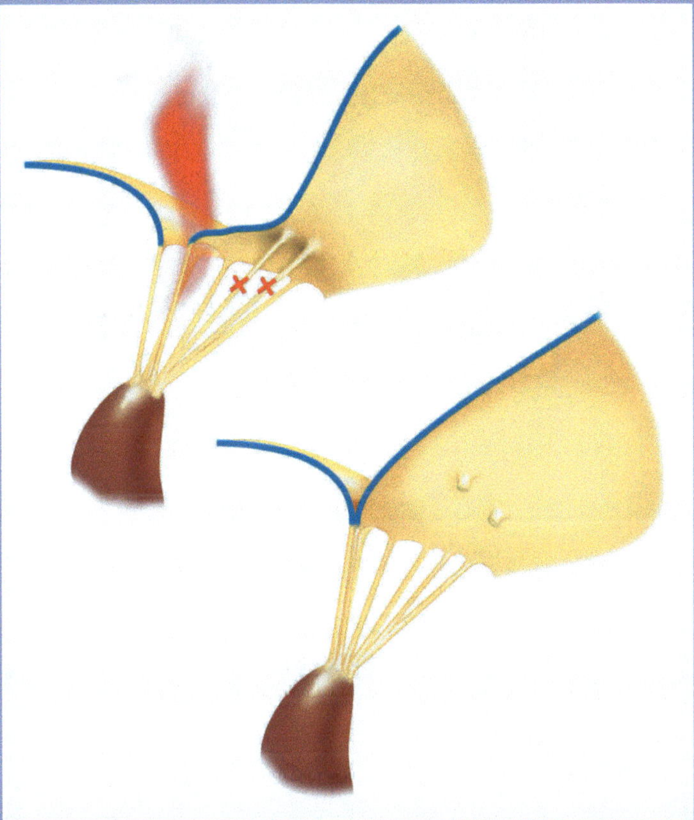

Fig. 6.59 Resection of secondary chordae causing retraction of anterior mitral leaflet

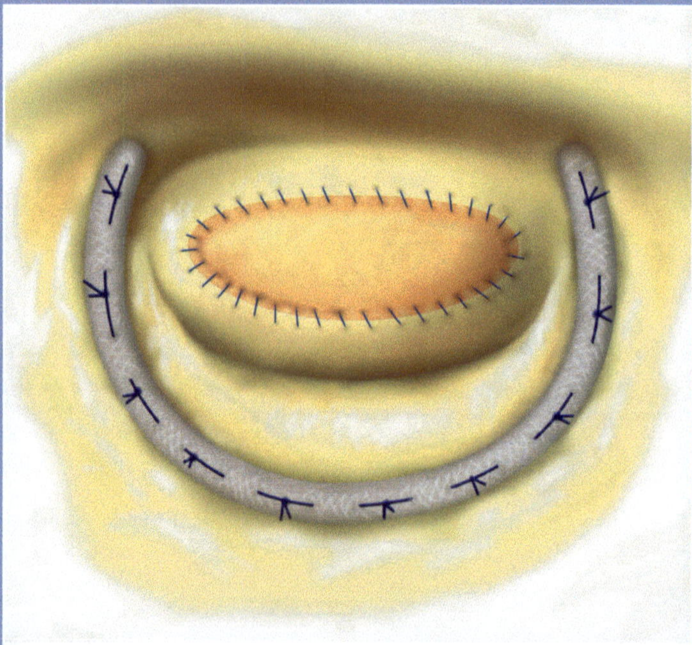

Fig. 6.60 Augmentation of the anterior leaflet by autologous pericardium

valve-sparing surgery be attempted (in spite of mitral valve replacement) dissection of the fused commissures, liberation of the thickened, fused, and shortened chordae, and dissection of the thickened papillary muscles is performed (see Fig. 6.10). Improved billowing of the retracted leaflets can be obtained by secondary chordae resection and by anterior leaflet augmentation with autologous pericardium (Fig. 6.60) [92–95]. The posterior leaflet can also be augmented in a similar manner, e.g., if retracted due to left ventricular dysfunction. The enlarged area of the posterior leaflet will enable its coaptation with the anterior leaflet.

References

1. Galloway AC, Schwartz CF, Ribakove GH et al. (2009) A decade of minimally invasive mitral repair: long-term outcomes. Ann Thorac Surg 88:1180–1184
2. Modi P, Hassan A, Chitwood WR Jr (2008) Minimally invasive mitral valve surgery: a systematic review and meta-analysis. Eur J Cardiothorac Surg 34:943–952
3. Seeburger J, Borger MA, Falk V et al. (2008) Minimal invasive mitral valve repair for mitral regurgitation: results of 1339 consecutive patients. Eur J Cardiothorac Surg 34:760–765
4. Suzuki Y, Pagani FD, Bolling SF (2008) Left thoracotomy for multiple-time redo mitral valve surgery using on-pump beating heart technique. Ann Thorac Surg 86:466–471
5. Thompson MJ, Behranwala A, Campanella C et al. (2003) Immediate and long-term results of mitral prosthetic replacement using a right thoracotomy beating heart technique. Eur J Cardiothorac Surg 24:47–51
6. Loulmet DF, Patel NC, Jennings JM et al. (2008) Less invasive intracardiac surgery performed without aortic clamping. Ann Thorac Surg 85:1551–1555

7. Umakanthan R, Leacche M, Petracek MR et al. (2008) Safety of minimally invasive mitral valve surgery without aortic cross-clamp. Ann Thorac Surg 85:1544–1550
8. Lazzara RR, Kidwell FE (1998) Right parasternal incision: a uniform minimally invasive approach for valve operations. Ann Thorac Surg 65:271–272
9. Nair RU, Sharpe DA (1998) Limited lower sternotomy for minimally invasive mitral valve replacement. Ann Thorac Surg 65:273–274
10. Pifarre R, Balderman S, Sullivan HJ et al. (1982) Technique to facilitate mitral valve exposure. Ann Thorac Surg 33:92–93
11. Alfieri O, Sandrelli L, Pardini A et al. (1991) Optimal exposure of the mitral valve through an extended vertical transeptal approach. Eur J Cardiothorac Surg 5:294–299
12. Guiraudon GM, Ofiesh JG, Kaushik R (1991) Extended vertical transatrial septal approach to the mitral valve. Ann Thorac Surg 52:1058–1062
13. Smith CR (1992) Septal–superior exposure of the mitral valve. The transplant approach. J Thorac Cardiovasc Surg 103:623–628
14. Berreklouw E, Ercan H, Schonberger JP (1991) Combined superior–transseptal approach to the left atrium. Ann Thorac Surg 51:293–295
15. Garcia-Villarreal OA, Gonzalez-Oviedo R, Rodriguez-Gonzalez H et al. (2003) Superior septal approach for mitral valve surgery: a word of caution. Eur J Cardiothorac Surg 24:862–867
16. Gaudino M, Alessandrini F, Glieca F et al. (1997) Conventional left atrial versus superior septal approach for mitral valve replacement. Ann Thorac Surg 63:1123–1127
17. Misawa Y, Fuse K, Kawahito K et al. (1999) Conduction disturbances after superior septal approach for mitral valve repair. Ann Thorac Surg 68:1262–1265
18. Dubost C, Guilmet D, Parades B de et al. (1966) New technic of opening of the left auricle in open-heart surgery: the transseptal bi-auricular approach. Presse Med 74:1607–1608 [in French]

19. Khonsari S, Sintek CF (1990) Transatrial approach revisited. Ann Thorac Surg 50:1002–1003
20. Zacek P, Harrer J, Dominik J et al. (2010) Modified hockey-stick approach to the mitral valve. J Card Surg 25:26–27
21. Legare JF, Buth KJ, Arora RC et al. (2003) The dome of the left atrium: an alternative approach for mitral valve repair. Eur J Cardiothorac Surg 23:272–276
22. Meyer BW, Verska JJ, Lindesmith GG et al. (1965) Open repair of mitral valve lesions: the superior approach. Ann Thorac Surg 92:453–457
23. Richi AA, Sade RM, May MG et al. (1981) Repair of left atrial abnormalities in children by the superior approach. Ann Thorac Surg 31:433–436
24. Vijayanagar R, Bognolo DA, Eckstein PF et al. (1985) Advantages of superior approach for mitral valve surgery. J Cardiovasc Surg (Torino) 26:426–432
25. Carmichael MJ, Cooley DA, Favor AS (1983) Aortic and mitral valve replacement through a single transverse aortotomy: a useful approach in difficult mitral valve exposure. Tex Heart Inst J 10:415–419
26. Bonow RO, Carabello BA, Kanu C et al. (2006) ACC/AHA 2006 guidelines for the management of patients with valvular heart disease. A report of the American College of Cardiology/ American Heart Association Task Force on Practice Guidelines (writing committee to revise the 1998 Guidelines for the Management of Patients With Valvular Heart Disease); developed in collaboration with the Society of Cardiovascular Anesthesiologists; endorsed by the Society for Cardiovascular Angiography and Interventions and the Society of Thoracic Surgeons. Circulation 114:e84–e231
27. Vahanian A, Baumgartner H, Bax J et al. (2007) Guidelines on the management of valvular heart disease: The Task Force on the Management of Valvular Heart Disease of the European Society of Cardiology. Eur Heart J 28:230–268
28. Westaby S (1997) Development of surgery for valvular heart disease. In: Westaby S (ed) Landmarks in cardiac surgery. ISIS Medical Media, Oxford

29. John S, Bashi VV, Jairaj PS et al. (1983) Closed mitral valvotomy: early results and long-term follow-up of 3724 consecutive patients. Circulation 68:891–896
30. Tutun U, Ulus AT, Aksoyek AI et al. (2003) The place of closed mitral valvotomy in the modern cardiac surgery era. J Heart Valve Dis 12:585–591
31. Carpentier A (1983) Cardiac valve surgery: the "French correction." J Thorac Cardiovasc Surg 86:323–337
32. Lillehei CW, Levy MJ, Bonnabeau RC Jr (1964) Mitral valve replacement with preservation of papillary muscles and chordae tendinae. J Thorac Cardiovasc Surg 47:532–543
33. David TE, Strauss HD, Mesher E et al. (1981) Is it important to preserve the chordae tendinae and papillary muscles during mitral valve replacement? Can J Surg 24:236–239
34. Hetzer R, Bougioukas G, Franz M et al. (1983) Mitral valve replacement with preservation of papillary muscles and chordae tendinae: revival of a seemingly forgotten concept. I. Preliminary clinical report. Thorac Cardiovasc Surg 31:291–296
35. Choh JH (1997) Preservation of anterior and posterior leaflet in mitral valve replacement with a tilting-disc valve. Ann Thorac Surg 64:271–273
36. Kuralay E, Demirkilic U, Gunay C et al. (2002) Mitral valve replacement with bileaflet preservation: a modified technique. Eur J Cardiothorac Surg 22:630–632
37. Miki S, Kusuhara K, Ueda Y et al. (1988) Mitral valve replacement with preservation of chordae tendinae and papillary muscles. Ann Thorac Surg 45:28–34
38. Sasaki H, Ihashi K (2003) Chordal-sparing mitral valve replacement: pitfalls and techniques to prevent complications. Eur J Cardiothorac Surg 24:650–652
39. Soga Y, Nishimura K, Yamazaki K et al. (2003) Simplified chordal reconstruction: "oblique" placement of artificial chordae tendinae in mitral valve replacement. Eur J Cardiothorac Surg 24:653–655
40. Vucinic M (1993) Suspension of the papillary muscles during valve replacement for mitral stenosis. J Heart Valve Dis 2:311–314

41. Dumesnil JG, Pibarot P (2006) Prosthesis–patient mismatch and clinical outcomes: the evidence continues to accumulate. J Thorac Cardiovasc Surg 131:952–955
42. Magne J, Mathieu P, Dumesnil JG et al. (2007) Impact of prosthesis–patient mismatch on survival after mitral valve replacement. Circulation 115:1417–1425
43. Azariades M, Lennox SC (1988) Rupture of the posterior wall of the left ventricle after mitral valve replacement: etiological and technical considerations. Ann Thorac Surg 46:491–494
44. Fuente A de la, Agudo O, Sanchez R et al. (1999) Repair of left ventricular rupture after mitral valve replacement: use of a Teflon patch and glue. Ann Thorac Surg 67:1802–1803
45. Gosalbez F, Linera FA de, Cofino JL et al. (1981) Isolated mitral valve replacement and ventricular rupture: presentation of 6 patients. Ann Thorac Surg 31:105–110
46. Bortolotti U, Livi U, Mazzucco A et al. (1981) Successful treatment of intraoperative rupture of the left ventricle after mitral valve replacement: report of a case and review of the literature. Int Surg 66:345–347
47. Deniz H, Sokullu O, Sanioglu S et al. (2008) Risk factors for posterior ventricular rupture after mitral valve replacement: results of 2560 patients. Eur J Cardiothorac Surg 34:780–784
48. Carpentier AF, Pellerin M, Fuzellier JF et al. (1996) Extensive calcification of the mitral valve anulus: pathology and surgical management. J Thorac Cardiovasc Surg 111:718–730
49. d'Alessandro C, Vistarini N, Aubert S et al. (2007) Mitral annulus calcification: determinants of repair feasibility, early and late surgical outcome. Eur J Cardiothorac Surg 32:596–603
50. Nili M, Salomon J, Halevi A et al. (1981) Left ventricular rupture after mitral valve replacement. Report of two cases and a review of the literature. Scand J Thorac Cardiovasc Surg 15:235–238
51. Craver JM, Jones EL, Guyton RA et al. (1985) Avoidance of transverse midventricular disruption following mitral valve replacement. Ann Thorac Surg 40:163–171
52. Levine RA, Schwammenthal E (2005) Ischemic mitral regurgitation on the threshold of a solution: from paradoxes to unifying concepts. Circulation 112:745–758

53. Yamaguchi H, Eishi K (2007) Surgical treatment of active infective mitral valve endocarditis. Ann Thorac Cardiovasc Surg 13:150–155
54. Chenot F, Montant P, Vancraeynest D et al. (2009) Long-term clinical outcome of mitral valve repair in asymptomatic severe mitral regurgitation. Eur J Cardiothorac Surg 36:539–545
55. Kang DH, Kim MJ, Kang SJ et al. (2006) Mitral valve repair versus revascularization alone in the treatment of ischemic mitral regurgitation. Circulation 114:I499–I503
56. Srivastava AR, Banerjee A, Jacob S et al. (2007) Should patients undergoing coronary artery bypass grafting with mild to moderate ischaemic mitral regurgitation also undergo mitral valve repair or replacement? Interact Cardiovasc Thorac Surg 6:538–546
57. Enriquez-Sarano M, Avierinos JF, Messika-Zeitoun D et al. (2005) Quantitative determinants of the outcome of asymptomatic mitral regurgitation. N Engl J Med 352:875–883
58. Otto CM, Salerno CT (2005) Timing of surgery in asymptomatic mitral regurgitation. N Engl J Med 352:928–929
59. Suri RM, Grewal J, Mankad S et al. (2009) Is the anterior intertrigonal distance increased in patients with mitral regurgitation due to leaflet prolapse? Ann Thorac Surg 88:1202–1208
60. Adams DH, Anyanwu AC, Rahmanian PB et al. (2006) Large annuloplasty rings facilitate mitral valve repair in Barlow's disease. Ann Thorac Surg 82:2096–2101
61. Silberman S, Klutstein MW, Sabag T et al. (2009) Repair of ischemic mitral regurgitation: comparison between flexible and rigid annuloplasty rings. Ann Thorac Surg 87:1721–1727
62. Fasol R, Meinhart J, Deutsch M et al. (2004) Mitral valve repair with the Colvin–Galloway Future Band. Ann Thorac Surg 77:1985–1988
63. Gorton ME, Piehler JM, Killen DA et al. (1993) Mitral valve repair using a flexible and adjustable annuloplasty ring. Ann Thorac Surg 55:860–863
64. McCarthy PM, McGee EC, Rigolin VH et al. (2008) Initial clinical experience with Myxo-ETlogix mitral valve repair ring. J Thorac Cardiovasc Surg 136:73–81

65. Gillinov AM, Tantiwongkosri K, Blackstone EH et al. (2009) Is prosthetic annuloplasty necessary for durable mitral valve repair? Ann Thorac Surg 88:76–82
66. Burr LH, Krayenbuhl C, Sutton MS (1977) The mitral plication suture: a new technique of mitral valve repair. J Thorac Cardiovasc Surg 73:589–595
67. Matsuda H, Shintani H, Taniguchi K et al. (1997) Semicircular suture annuloplasty for mitral regurgitation: appraisal of the Paneth–Burr method. J Heart Valve Dis 6:48–53
68. Nagy ZL, Peterffy A (2000) Mitral annuloplasty with a suture technique. Eur J Cardiothorac Surg 18:739–741
69. Kay EB, Nogueira C, Head LR et al. (1958) Surgical treatment of mitral insufficiency. J Thorac Surg 36:677–690
70. Wooler GH, Nixon PG, Grimshaw VA et al. (1962) Experiences with the repair of the mitral valve in mitral incompetence. Thorax 17:49–57
71. Gillinov AM, Cosgrove DM III (2001) Modified quadrangular resection for mitral valve repair. Ann Thorac Surg 72:2153–2154
72. Gillinov AM, Cosgrove DM III (1999) Modified sliding leaflet technique for repair of the mitral valve. Ann Thorac Surg 68:2356–2357
73. Calafiore AM, Mauro M di, Actis Dato G et al. (2006) Longitudinal plication of the posterior leaflet in myxomatous disease of the mitral valve. Ann Thorac Surg 81:1909–1910
74. Perier P, Hohenberger W, Lakew F et al. (2008) Toward a new paradigm for the reconstruction of posterior leaflet prolapse: midterm results of the "respect rather than resect" approach. Ann Thorac Surg 86:718–725
75. Tabata M, Ghanta RK, Shekar PS et al. (2008) Early and midterm outcomes of folding valvuloplasty without leaflet resection for myxomatous mitral valve disease. Ann Thorac Surg 86:1388–1390
76. Crescenzi G, Landoni G, Zangrillo A et al. (2009) Management and decision-making strategy for systolic anterior motion after mitral valve repair. J Thorac Cardiovasc Surg 137:320–325

77. Filsoufi F, Carpentier A (2007) Systolic anterior motion of the mitral valve. J Thorac Cardiovasc Surg 134:265–266
78. Zegdi R, Carpentier A, Doguet F et al. (2005) Systolic anterior motion after mitral valve repair: an exceptional cause of late failure. J Thorac Cardiovasc Surg 130:1453–1454
79. Quigley RL (2005) Prevention of systolic anterior motion after repair of the severely myxomatous mitral valve with an anterior leaflet valvuloplasty. Ann Thorac Surg 80:179–182
80. Brown ML, Abel MD, Click RL et al. (2007) Systolic anterior motion after mitral valve repair: Is surgical intervention necessary? J Thorac Cardiovasc Surg 133:136–143
81. George KM, Gillinov AM (2008) Posterior leaflet shortening to correct systolic anterior motion after mitral valve repair. Ann Thorac Surg 86:1699–1700
82. Mascagni R, Al Attar N, Lamarra M et al. (2005) Edge-to-edge technique to treat post-mitral valve repair systolic anterior motion and left ventricular outflow tract obstruction. Ann Thorac Surg 79:471–474
83. Alfieri O, Bonis M de, Lapenna E et al. (2004) "Edge-to-edge" repair for anterior mitral leaflet prolapse. Semin Thorac Cardiovasc Surg 16:182–187
84. Maisano F, Torracca L, Oppizzi M et al. (1998) The edge-to-edge technique: a simplified method to correct mitral insufficiency. Eur J Cardiothorac Surg 13:240–246
85. Fundaro P, Mattia DG di, Salati M et al. (1997) Free edge suture plication and remodeling: a technique for anterior mitral leaflet prolapse repair. Ann Thorac Surg 63:1186–1188
86. Fundaro P, Moneta A, Villa E et al. (2001) Chordal plication and free edge remodeling for mitral anterior leaflet prolapse repair: 8-year follow-up. Ann Thorac Surg 72:1515–1519
87. Fattouch K, Bianco G, Sbraga F et al. (2007) Simple, safe and easy technique to ensure the correct length of artificial chordae in mitral valve repair. Ann Thorac Surg 83:1902–1903
88. Kasegawa H, Shimokawa T, Shibazaki I et al. (2006) Mitral valve repair for anterior leaflet prolapse with expanded polytetrafluoroethylene sutures. Ann Thorac Surg 81:1625–1631

89. Kuntze T, Borger MA, Falk V et al. (2008) Early and mid-term results of mitral valve repair using premeasured Gore-Tex loops ("loop technique"). Eur J Cardiothorac Surg 33:566–572
90. Ishikawa S, Ueda K, Kawasaki A et al. (2008) Papillary muscle sandwich plasty for ischemic mitral regurgitation: a new simple technique. J Thorac Cardiovasc Surg 135:1384–1386
91. Tanemoto K (2005) Surgical treatment of ischemic mitral valve regurgitation. Ann Thorac Cardiovasc Surg 11:228–231
92. Acar C, Ibarra JS de, Lansac E (2004) Anterior leaflet augmentation with autologous pericardium for mitral repair in rheumatic valve insufficiency. J Heart Valve Dis 13:741–746
93. Aubert S, Flecher E, Rubin S et al. (2007) Anterior mitral leaflet augmentation with autologous pericardium. Ann Thorac Surg 83:1560–1561
94. Chauvaud S, Fuzellier JF, Berrebi A et al. (2001) Long-term (29 years) results of reconstructive surgery in rheumatic mitral valve insufficiency. Circulation 104:I12–I15
95. Romano MA, Patel HJ, Pagani FD et al. (2005) Anterior leaflet repair with patch augmentation for mitral regurgitation. Ann Thorac Surg 79:1500–1504

Tricuspid Valve Surgery

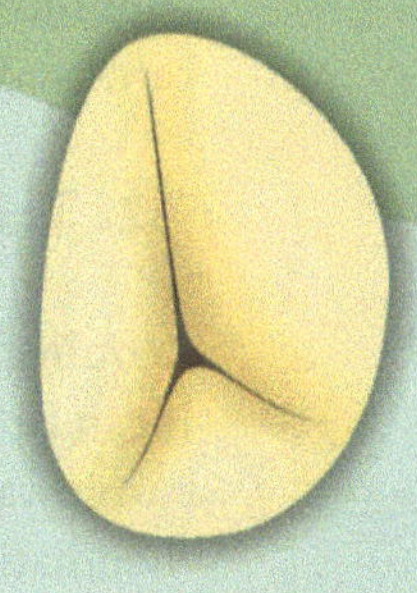

7 Tricuspid Valve Surgery

7.1 Introduction

Similarly to aortic and mitral valve disease, both tricuspid stenosis and tricuspid regurgitation can be treated surgically. In clinical practice, however, surgical procedures for tricuspid stenosis are extremely rare. Numerous techniques for correction of tricuspid regurgitation have been elaborated since the 1960s but for decades surgeons have remained rather conservative in indications for tricuspid valve repair. Tricuspid regurgitation was traditionally believed to ameliorate spontaneously after surgical correction of left-sided heart valve disease and, in general, to be well tolerated by the patient. A shift in the paradigm towards a more aggressive surgical approach to secondary tricuspid regurgitation has been advocated by many in recent years in order to prevent further worsening of regurgitation and to avoid late reoperations with unfavorable results [1–4]. The number of surgical corrections of tricuspid regurgitation has been increasing because modern indication criteria do rightly suggest surgical intervention, even in less-significant tricuspid regurgitation, as part of a combined cardiac operation.

7.2 Tricuspid Stenosis

Acquired organic stenosis of the tricuspid valve is very rare. It can be caused by rheumatic disease as a part of mitro-tricuspid valve involvement or even more rarely as an isolated rheumatic tricuspid stenosis. Similarly rare is the carcinoid

J. Dominik and P. Zacek, *Heart Valve Surgery: An Illustrated Guide*,
DOI 10.1007/978-3-642-12206-4_7,

that requires operation because of causing tricuspid stenosis. Right atrial tumors may almost completely occlude the tricuspid orifice and thereby imitate tricuspid stenosis.

Operations of tricuspid stenosis as a part of mitro-tricuspid rheumatic valve disease are currently extremely rare in developed countries. Indication for surgical intervention is justified in symptomatic patients with hemodynamically significant tricuspid stenosis (diastolic gradient ≥5 mmHg and orifice area ≤1.0–1.5 cm^2). Treatment is either a valve-sparing procedure (dissection of the fused commissures, eventually followed by valvular repair) or valve replacement in cases of rigid circular orifice with calcifications.

7.3 Tricuspid Regurgitation

7.3.1 Etiology of Tricuspid Regurgitation

Secondary (functional, non-organic) tricuspid regurgitation caused by dilation of the tricuspid annulus is the most frequent reason for surgical intervention on the tricuspid valve. Secondary tricuspid regurgitation evolves as a result of long-term elevated right ventricular pressure caused most often by pulmonary hypertension. Pressure or volume right ventricular overload leads to right ventricular hypertrophy and dilation together with the tricuspid annular dilation (Fig. 7.1). Primary causes of development of secondary tricuspid regurgitation are left heart valve disease (tricuspidalized disease), pulmonary stenosis, or regurgitation or congenital heart defects with left-to-right shunt.

Acquired organic tricuspid regurgitation is less frequent and may be caused by myxomatous degeneration, infective endocarditis (Figs. 7.2, 7.3), trauma, and carcinoid. Ebstein's anomaly and various forms of atrioventricular

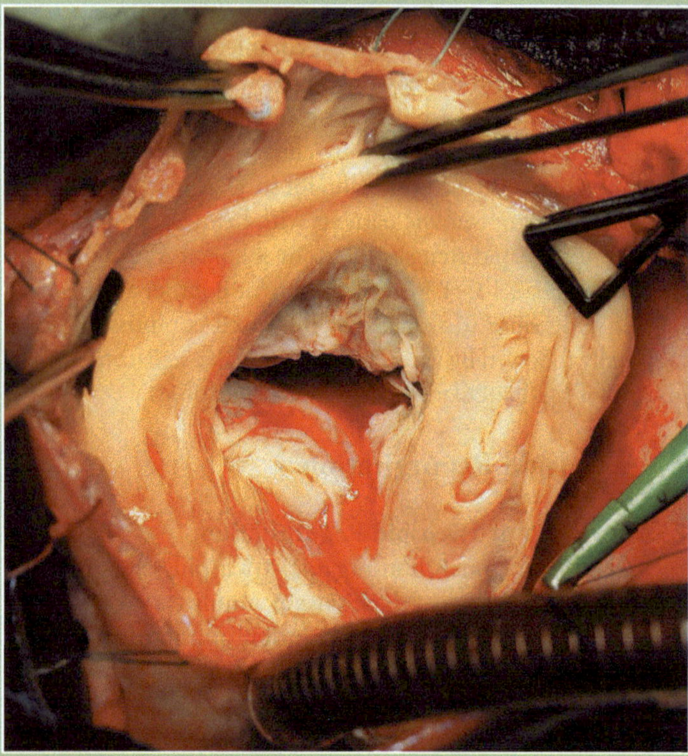

Fig. 7.1 Dilation of the tricuspid annulus causing secondary tricuspid regurgitation

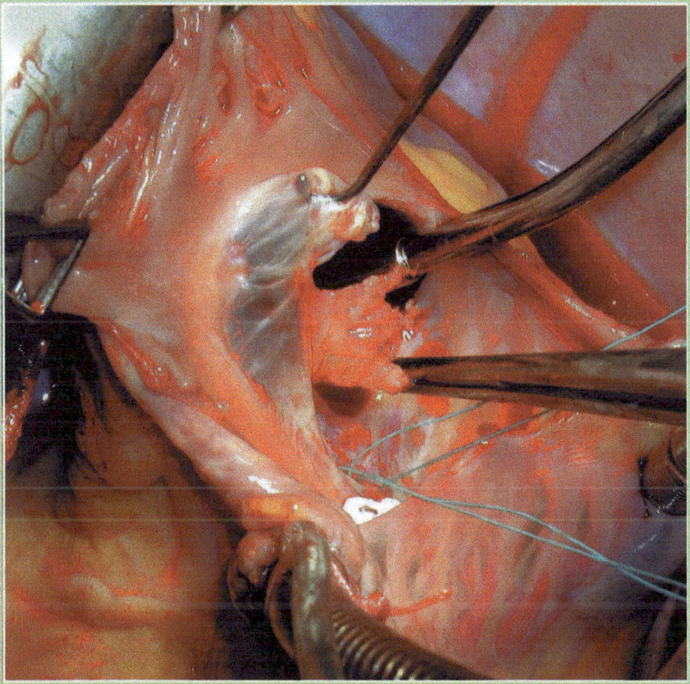

Fig. 7.2 Infective endocarditis of the tricuspid valve. Vegetation on the anterior leaflet

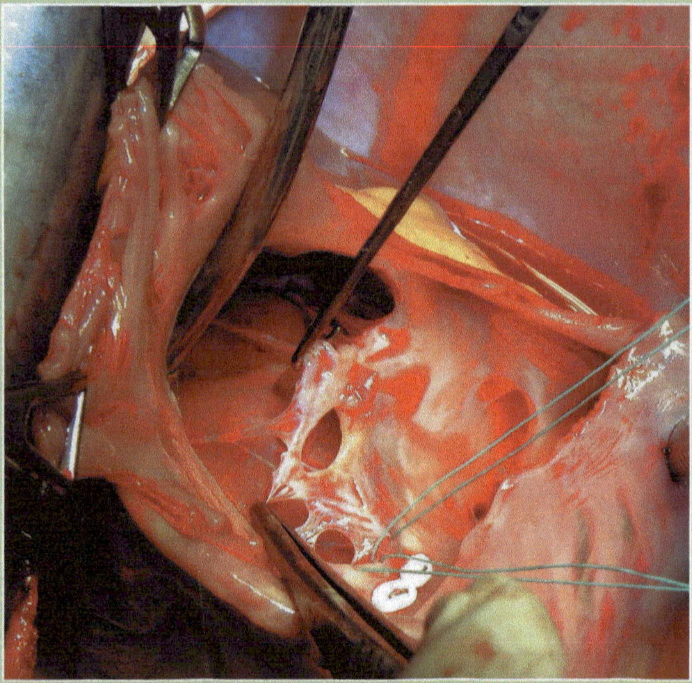

Fig. 7.3 Infective endocarditis of the tricuspid valve. Defects and vegetation at the septal leaflet

septal defect are the main instances of congenital tricuspid regurgitation.

Echocardiography examination offers precise morphological analysis of tricuspid regurgitation and evaluation of its hemodynamic significance.

7.3.2 Indications for Surgery

Surgical procedure for tricuspid regurgitation is most often undertaken due to tricuspid annular dilation or more rarely due to organic changes resulting from endocarditis or congenital cardiac defects.

Isolated tricuspid valve procedure is relatively rare, accounting for 5–10% of all tricuspid valve procedures. It is indicated in symptomatic patients [fatigue, dyspnea, symptoms of low cardiac output, hepatomegaly, edema of low extremities, New York Heart Association (NYHA) stages III–IV] and also in those in whom clear progression of right-sided heart chambers can be evidenced together with impairment of right ventricular systolic function. Uncontrolled sepsis and development of right ventricular failure in tricuspid valve infective endocarditis is also an indication for surgery.

Surgery for tricuspid regurgitation as a part of multiple-valve procedure (together with interventions on the left heart valves) is unequivocally indicated not only for severe tricuspid regurgitation (vena contracta >6–7 mm, reversal of flow in the hepatic veins) but also for moderate regurgitation with dilation of the tricuspid annulus (echocardiographically documented dilation >40 mm or >21 mm/m^2) [1]. The most recent recommendation for tricuspid annuloplasty suggests a cut-off value of the annular dilation over 35 mm [2]. The rationale for such strategy is based on a history of unpredictable course of mild to moderate tricuspid regurgitation that was left untreated at the time of mitral procedure [2, 3]. This is also supported by poor results of reoperations of patients with advanced severe tricuspid regurgitation many years after isolated mitral procedure.

With regard to all these factors, performance of tricuspid repair as part of a combined procedure must be justified, even in cases of mild tricuspid regurgitation if annular dilation or pulmonary hypertension are present. Dreyfus et al. recommend tricuspid valve repair should the intraoperative anteroposterior tricuspid diameter measurement exceed 7 cm (even in trivial regurgitation) [4]. Such advanced annular dilation will not regress, even after left heart valve surgery, but will most likely advance progress.

7.3.3 Surgical Procedures on the Tricuspid Valve

There are three types of surgical interventions on the tricuspid valve: (1) repair; (2) replacement; and (3) excision.

7.3.3.1 Tricuspid Valve Repair for Secondary Regurgitation

Valve-sparing procedures (repairs) are the most often performed operations on the tricuspid valve. The most frequent reason for the repair is annular dilation causing secondary tricuspid regurgitation. Tricuspid annulus typically dilates only in the area of the anterior and posterior leaflet, whereas its septal-leaflet length remains unchanged (Fig. 7.4) [4, 5]. This fact is the key feature of all tricuspid annuloplasty techniques: shortening of the tricuspid annulus in the area of the anterior and posterior leaflets. The shortening can be achieved by suture repairs or by annuloplasty ring implantation.

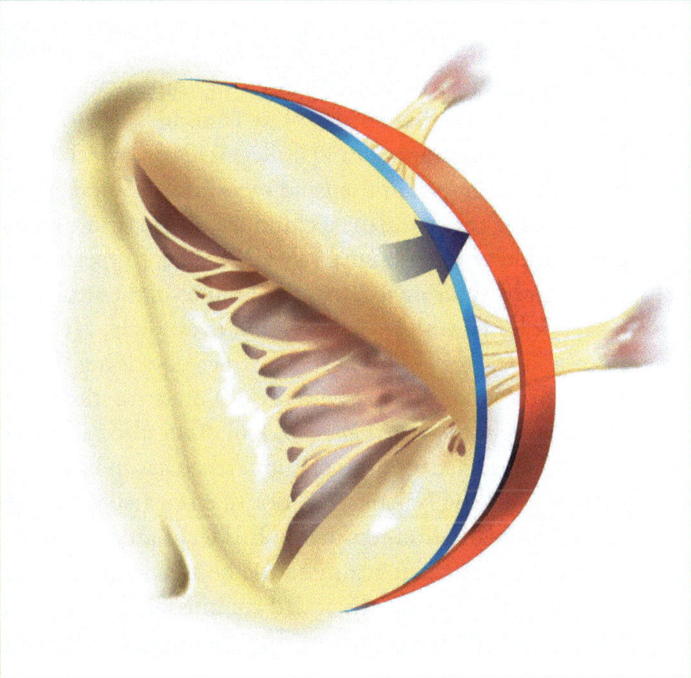

Fig. 7.4 Disproportional dilation of tricuspid annulus in secondary tricuspid regurgitation. Dilation develops in the area of anterior and posterior leaflets. Annulus does not dilate in the area of septal leaflet

A variety of suture techniques have been described and introduced into clinical practice despite recent decline in their use in favor of annuloplasty ring implantation. The oldest repair was described by Kay et al. in 1965 [6]. The principle is posterior tricuspid leaflet exclusion, which transforms the incompetent tricuspid valve into a competent bicuspid valve; therefore, the technique is called suture bicuspidalization of the tricuspid valve. Kay et al. [6] performed the repair by suturing together the annulus in the area of the posterior leaflet with several over-and-over stitches. In 1967 Reed and Cortes [7] published a paper describing the bicuspidalization technique with use of a mattress stitch with pledgets on both sides (Figs. 7.5, 7.6). They also calculated that the shortened annulus circumference has to be at least 8 cm [7]. In 1984 Nakano et al. described an analogous type of a bicuspidalization repair [8]. This technique is suitable for those valves where regurgitation occurs predominantly through pathologically distended commissure between the anterior and posterior leaflets. The commissure is sutured and then Kay's plasty is added to a somewhat lesser extent (Figs. 7.7, 7.8) [9].

The most popular and widely used suture technique is DeVega annuloplasty (described in 1972) [10]. The principle of this technique lies in shortening the tricuspid annulus in the area corresponding to the anterior and posterior leaflets. Two pledgeted parallel running stitches are placed in semicircular manner from the anterolateral to the posteroseptal commissure and tied (Figs. 7.9, 7.10). The possibility of failure of this repair, however, has been also described. One of the reasons for failure is cutting through of the stitches placed in a fragile tricuspid annulus (Fig. 7.11). To avoid this potential risk, Antunes and Girdwood in

1983 suggested modification of DeVega technique [11]. The semicircular stitch is passed through a pledget between every bit of annular tissue (Figs. 7.12, 7.13). Revuelta and Garcia-Rinaldi in 1989 published a different solution: for annular shortening they used separate pledgeted mattress stitches [12]. Another advantage of this technique is the possibility to affect selectively the degree of reduction in different portions of the annulus by the width of the mattress stitches (Figs. 7.14, 7.15).

Modification of the classic DeVega technique, enabling selective regulation of the reduction of the anterior and posterior portions of the tricuspid annulus, was used by Senning and published by Brugger et al. in 1982 [13]. The stitch is first tied in the area of anteroposterior commissure and then its arms are passed through the tricuspid annulus in opposite directions analogous to the DeVega technique (Fig. 7.16). It is interesting that even in the current era of annuloplasty rings Sarraj et al. published in 2007 a very similar technique, which they named adjustable segmental tricuspid annuloplasty (Fig. 7.17) [14, 15].

In 1987 Kurlansky et al. described an interesting modification of the DeVega technique [16]. Placement of two rows of stitches along the annulus from the anteroseptal commissure to the posteroseptal commissure is the same, but then the stitches are led out through the right atrial wall and snared through a tourniquet. After restoration of the heart rhythm and weaning off the cardiopulmonary bypass, the surgeon evaluates regurgitation with a forefinger inserted through the right atrial appendage (Fig. 7.18). The stitches are tightened until the moment of cessation of regurgitation. An identical principle can be applied with the aid of peroperative echocardiography (published by Cook

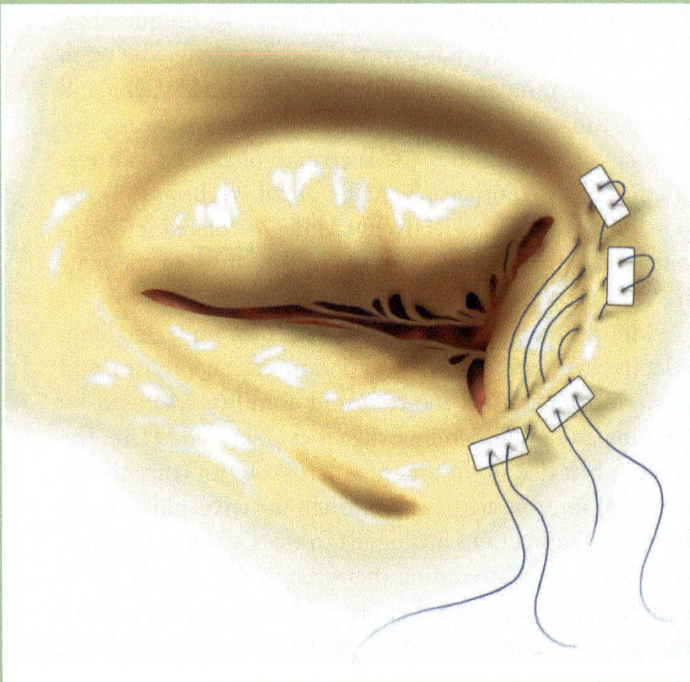

Fig. 7.5 Placement of sutures in tricuspid repair. (According to Kay et al. [6] and Reed and Cortes [7])

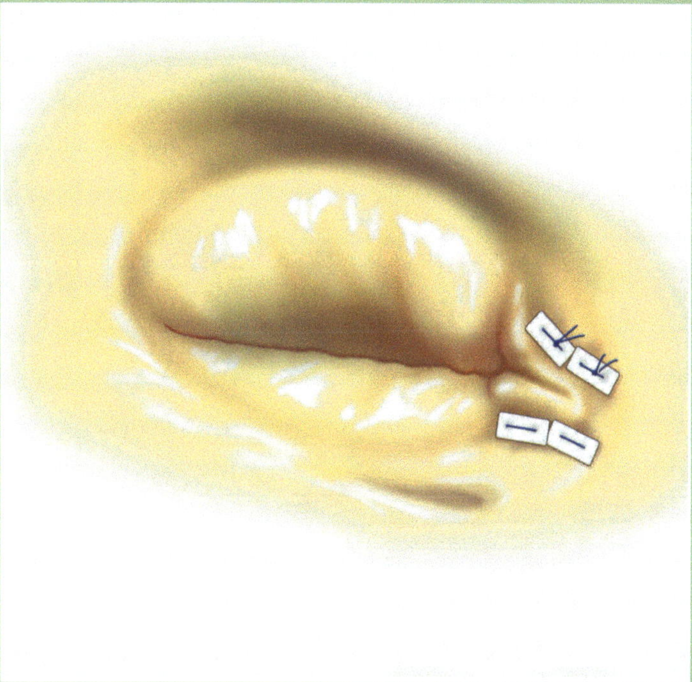

Fig. 7.6 Result of tricuspid repair (bicuspidalization of the tricuspid valve). (According to Kay et al. [6] and Reed and Cortes [7])

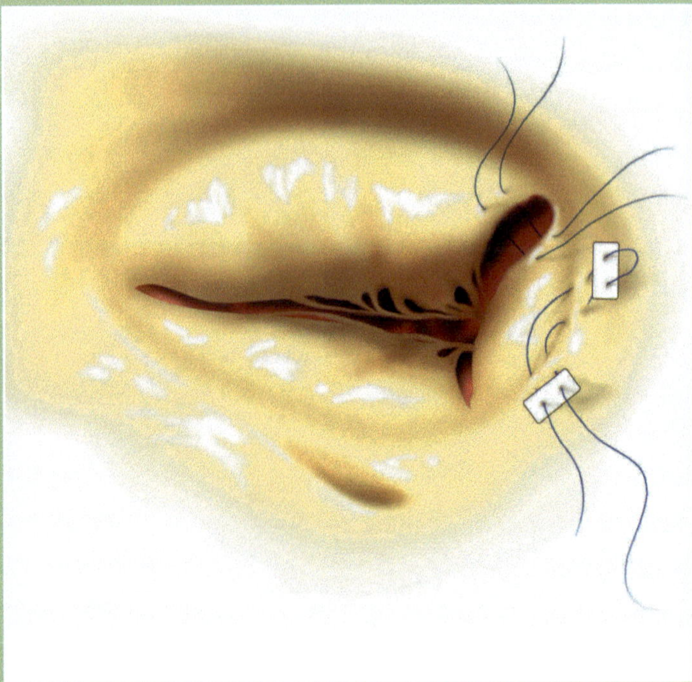

Fig. 7.7 Placement of sutures in tricuspid repair. (According to Nakano et al. [8])

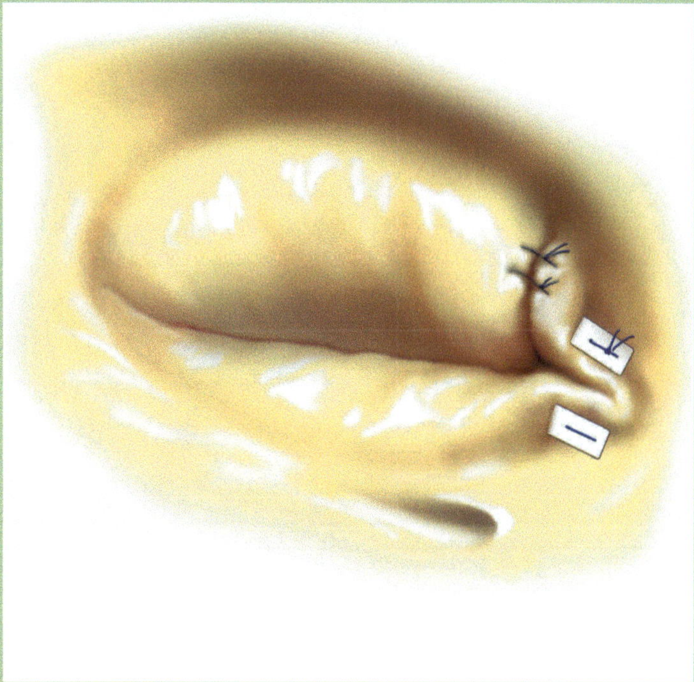

Fig. 7.8 Result of tricuspid repair. (According to Nakano et al. [8])

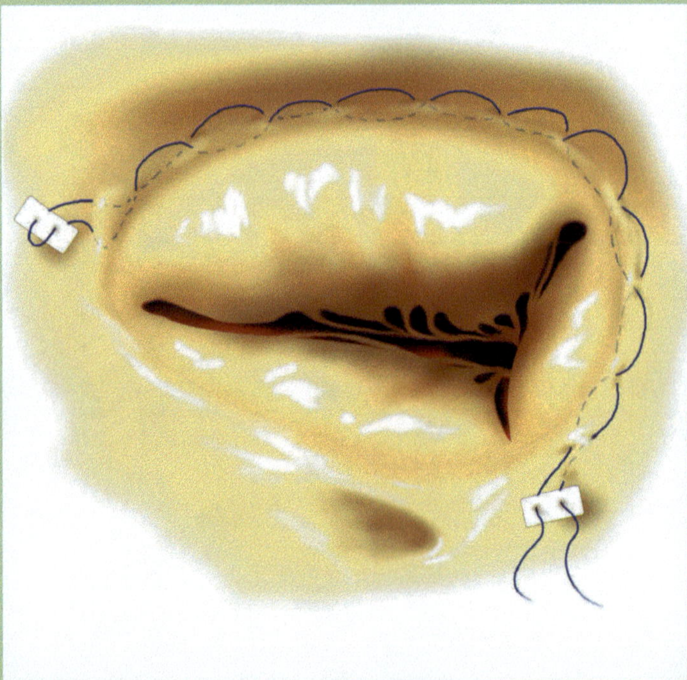

Fig. 7.9 Placement of two suture lines in tricuspid annuloplasty. (According to DeVega [10])

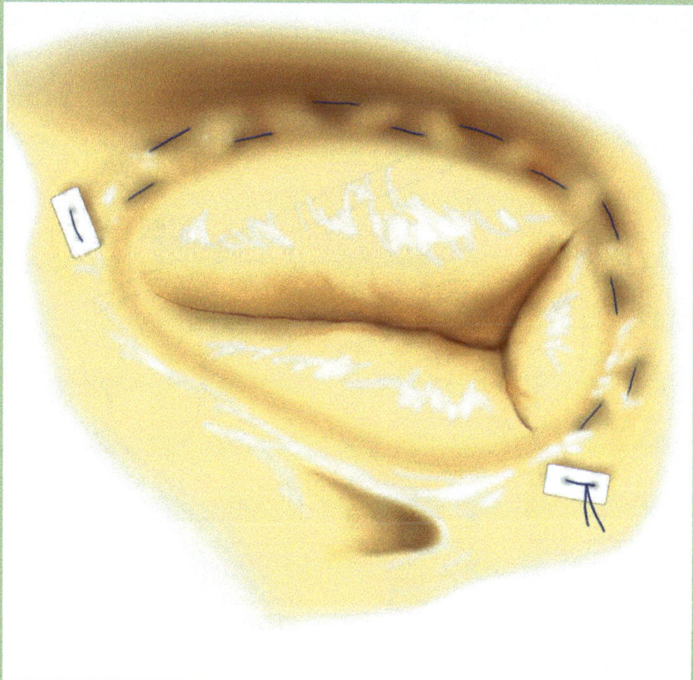

Fig. 7.10 Result of suture tricuspid annuloplasty. (According to DeVega [10])

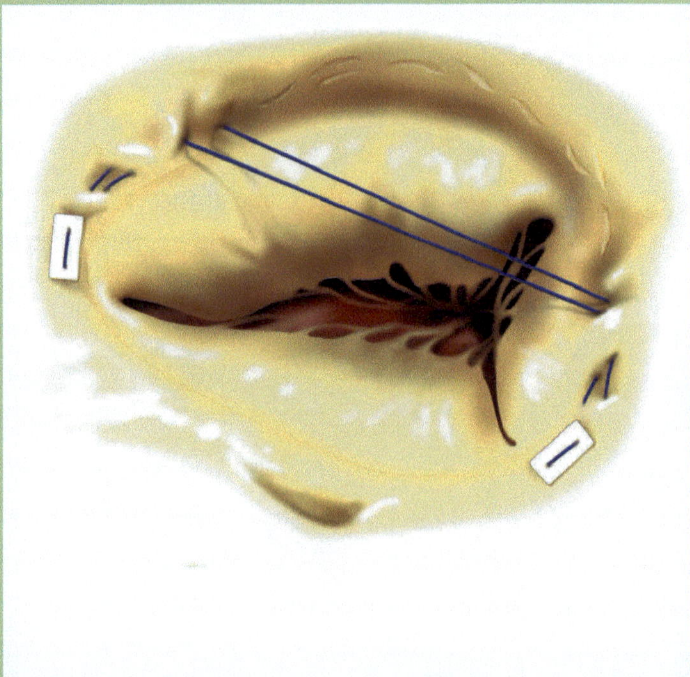

Fig. 7.11 Failure of DeVega annuloplasty: cutting through of the stitches in a fragile tricuspid annulus ("guitar-string syndrome")

in 1994). The tightening proceeds until the echocardiography confirms cessation of regurgitation and simultaneously excludes creation of tricuspid stenosis [17].

The overview of suture-repair techniques should include also the less frequently used technique described by Minale et al. in 1987 [18]. With this technique the anterior and posterior leaflets are partially detached from the tricuspid annulus in the area of anteroposterior commissure to allow their central coaptation. The isolated portion of the annulus is reduced by its plication and exclusion. The cut edges of the leaflets are then readapted to the shortened annulus (Figs. 7.19–7.21).

Finally, there exists a "triple-orifice" method termed also a trefoil or "edge-to-edge" repair of the tricuspid valve. This technique was first performed by Giedrius in 2000 and published by DeBonis in 2004 [19]. Tricuspid regurgitation caused by myxomatous degeneration and leaflet prolapse can be treated in addition to the annuloplasty ring implantation by suturing the midpoints of all three leaflets together, thus creating three orifices (Fig. 7.22) [20].

Competence of the tricuspid valve can also be restored by implantation of the annuloplasty rings that have the ideal shape of tricuspid annulus (Fig. 7.23) [5]. The implanted ring not only reduces the annular circumference within the extent of the anterior and posterior leaflet, but also enforces its proper shape and guarantees annular shape and size retainment in the long term. Implantation is performed with mattress sutures placed proportionally in the non-dilated septal portion of the annulus, whereas in the dilated anteroposterior circumference the sutures bite more of the annulus and are passed in narrower intervals through the ring fabric (Fig. 7.24). This results in controlled plication

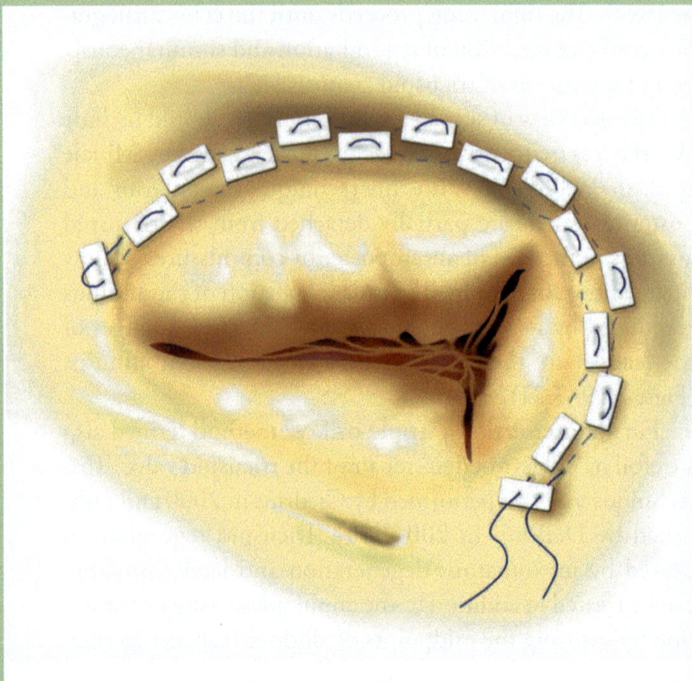

Fig. 7.12 Tricuspid valve annuloplasty. Placement of two semicircular suture lines with pledgets. (According to Antunes and Girdwood [11])

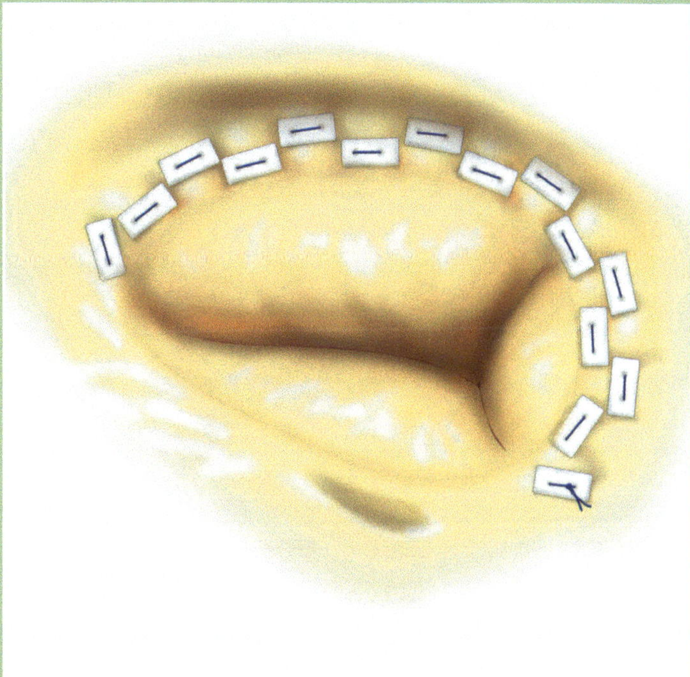

Fig. 7.13 Result of tricuspid valve annuloplasty. Pledgets prevent cutting through of the sutures. (According to Antunes and Girdwood [11])

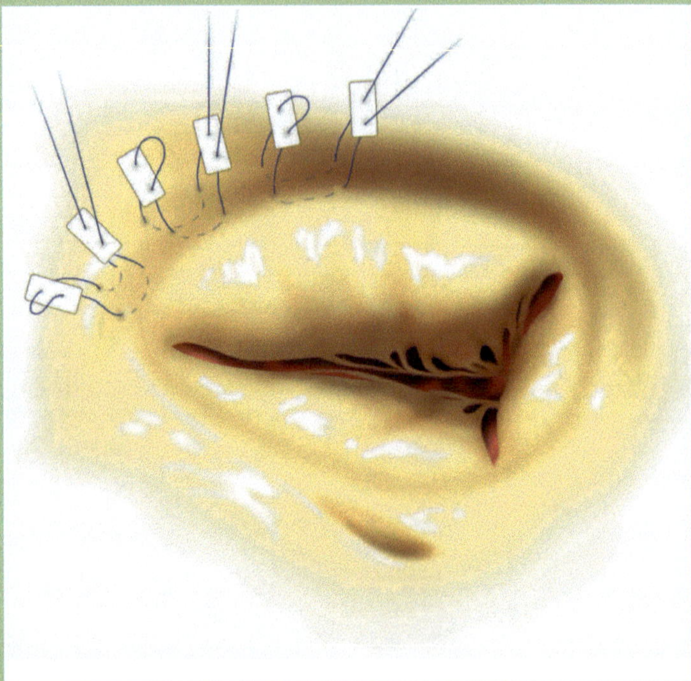

Fig. 7.14 Tricuspid valve annuloplasty. Placement of pledgeted mattress sutures. (According to Revuelta and Garcia-Rinaldi [12])

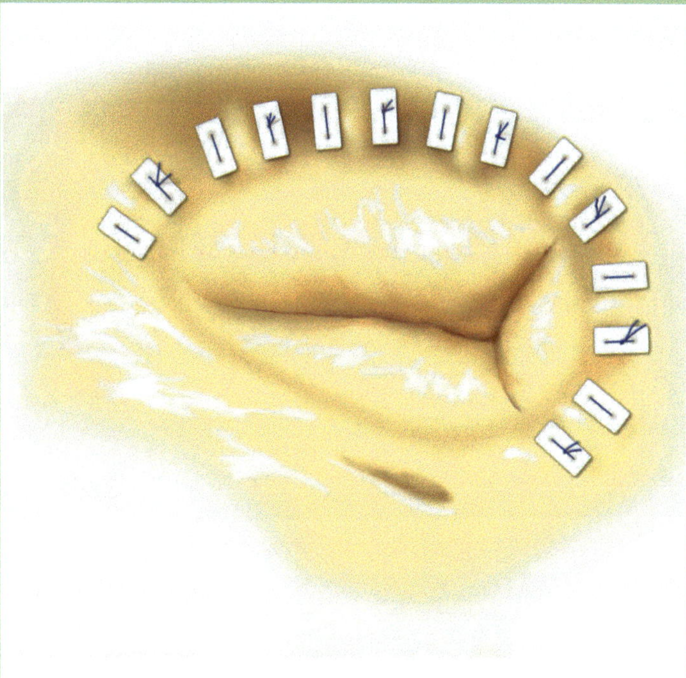

Fig. 7.15 Result of tricuspid annuloplasty. (According to Revuelta and Garcia-Rinaldi [12])

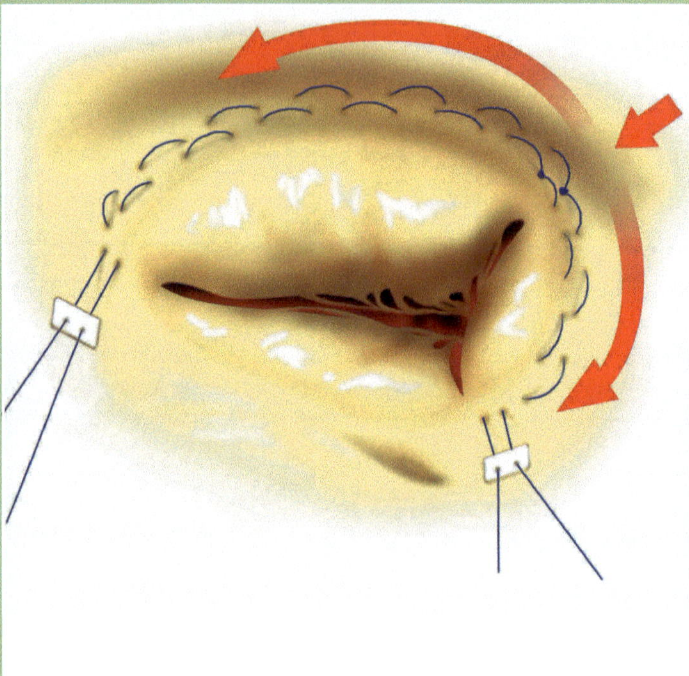

Fig. 7.16 Suture annuloplasty of tricuspid valve. (According to Brugger et al. [13])

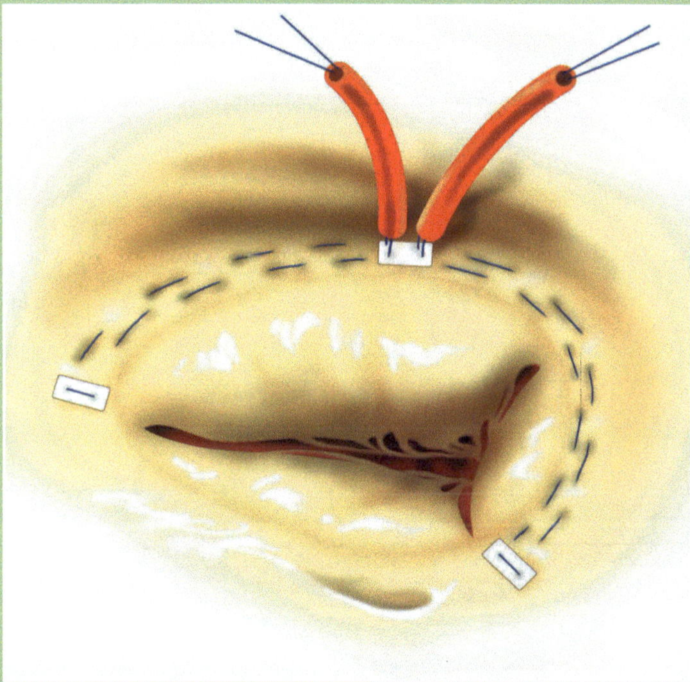

Fig. 7.17 Adjustable segmentary tricuspid annuloplasty. (According to Sarraj and Duarte [14])

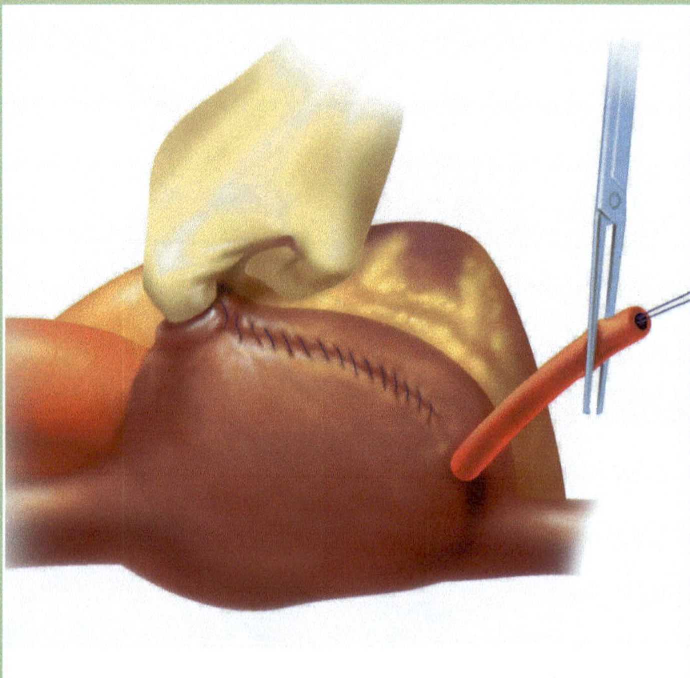

Fig. 7.18 Principle of modification of DeVega tricuspid annuloplasty (tightening of suture repair as much as required for cessation of regurgitation). (According to Kurlansky et al. [16])

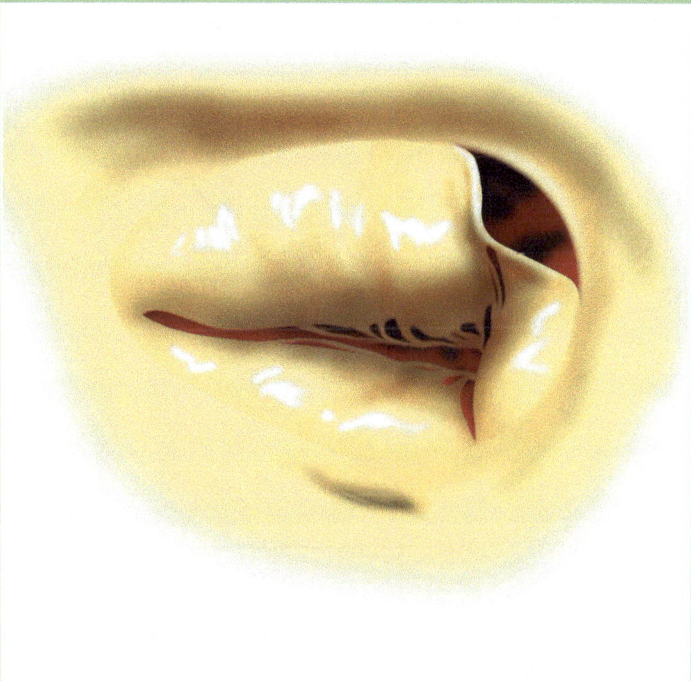

Fig. 7.19 Tricuspid valve repair. Detachment of the valve from annulus in the area between posterior and anterior leaflets. (According to Minale et al. [18])

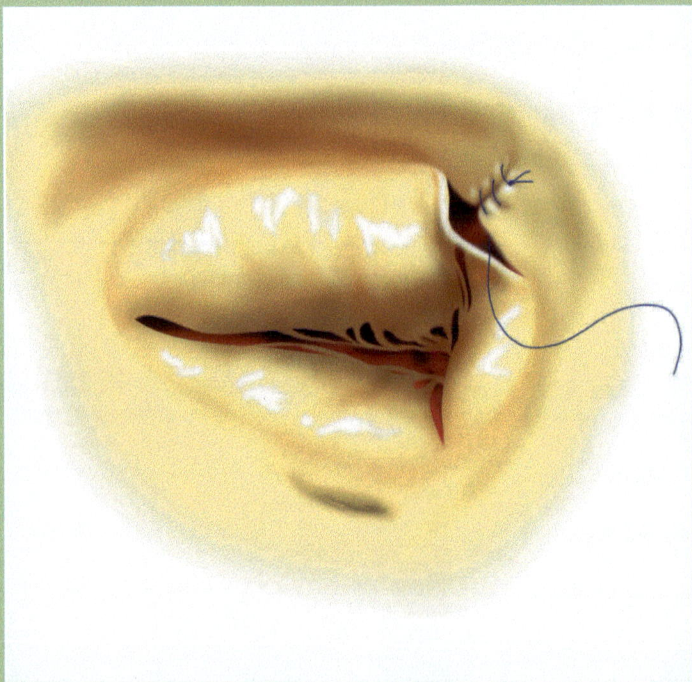

Fig. 7.20 Tricuspid valve repair. Shortening of the annular circumference. (According to Minale et al. [18])

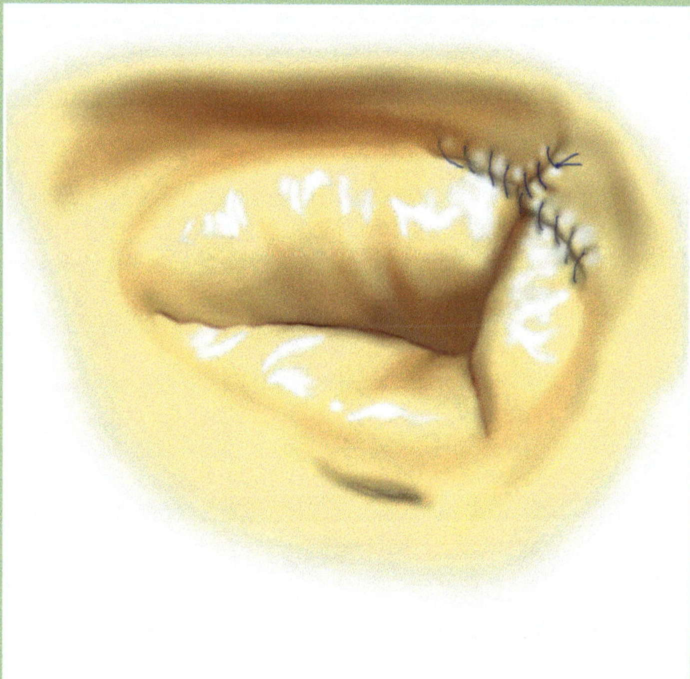

Fig. 7.21 Result of tricuspid valve repair. (According to Minale et al. [18])

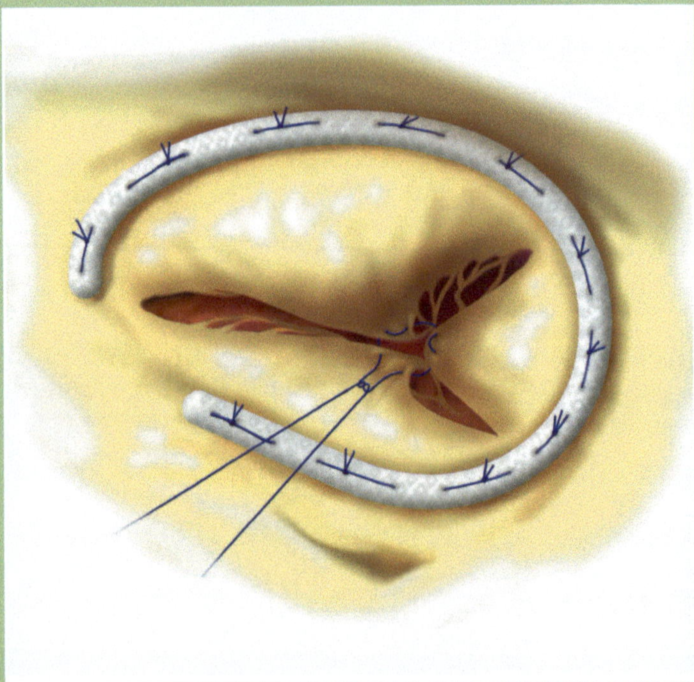

Fig. 7.22 Tricuspid valve repair ("triple orifice," "edge to edge," and "trefoil method"). (According to DeBonis [19])

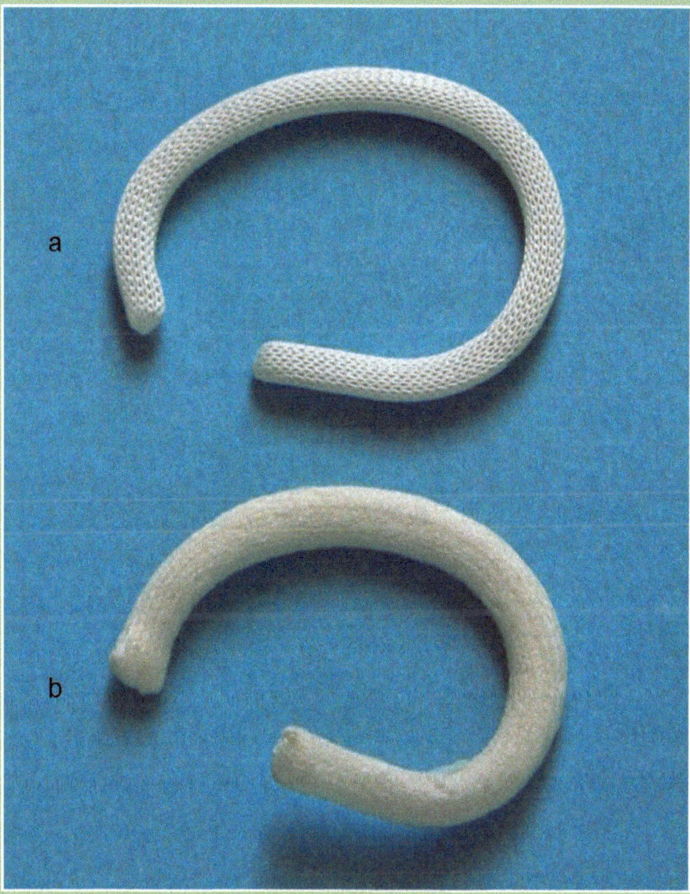

Fig. 7.23 Annuloplasty ring for tricuspid valve repair. **a** Standard Carpentier–Edwards. **b** Edwards MC3

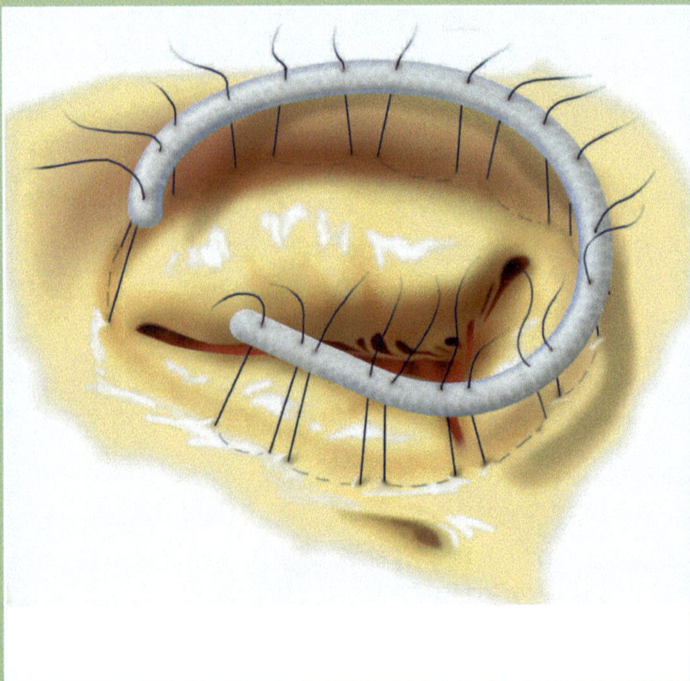

Fig. 7.24 Principle of tricuspid annuloplasty ring implantation for secondary tricuspid regurgitation

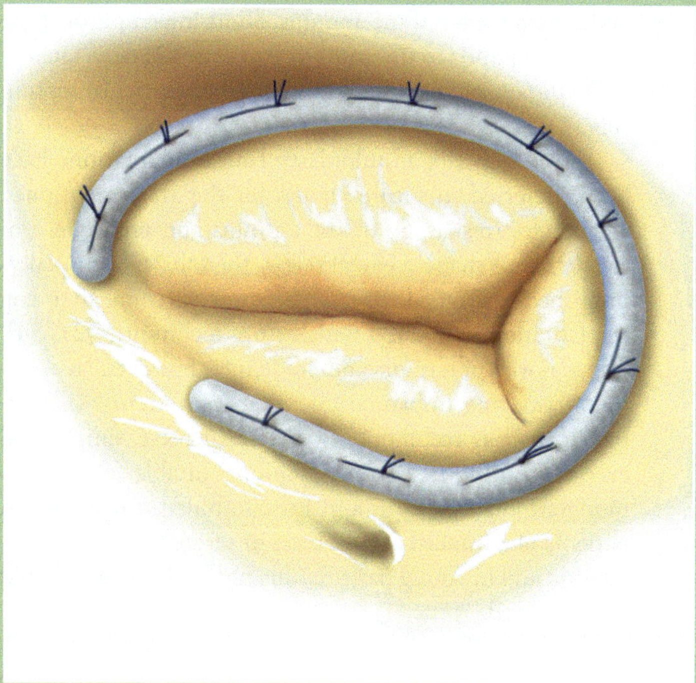

Fig. 7.25 Competent tricuspid valve after implantation of annuloplasty ring

and remodelation of the annulus. Short interruption of the ring corresponds to the anterior septal area in close vicinity of the bundle of His penetration into the ventricular septum (Fig. 7.25).

In recent years annuloplasty ring implantations have been preferred to suture repairs for the abovementioned advantages (reshaping of the annulus and retainment of the achieved shape). Nonetheless, there have been papers published that failed to prove superior outcome after ring implantation compared with suture techniques [21–24]. The majority of authors and guidelines, however, favor annuloplasty ring implantation [25]. Suture repair (in particular the Kay technique) is fast, inexpensive, simple, and even, according to current opinion, suitable for mild to moderate regurgitation and for combined procedures in patients of advanced age. In cases of severe tricuspid regurgitation and in young patients, an annuloplasty ring should be implanted.

Selection of a given type of repair or preference of annuloplasty ring depends on the customary practice of the institution, the surgeon's experience, as well as valve pathology and severity of tricuspid regurgitation. In the present authors' opinion, the decision to implant annuloplasty rings in all patients with secondary tricuspid regurgitation is justifiable and perhaps the correct strategy, although suture repair in mild to moderate regurgitation cannot be considered a fault.

Tricuspid valve repairs are seldom performed as isolated procedures. Most often they are part of the complex treatment of mitro-tricuspid valve disease together with mitral valve replacement or repair. The majority of these patients are indicated too late for mitral valve surgery. Patients with mitral valve disease should be indicated for surgery before development of secondary tricuspid regurgitation [26].

7.3.3.2 Repair for Ebstein's Anomaly

Ebstein's anomaly is characterized by downward displacement of the septal and posterior tricuspid leaflet attachment toward the right ventricular apex. The trabeculized portion of the right ventricle beneath the valve is small and dysfunctional. The atrialized portion of the right ventricle above the valve is thin-walled and belongs to the dilated right atrium (Fig. 7.26) [27]. Hemodynamically the situation is characterized by decreased pulmonary blood flow, tricuspid regurgitation, and in the presence of atrial septal defect (in 50%), by a right-to-left shunt with cyanosis. Clinical symptoms may be striking in infancy or childhood, but often problems present only in adulthood (fatigue, cyanosis, signs of tricuspid regurgitation). Dysrhythmias occur frequently (supraventricular tachycardia, Wolff-Parkinson-White syndrome).

Indications for surgery are worsening of exercise tolerance, progression of cyanosis, congestive right-sided heart failure, and NYHA stages III–IV. Surgery is aimed at improvement of pulmonary blood flow, correction of tricuspid regurgitation, and closure of the right-to-left shunt (if present).

In case the anterior leaflet of the tricuspid valve is sufficiently developed, there exists a good chance for correction by Danielson repair (first performed in 1972) [28, 29] or by Carpentier repair (published in 1988) [30]. The principle of both techniques is based on reduction of the dilated right atrium by plication of the atrialized right ventricular wall, reduction of the tricuspid annulus, and creation of a com-

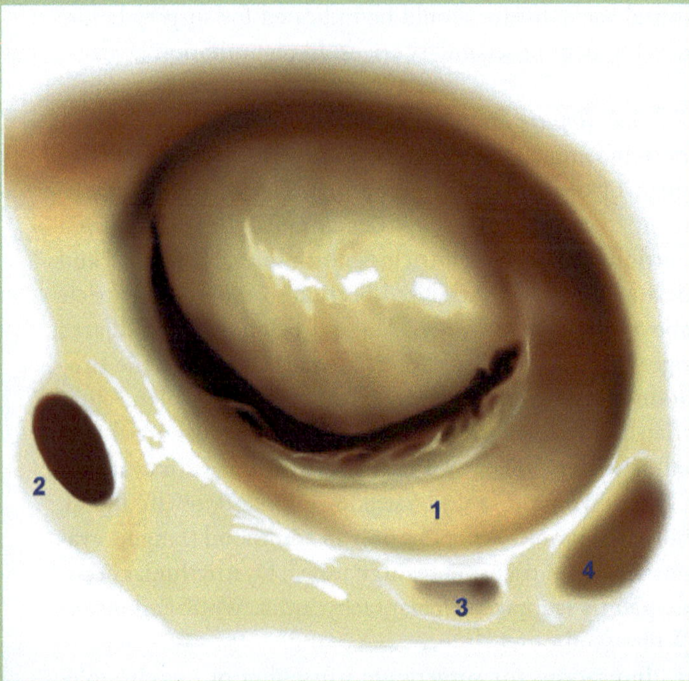

Fig. 7.26 Ebstein's anomaly of the tricuspid valve (type A) with a well-developed mobile anterior leaflet. *1* Atrialized portion of the right ventricle, *2* atrial septal defect, *3* sinus coronarius, *4* inferior vena cava

petent monocuspid orifice from the anterior leaflet. Forms with severe malformation of the anterior leaflet require valve replacement usually with a bioprosthesis. Bidirectional cavopulmonary connection has to be performed sometimes in the most severe cases [31].

With the Danielson technique [28, 29], plication of the atrialized right ventricular wall is achieved by a series of interrupted pledgeted mattress sutures. After the sutures are tied, the atrialized right ventricular wall is obliterated, which results in lowering the dilated right atrial capacity. The annulus in the area of dysplastic posterior leaflet is moved toward the septum by another stitch. This results in reduction of tricuspid annular circumference. The valve itself consists of the anterior tricuspid leaflet only (Figs. 7.27, 7.28).

The Carpentier technique is anterior leaflet rotating plasty [30]. The anterior leaflet is first detached from the tricuspid annulus, and then vertical (perpendicular to the annular plane) plication of the atrialized right ventricular wall is performed in the area of posterior leaflet. The anterior leaflet is reattached with simultaneous clockwise rotatory shift to the area corresponding normally to the posteroseptal leaflet commissure (Figs. 7.29, 7.30). Carpentier finally adds annuloplasty ring implantation. The atrial septal defect is closed with a pericardial patch.

7.3.3.3 Tricuspid Valve Replacement

The decision for tricuspid valve replacement is the ultimate solution in case the valve cannot be repaired. This situation occurs most often for advanced organic changes at rheumatic tricuspid stenosis, in heavily damaged valves due to endocarditis, and in severe forms of Ebstein's anomaly. The problem of selecting the optimal valve for replacement has

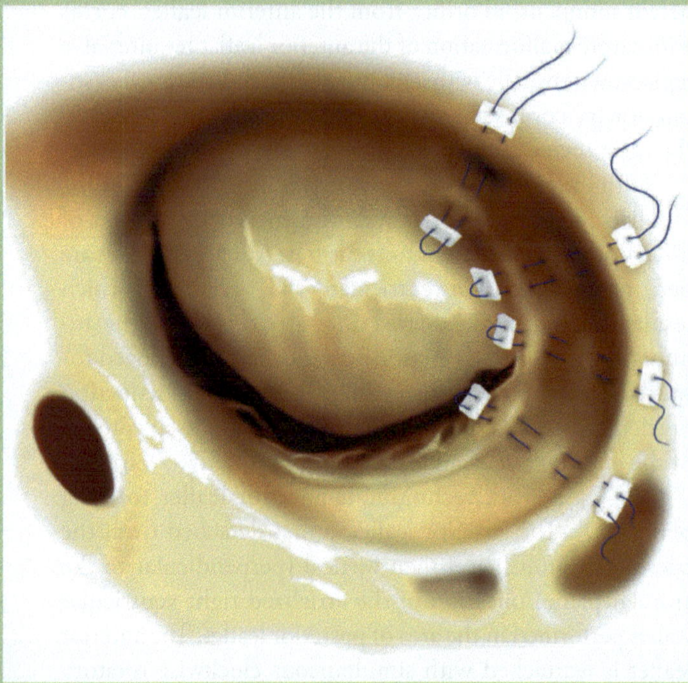

Fig. 7.27 Repair of Ebstein's anomaly. Placement of sutures for obliteration of the atrialized portion of the right ventricle. (According to Danielson et al. [28, 29])

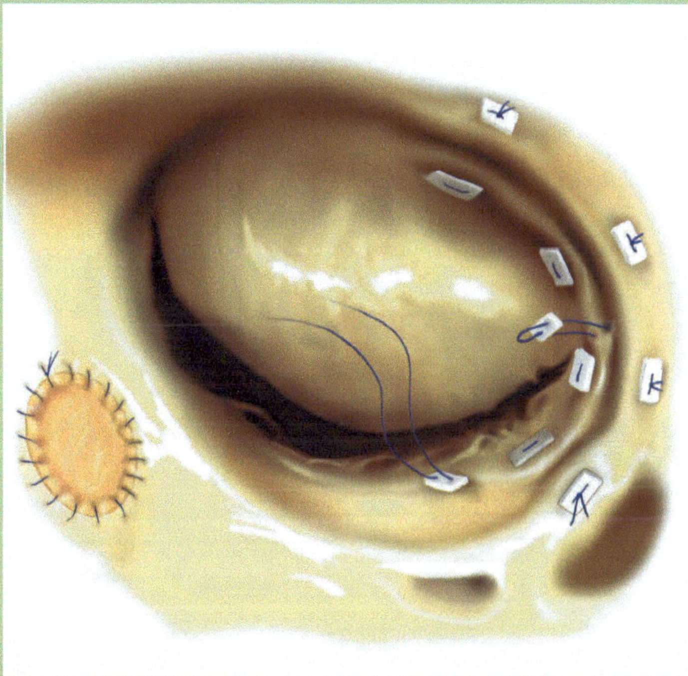

Fig. 7.28 Repair of Ebstein's anomaly. Atrialized portion of the right ventricle is obliterated by tying of the sutures. Closure of the atrial septal defect. Placement of the suture for shortening of the tricuspid annulus in the area of the dysplastic and downward displaced posterior leaflet. After tying of the suture, a functionally monocuspid valve will be created. (According to Danielson et al. [28, 29])

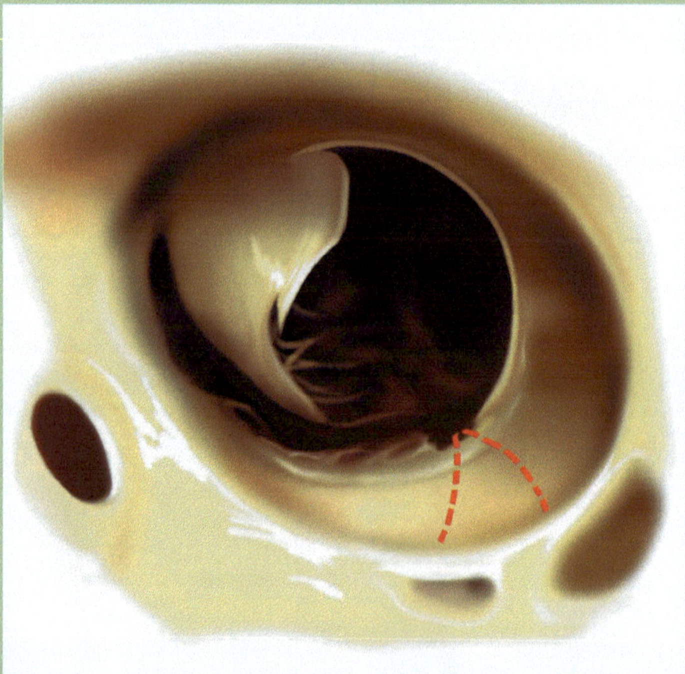

Fig. 7.29 Repair of Ebstein's anomaly. Detachment of most of the anterior leaflet from the annulus. Marked in *red* is the zone of plication (perpendicular to annulus in the area of dysplastic posterior leaflet). (According to Carpentier et al. [30])

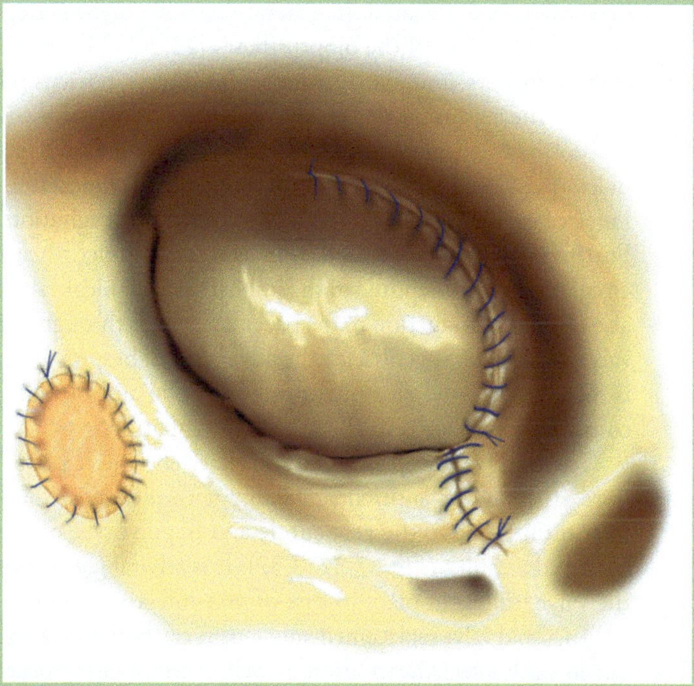

Fig. 7.30 Repair of Ebstein's anomaly. Rotatory plasty of the anterior leaflet (which results in a monocuspid valve). Vertical plication of the atrialized right ventricle. Closure of the atrial septal defect. (According to Carpentier et al. [30])

been extensively debated. In general, there is a slight preference implantation of the bioprostheses [23, 32–35]. In the present authors' unit, we implant bioprostheses in tricuspid orifice. The reason for this strategy is the very slow course of bioprosthesis degeneration thanks to lesser mechanical stress in low-pressure right-heart circulation and good clinical tolerance of eventually developed mild tricuspid regurgitation. Furthermore, mechanical valves in low-pressure right-heart circulation are susceptible to thrombosis. Mechanical valves also disable introduction of the pacemaker leads through the valve into the right ventricle. The advantage of bioprosthesis is, of course, avoidance of thromboembolic and bleeding complications related to chronic anticoagulation.

Tricuspid valve replacement is a relatively simple procedure. The valve is sutured preferably with pledgeted mattress sutures due to the very subtle and fragile tissue of the tricuspid annulus (Figs. 7.31, 7.32). It is advisable to leave the valve leaflets in place in case of non-infective lesion.

Tricuspid valve replacement and repairs can both be carried out in cardioplegic heart arrest as well as on a beating heart after release of aortic cross-clamping. Choice of the strategy is influenced by the surgeon's customary practice, accessibility of the tricuspid valve, and overall length of aortic cross-clamping. A compromise procedure can also be chosen, i.e., placement of the principal and most difficult stitches during asystole and then, after aortic declamping, accomplishment of the rest of the valve implantation on an already beating heart.

7.3.3.4 Tricuspid Valve Excision

In certain circumstances the tricuspid valve can be excised and left unreplaced. This option has been known since 1981, when Arbulu et al. reported on 55 intravenous heroin

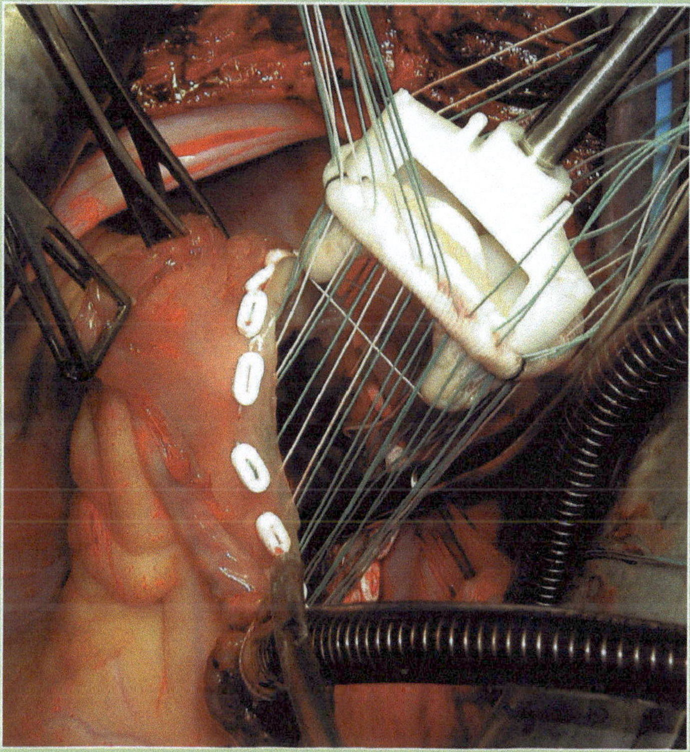

Fig. 7.31 Tricuspid valve replacement by a bioprosthesis. Pledgeted mattress sutures are placed in the tricuspid annulus and the sewing ring of the bioprosthesis

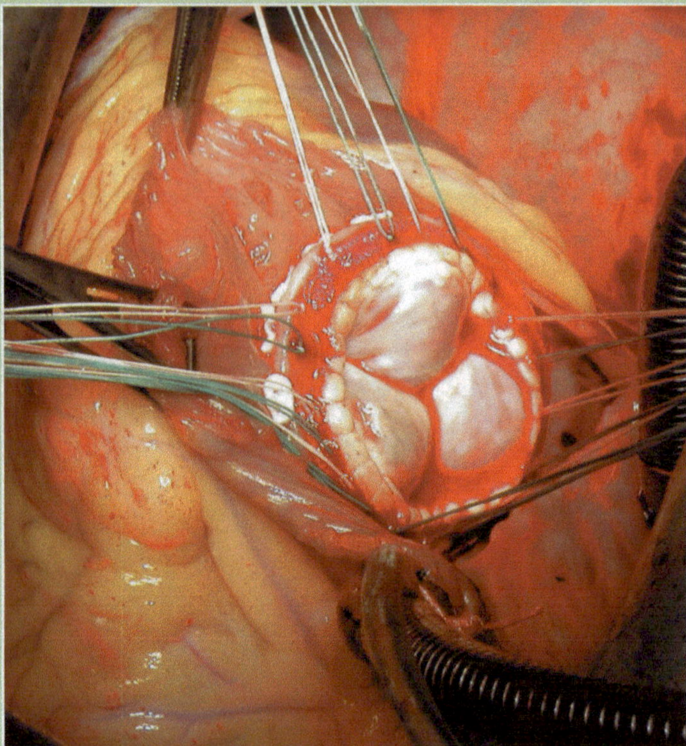

Fig. 7.32 Bioprosthesis St. Jude Medical Epic implanted into the tricuspid orifice

addicts operated for endocarditis in whom the tricuspid valve was excised without replacement [36, 37]. Only 6 of them required prosthetic valve insertion from 2 days to 13 years after excision of the valve. A prerequisite for this procedure is low or normal pulmonary pressure, i.e., the absence of pulmonary hypertension. Postoperatively, an intensive volumotherapy is mandatory to maintain elevated right atrial pressure (systole >25 mmHg). The rationale for this rather dubious strategy lies in the fear of prosthetic endocarditis, which is very likely in patients who continue intravenous drug abuse. The authors have never chosen this method of treatment. Perhaps it might be considered in those addicts whose personal posture and history are unequivocally predictive of continuing the intravenous drug abuse. Another cause might be excessive infective annular destruction, in which fear of sewing-ring infection would justify choice of this procedure with the possibility to replace the valve later, after curing the infection.

References

1. Vahanian A, Baumgartner H, Bax J et al. (2007) Guidelines on the management of valvular heart disease: The Task Force on the Management of Valvular Heart Disease of the European Society of Cardiology. Eur Heart J 28:230–268
2. Shiran A, Sagie A (2009) Tricuspid regurgitation in mitral valve disease incidence, prognostic implications, mechanism, and management. J Am Coll Cardiol 53:401–408
3. Wechsler AS (2009) Mitral valve surgery for functional mitral regurgitation: Should moderate to severe tricuspid regurgitation be treated? A propensity score analysis. J Thorac Cardiovasc Surg 137:267–268

4. Dreyfus GD, Corbi PJ, Chan KM et al (2005) Secondary tricuspid regurgitation or dilatation: which should be the criteria for surgical repair? Ann Thorac Surg 79:127–32
5. Carpentier A, Deloche A, Hanania G et al. (1974) Surgical management of acquired tricuspid valve disease. J Thorac Cardiovasc Surg 67:53–65
6. Kay JH, Maselli-Campagna G, Tsuji KK (1965) Surgical treatment of tricuspid insufficiency. Ann Surg 162:53–58
7. Reed GE, Cortes LE (1976) Measured tricuspid annuloplasty: a rapid and reproducible technique. Ann Thorac Surg 21:168–169
8. Nakano S, Kawashima Y, Hirose H et al. (1984) An effective adjunct to tricuspid annuloplasty. Ann Thorac Surg 38:68–69
9. Nakano S, Kawashima Y, Hirose H et al. (1988) Evaluation of long-term results of bicuspidalization annuloplasty for functional tricuspid regurgitation. A seventeen-year experience with 133 consecutive patients. J Thorac Cardiovasc Surg 95:340–345
10. Vega NG de (1972) Selective, adjustable and permanent annuloplasty. An original technique for the treatment of tricuspid insufficiency. Rev Esp Cardiol 25:555–556 [in Spanish]
11. Antunes MJ, Girdwood RW (1983) Tricuspid annuloplasty: a modified technique. Ann Thorac Surg 35:676–678
12. Revuelta JM, Garcia-Rinaldi R (1989) Segmental tricuspid annuloplasty: a new technique. J Thorac Cardiovasc Surg 97:799–801
13. Brugger JJ, Egloff L, Rothlin M et al. (1982) Tricuspid annuloplasty. Results and complications. Thorac Cardiovasc Surg 30:284–287
14. Sarraj A, Duarte J (2007) Adjustable segmental tricuspid annuloplasty: a new modified technique. Ann Thorac Surg 83:698–699
15. Sarraj A, Nuche JM, Dominguez L et al. (2009) Adjustable segmental tricuspid annuloplasty: technical advantages and midterm results. Ann Thorac Surg 87:1148–1153
16. Kurlansky P, Rose EA, Malm JR (1987) Adjustable annuloplasty for tricuspid insufficiency. Ann Thorac Surg 44:404–406
17. Cook JW (1994) Accurate adjustment of de Vega tricuspid annuloplasty using transesophageal echocardiography. Ann Thorac Surg 58:570–572

18. Minale C, Lambertz H, Nikol S et al. (1987) New developments for reconstruction of the tricuspid valve. Helv Chir Acta 54:295–301
19. Bonis M de, Lapenna E, La Canna G et al. (2004) A novel technique for correction of severe tricuspid valve regurgitation due to complex lesions. Eur J Cardiothorac Surg 25:760–765
20. Lai YQ, Meng X, Bai T et al. (2006) Edge-to-edge tricuspid valve repair: an adjuvant technique for residual tricuspid regurgitation. Ann Thorac Surg 81:2179–2182
21. Bernal JM, Gutierrez-Morlote J, Llorca J et al. (2004) Tricuspid valve repair: an old disease, a modern experience. Ann Thorac Surg 78:2069–2075
22. Ghanta RK, Chen R, Narayanasamy N et al. (2007) Suture bicuspidization of the tricuspid valve versus ring annuloplasty for repair of functional tricuspid regurgitation: midterm results of 237 consecutive patients. J Thorac Cardiovasc Surg 133:117–126
23. Guenther T, Noebauer C, Mazzitelli D et al. (2008) Tricuspid valve surgery: a thirty-year assessment of early and late outcome. Eur J Cardiothorac Surg 34:402–409
24. Peterffy A, Szentkiralyi I, Galajda Z (2007) Tricuspid valve repair: indication and type of repair. J Thorac Cardiovasc Surg 134:266–267
25. Tang GH, David TE, Singh SK et al. (2006) Tricuspid valve repair with an annuloplasty ring results in improved long-term outcomes. Circulation 114:I577–I581
26. Filsoufi F, Anyanwu AC, Salzberg SP et al. (2005) Long-term outcomes of tricuspid valve replacement in the current era. Ann Thorac Surg 80:845–850
27. Frescura C, Angelini A, Daliento L et al. (2000) Morphological aspects of Ebstein's anomaly in adults. Thorac Cardiovasc Surg 48:203–208
28. Danielson GK, Maloney JD, Devloo RA (1979) Surgical repair of Ebstein's anomaly. Mayo Clin Proc 54:185–192
29. Danielson GK, Driscoll DJ, Mair DD et al. (1992) Operative treatment of Ebstein's anomaly. J Thorac Cardiovasc Surg 104:1195–1202

30. Carpentier A, Chauvaud S, Mace L et al. (1988) A new reconstructive operation for Ebstein's anomaly of the tricuspid valve. J Thorac Cardiovasc Surg 96:92–101
31. Chauvaud S, Berrebi A, d'Attellis N et al. (2003) Ebstein's anomaly: repair based on functional analysis. Eur J Cardiothorac Surg 23:525–531
32. Kawano H, Oda T, Fukunaga S et al. (2000) Tricuspid valve replacement with the St. Jude Medical valve: 19 years of experience. Eur J Cardiothorac Surg 18:565–569
33. Kunadian B, Vijayalakshmi K, Balasubramanian S et al. (2007) Should the tricuspid valve be replaced with a mechanical or biological valve? Interact Cardiovasc Thorac Surg 6:551–557
34. Peterffy A, Szentkiralyi I (2001) Mechanical valves in tricuspid position: cause of thrombosis and prevention. Eur J Cardiothorac Surg 19:735–736
35. Rizzoli G, Vendramin I, Nesseris G et al. (2004) Biological or mechanical prostheses in tricuspid position? A meta-analysis of intra-institutional results. Ann Thorac Surg 77:1607–1614
36. Arbulu A, Asfaw I (1981) Tricuspid valvulectomy without prosthetic replacement. Ten years of clinical experience. J Thorac Cardiovasc Surg 82:684–691
37. Arbulu A, Holmes RJ, Asfaw I (1991) Tricuspid valvulectomy without replacement. Twenty years' experience. J Thorac Cardiovasc Surg 102:917–922

Pulmonary Valve Surgery

8 Pulmonary Valve Surgery

Surgery for isolated pulmonary stenosis or pulmonary regurgitation is extremely rare in adulthood. Etiology of the isolated pulmonary stenosis is almost always congenital. Hemodynamically severe pulmonary stenosis is in most cases resolved in childhood by a percutaneous balloon valvuloplasty. Surgery is indicated in children with dysplastic pulmonary valve or infundibular stenosis. Other reasons of pulmonary stenosis (acquired) are mentioned in the literature (e.g., carcinoid or rheumatic etiology, obstruction by a vegetation), but incidence is very seldom and indication for surgery results extremely rarely.

Congenital pulmonary stenosis may be diagnosed even in adulthood as either a valve disease not yet treated or a valve stenosis after inadequate percutaneous or surgical treatment. Adult patients with pulmonary stenosis are indicated for percutaneous balloon valvuloplasty if their peak gradient exceeds 50 mmHg, even when they are asymptomatic. Young patients, athletes, and women before planned pregnancy are indicated at the gradient of 40 mmHg, as is anyone who has become symptomatic (dyspnea, angina, presyncope, and syncope). If percutaneous intervention is not amenable, surgical treatment is required. At operation, the valve usually cannot be salvaged and valve replacement is performed, optimally with allograft or bioprosthesis that displays low rate of degeneration in the low-pressure right-sided circulation. Use of mechanical valve is also an option, which almost guarantees freedom from reoperation but necessitates lifelong anticoagulation with all related risks.

Pulmonary regurgitation in adulthood usually has also congenital etiology. It may be either pulmonary regurgi-

J. Dominik and P. Zacek, *Heart Valve Surgery: An Illustrated Guide*,
DOI 10.1007/978-3-642-12206-4_8,

tation resulting from balloon or surgical valvulotomy of a congenital, isolated pulmonary stenosis, or more often regurgitation after radical correction of tetralogy of Fallot where a narrow right-ventricular outflow tract, pulmonary annulus, and pulmonary trunk were enlarged with an oval-shaped patch [1]. Pulmonary regurgitation is well tolerated in the beginning, but a severe regurgitation within several decades leads to right ventricular dilation and dysfunction together with development of tricuspid regurgitation. Surgery is indicated in such cases and should not be delayed to prevent right ventricular failure due to irreversible right ventricular dysfunction. Usually, for pulmonary valve replacement, an allograft or bioprosthesis is used. In case the pulmonary annulus and pulmonary trunk are narrow, they can be enlarged with use of allograft tissue, or a fabric patch should it be decided to implant the bioprosthesis (Fig. 8.1); however, the use of mechanical valves might be considered, especially in patients who have had multiple prior operations and require anticoagulation treatment for additional mechanical valve or rhythm disturbances. This idea is supported by a study that reports very good long-term results with mechanical prostheses [2].

Pulmonary regurgitation that developed due to dilation of the annulus and pulmonary trunk is usually hemodynamically less significant and is managed by operation on the left heart valves, which will alleviate pulmonary hypertension.

A recently available option is catheterization implantation of a stent with tissue valve into pulmonary position ("valve into valve"). This method will probably prove to be efficient not only in patients with pulmonary regurgitation after correction of tetralogy of Fallot, but also in patients with pulmonary allograft failure after Ross procedure.

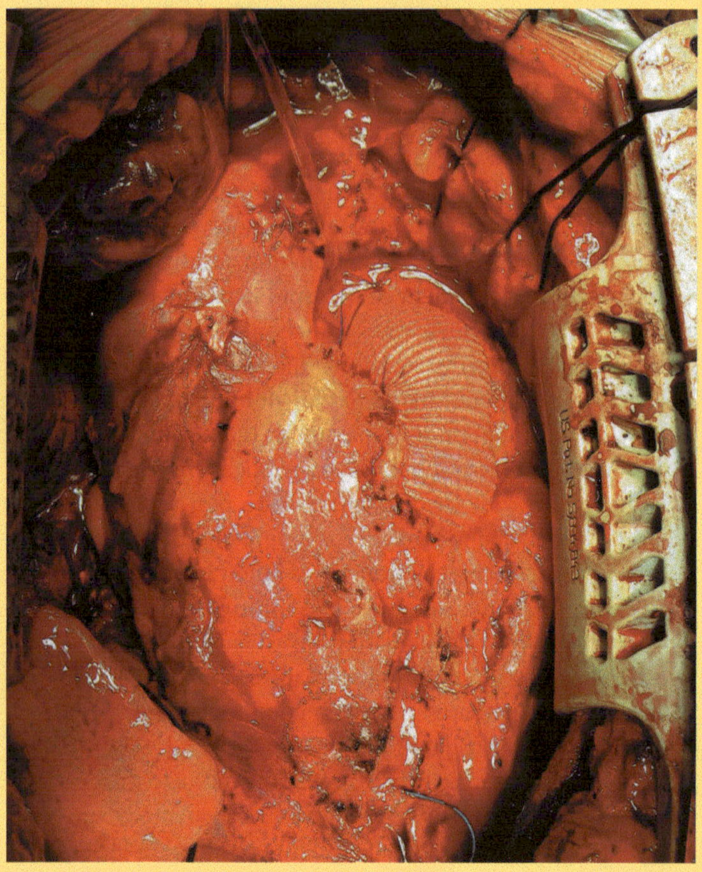

Fig. 8.1 Reoperation 33 years after radical correction of tetralogy of Fallot. Incompetent pulmonary valve was replaced by a bioprosthesis, and the right ventricular outflow tract and the pulmonary artery trunk were enlarged by a vascular graft

References

1. Hickey EJ, Veldtman G, Bradley TJ et al. (2009) Late risk of outcomes for adults with repaired tetralogy of Fallot from an inception cohort spanning four decades. Eur J Cardiothorac Surg 35:156–164
2. Waterbolk TW, Hoendermis ES, den Hamer IJ et al. (2006) Pulmonary valve replacement with a mechanical prosthesis. Promising results of 28 procedures in patients with congenital heart disease. Eur J Cardiothorac Surg 30:28–32

Dysfunction of Implanted Heart Valves

9 Dysfunction of Implanted Heart Valves

9.1 Introduction

After valve replacement, patients are never healed completely. Cardiac operation restores their hemodynamics and improves, both subjectively and objectively, their functional status. The patients, however, become the carriers of a valve prosthesis, and as such they are exposed to a lifelong risk of postoperative complications caused by potential valve dysfunctions. Anticoagulation therapy, which is inevitable in all patients after implantation of mechanical prostheses, is associated with bleeding complications (resulting mostly from overdose) as well as thromboembolic events (due to ineffective anticoagulation).

If the implanted cardiac valve does not work well for whatever reason, the clinical situation is termed dysfunction (malfunction) of the implanted valve. Dysfunctions include mechanical dysfunctions of the implanted valve due to defects and wear of material or failure of valve mechanism. These are true mechanical dysfunctions, so-called structural dysfunctions, caused by intrinsic factors. Valve malfunction can also be caused by external factors that interfere with the free motion of the occluder. This results usually from valve thrombosis, tissue overgrowth (pannus), interference of disc-tilting motion with myocardium, sutures, chordae, vegetations, etc.

Paraprosthetic leak, a situation when part of the valve ring remains disconnected from the recipient's annulus, can also be counted among valve dysfunctions. The valve itself

J. Dominik and P. Zacek, *Heart Valve Surgery: An Illustrated Guide*,
DOI 10.1007/978-3-642-12206-4_9,

works properly, but the leak causes regurgitation of variable severity, which sometimes requires reoperation. Paravalvular leak and some structural mechanical dysfunctions may cause significant hemolysis. Infective endocarditis located on an implanted valve (i.e., prosthetic endocarditis) used to also be included in valve dysfunctions and in most instances necessitates explantation of the infected prosthesis and re-implantation of a new valve.

All of the aforementioned dysfunctions of implanted valves are mostly life-threatening complications that may occur both in early- and long-term postoperative course. They usually require difficult reoperation (Fig. 9.1).

Incidence of any of the potential valve-related complications (including thromboembolic and bleeding events) ranges between 2 and 4% per patient-year. Risk of death ("prosthesis-related" mortality) is about 1% per year of life with prosthesis. The majority of these complications can be avoided by correct indications for surgery, choice of the optimal valve for replacement, proper surgical fixation of the valve, meticulous anticoagulation therapy management, and strict prevention of infective endocarditis.

9.2 Structural Dysfunction of Implanted Heart Valves

Structural dysfunction of the implanted mechanical valves is defined as valve failure resulting from unfavorable changes of the valve material. These events occurred formerly after implantation of "historic" valves (Figs. 9.2, 9.3) [1–7]. In most cases the reason was material defect, unsuitable material properties, or a construction defect in the valve mechanism. All currently used mechanical valves, however,

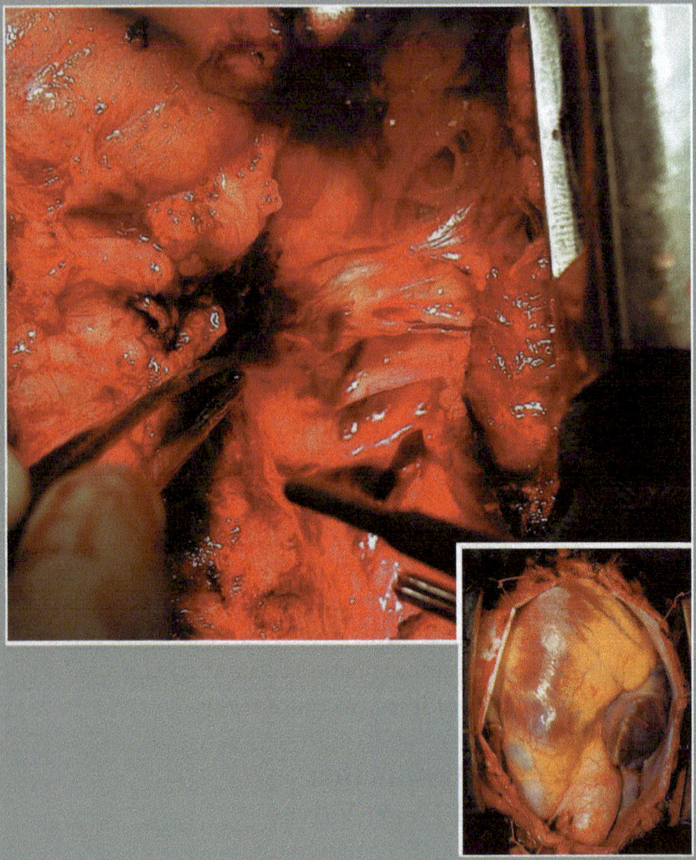

Fig. 9.1 Adhesions encountered in the anterior mediastinum at reoperation. *Inset* shows the situation at initial operation

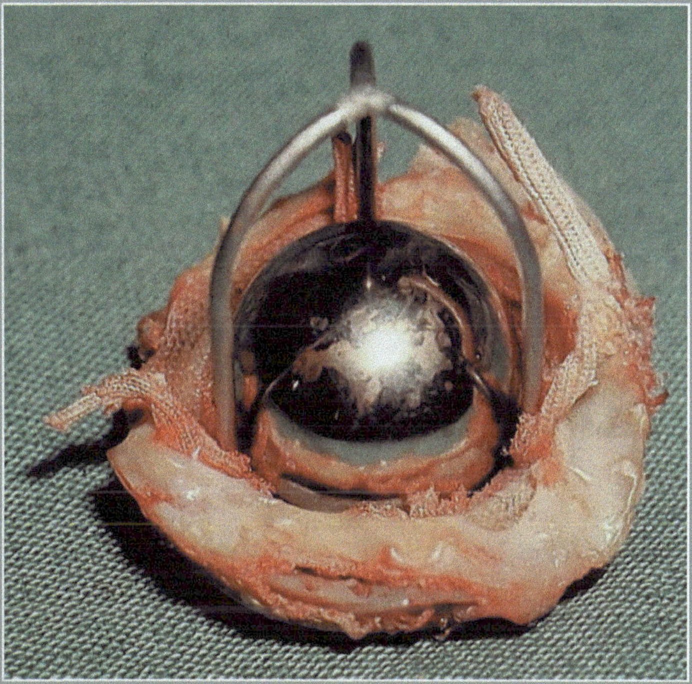

Fig. 9.2 Cloth-covered caged-ball valve Starr–Edwards (model 2320) explanted due to structural dysfunction 22 years after implantation

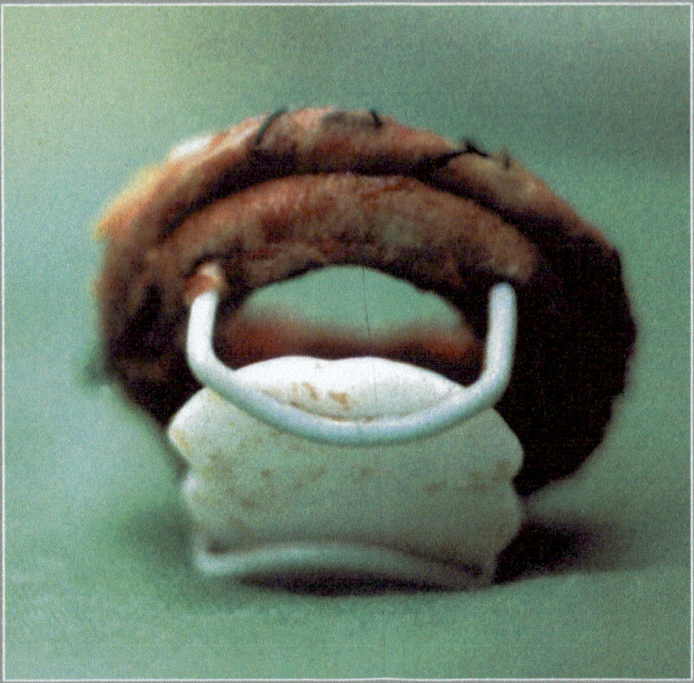

Fig. 9.3 Disc valve Beall explanted due to structural dysfunction 16 years after implantation. Uneven wearing of the disc

work without structural deterioration and their durability is unlimited (valve lasts for the rest of the patient's life).

Many mechanical heart valves have been replaced over the years by newly developed types, regardless of any structural dysfunction but as a result of improved construction, better hemodynamics, or superior materials. Some types, however, were withdrawn from production and the market due to higher incidence of structural deterioration.

The most serious structural dysfunction was the escape of the occluder (disc) from the valve housing. Acute aortic or mitral regurgitation was a lethal condition unless an urgent reoperation was performed immediately. This sudden and catastrophic structural failure of mechanical valves was reported with several types of disc valves (monodiscs and bileaflet valves) as an extremely rare and strange occurrence. In the 1980s, however, a higher incidence of disc escapes due to strut fracture was noticed with popular and widely implanted convex–concave Björk–Shiley valves after 2–3 years of proper postoperative function. The reason was imperfect weld between the valve housing and ring [8–10]. Currently all valves have their housing manufactured from a single block of metal (or plastic). New valve models are subjected to long-term testing in pulsators at high frequency and overload in order to detect the hidden material defects. All types of currently used mechanical valves should have lifelong durability without development of serious structural changes.

On the other hand, structural deterioration is encountered even with modern bioprostheses. Structural failure of bioprostheses is caused mainly by the development of degenerative changes in the leaflets of biological valves. Calcification is the most frequent and serious feature (Fig. 9.4).

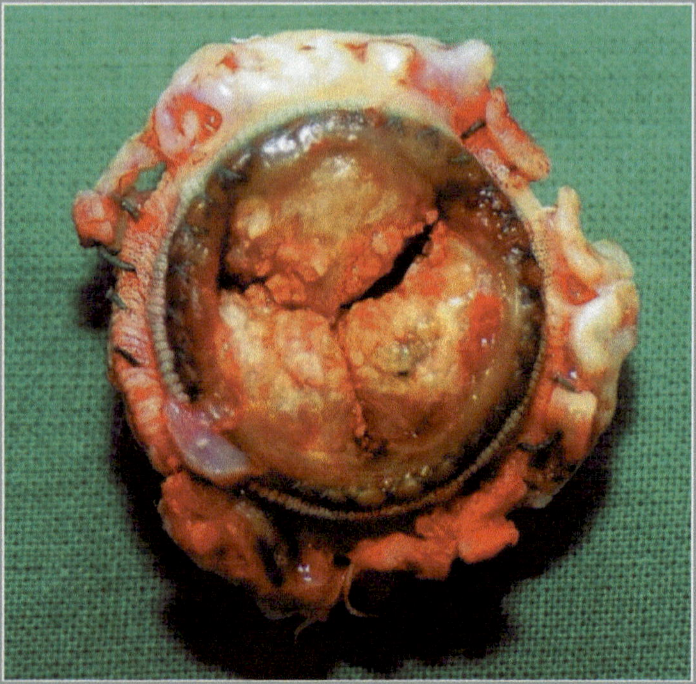

Fig. 9.4 Structural failure of bioprosthesis. The leaflets are stiff and diffusely calcified (8 years after implantation)

Leaflet tears and perforations also occur often, and occasionally a whole leaflet tears off the sewing ring (Fig. 9.5). Structural failure of bioprosthesis that requires reoperation appears usually several years after valve implantation. The rate of degeneration depends predominantly on the patient's age and valve stress load (see Chap. 4).

New modifications of bioprostheses are under constant development as well as the procedures focused on blocking the onset of degenerative changes and calcifications in the valve leaflets (e.g., detoxification, antimineralization, anticalcification, and antidegeneration treatments).

Indications for reoperation for tissue-valve failure are based on hemodynamic parameters and the patient's clinical status, and do not differ from indications for primary valve replacement. Operative risk of a planned reoperation is generally higher for 2–3% of cases than the risk of initial operation. Nevertheless, reoperation for tissue-valve failure is usually required in a patient of advanced age and with many concomitant diseases, which makes the actual risk of reoperation much higher than the risk of initial operation.

9.3 Thrombosis of Implanted Heart Valves

Thrombosis of implanted heart valve is a rare but lethal complication unless prompt and correct diagnosis is established and treatment undertaken. Its incidence with currently used mechanical valves is reported to be 0.2–0.5% per patient-year with the implanted valve. History of inadequate anticoagulation therapy has been documented in about 70% of patients with mechanical valve thrombosis, with the greatest risk resulting from international normalized ratio (INR) value fluctuation.

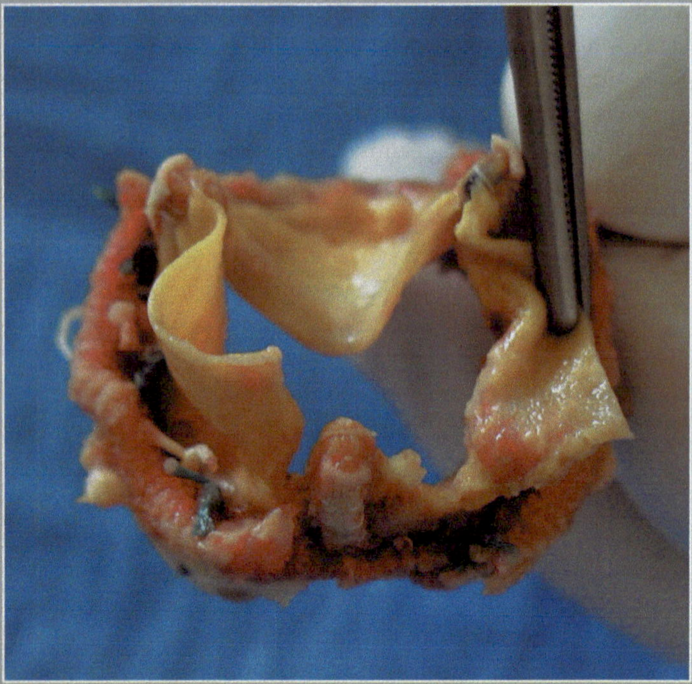

Fig. 9.5 Pericardial bioprosthesis Ionescu–Shiley explanted due to structural dysfunction 22 years after implantation. Tearing of the leaflets at a commissure

Thrombus formation restricts the disc opening or closure, or leads to complete disc immobilization (Figs. 9.6–9.9). Obstruction of the valve orifice is the dominant feature, but regurgitation also may be present. Similar clinical condition may result from pannus formation, a tissue overgrowing the valve ring [11–14]. In some cases, the thrombus is superimposed on pannus and thereby accelerates the acute clinical symptomatology (Figs. 9.10–9.13).

Diagnosis can be established based on the patient's history, auscultatory findings, diagnostic imaging, and coagulation tests. At auscultation, absence or decrease in intensity of the opening and closing click is a pathognostic sign. With some types of disc valves, the patient may witness the cessation of the "valve beat." Cinefluoroscopy can confirm the diagnosis of incomplete closure or opening of the poppet, or sometimes the poppet blockade. Transthoracic and, preferentially, transesophageal echocardiography is also diagnostic, providing information on the transvalvular gradient based on obstructing tissue echogeneity, and also discrimination between thrombus and pannus (not feasible in every case) [11, 14].

Treatment has to be started promptly after diagnosis is established. There is no consensus as to which treatment strategy is superior. The options are either surgically demanding reoperation with cardiopulmonary bypass or thrombolysis with unpredictable efficacy and indispensable risks, or, rarely, effective administration of anticoagulation therapy only.

The mortality rate for acute reoperation in hemodynamically stable patients [New York Heart Association (NYHA) stages I–III] without serious comorbidities is below 10% but varies widely (15–46%) in patients in NYHA stage IV

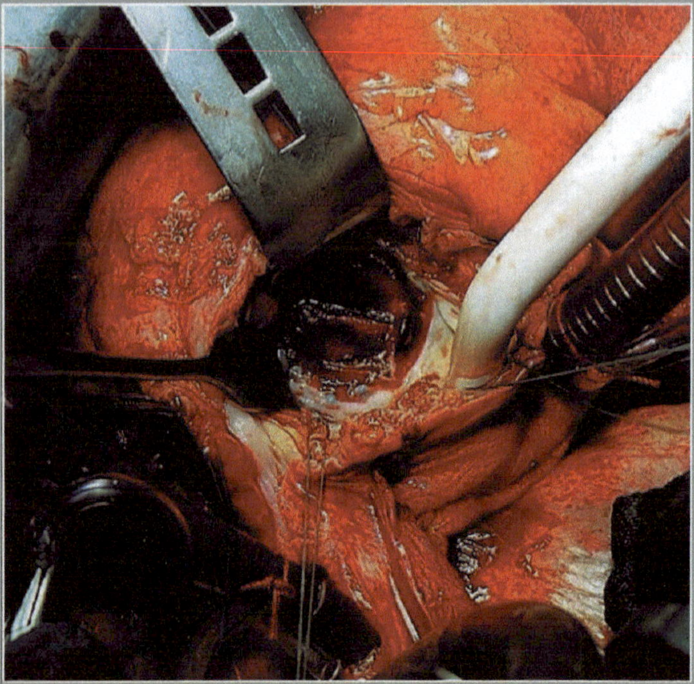

Fig. 9.6 Acute thrombosis of bileaflet mitral valve St. Jude Medical

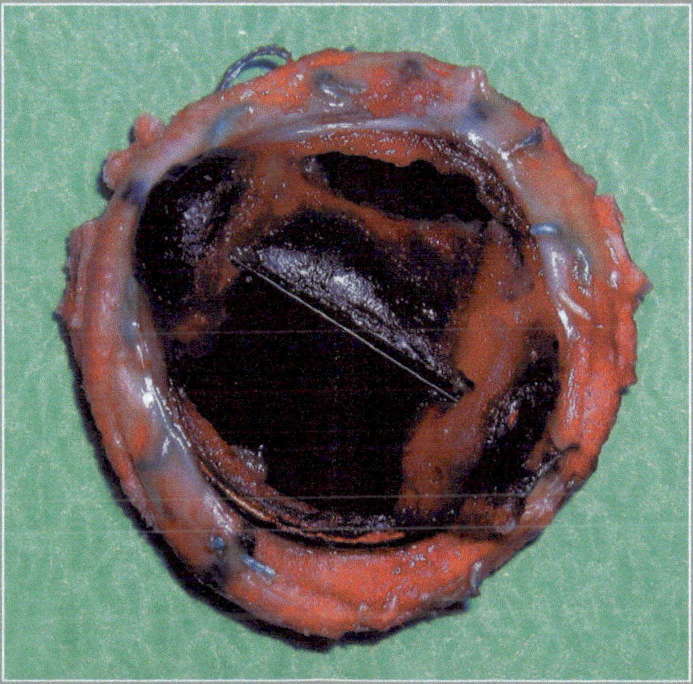

Fig. 9.7 Explanted bileaflet mitral valve (viewed from the left atrium). Thrombosis has caused immobilization of both leaflets

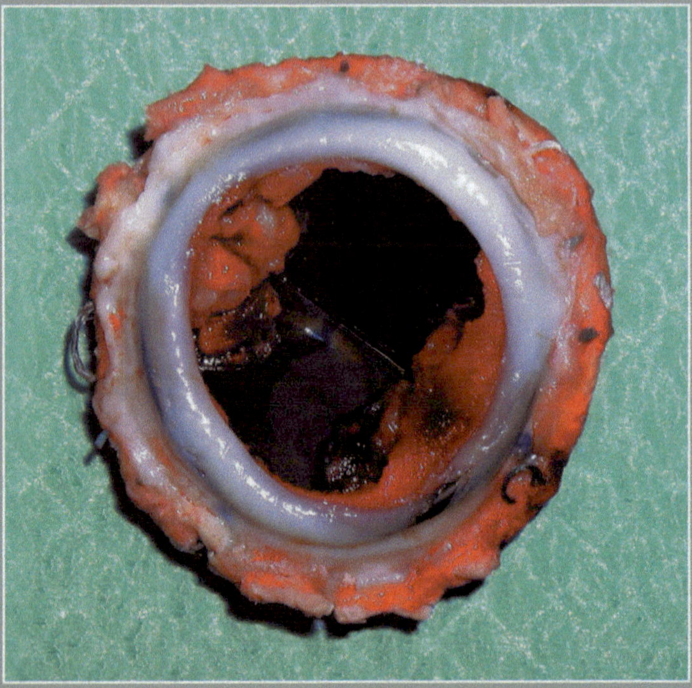

Fig. 9.8 Explanted bileaflet mitral valve (viewed from the left ventricle). Thrombi of various age together with originating circular pannus restrict tilting of the semilunar discs

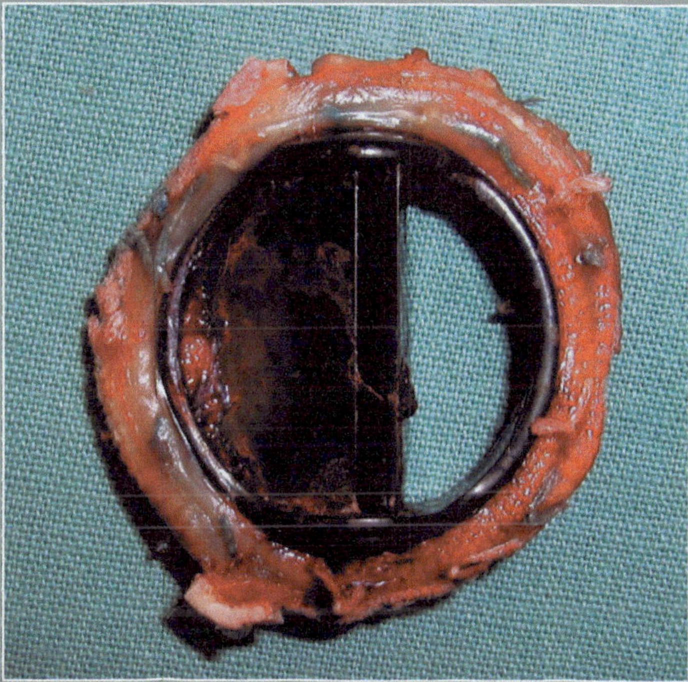

Fig. 9.9 Mitral valve St. Jude Medical explanted due to thrombosis. Thrombolysis was successful in mobilization of only one leaflet

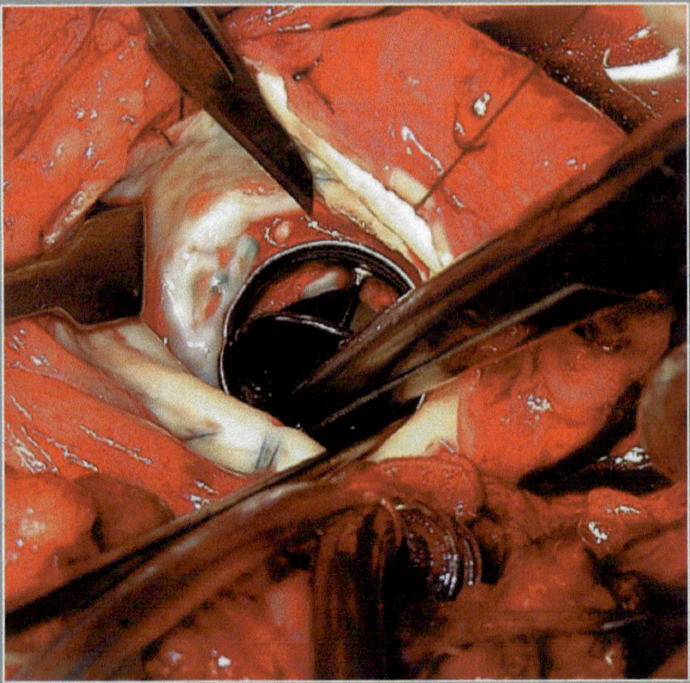

Fig. 9.10 Pannus beneath mechanical disc aortic valve Medtronic–Hall reduces effective orifice area and can even restrict tilting of the disc

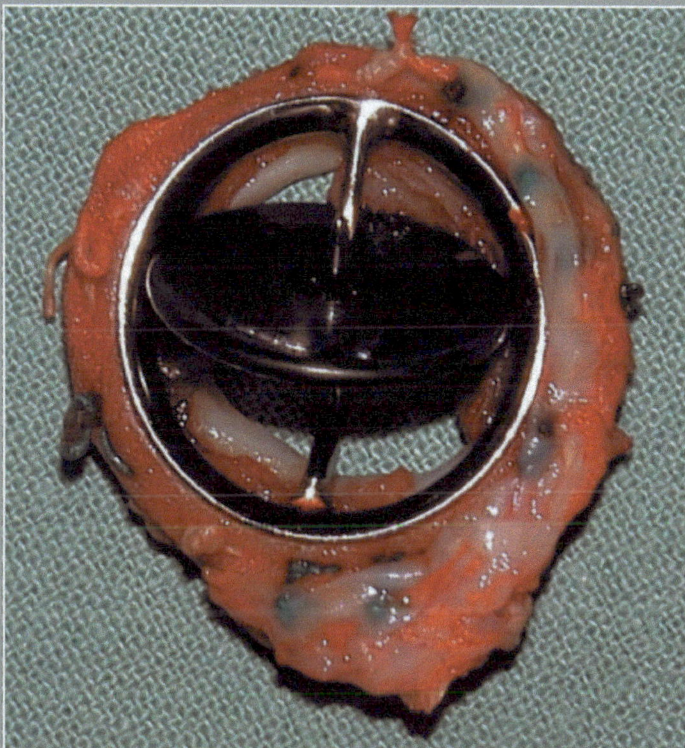

Fig. 9.11 Aortic disc valve Medtronic–Hall explanted due to dysfunction resulting from tissue overgrowing from beneath the valve

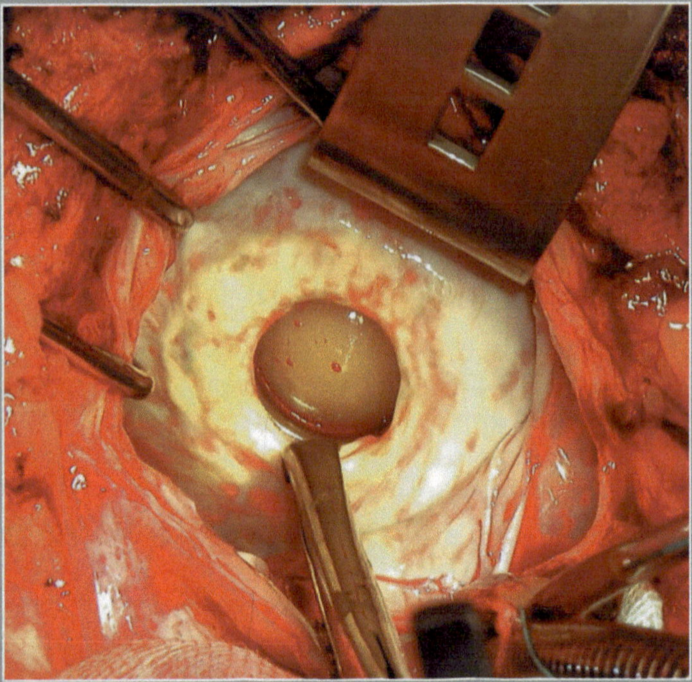

Fig. 9.12 Tissue overgrowing (pannus) mitral annulus after implantation of caged-ball valve Starr–Edwards

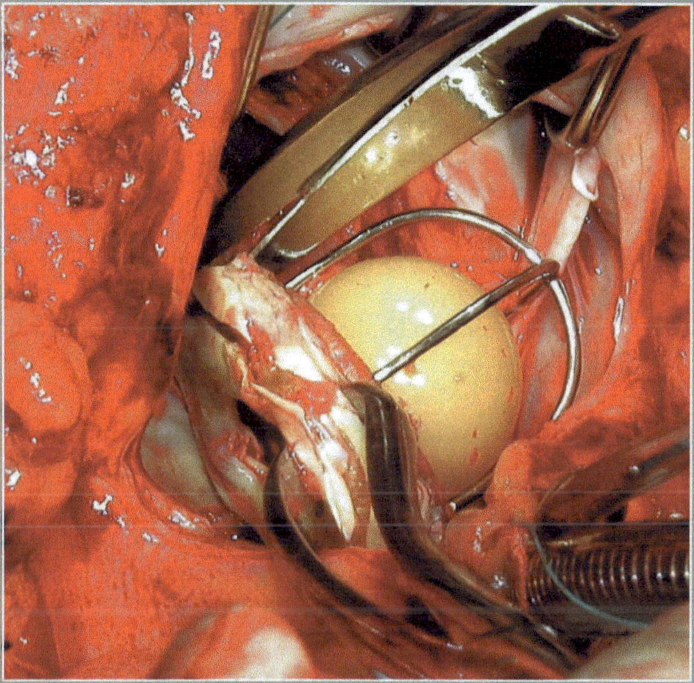

Fig. 9.13 Explantation of the valve Starr–Edwards due to dysfunction resulting from tissue overgrowing into the mitral orifice

[15, 16]. Thrombolysis carries risk of serious complications (e.g., embolizations, bleeding) that result in mortality in about 10% of cases, as reported in large cohorts. Failure of thrombolysis ranges between 10 and 15% [16, 17]. Choice of optimal treatment strategy is individual and is influenced by the given situation [18–23].

Surgery is necessary in cases of failure or contraindication of thrombolysis.

Surgery seems to be the most appropriate treatment in the following cases:

1. In patients with a large (>8 mm) billowing thrombus on left-sided prosthetic valves, which presents significant potential for embolization at thrombolysis
2. In critically ill patients without comorbidities
3. In patients in good clinical condition (risk of surgery does not exceed risk of thrombolysis)
4. When the presence of pannus or organized thrombus is suspected (ineffectiveness of thrombolysis)

Thrombolysis is advisable in the following cases:

1. In patients with a short history of disease (fresh thrombus is expected)
2. In high-risk patients (comorbidities)
3. In patients with echocardiographic findings of firmly seated, non-billowing thrombus
4. In those who refuse surgery
5. In cases of thrombosis of implanted tricuspid valve
6. In situations in which surgery is not immediately available and the patient cannot be transferred

Thrombolysis tends to be preferred in recent years. Many authors recommend thrombolysis as the first-line treatment in all patients with obstructive prosthetic valve thrombosis, independent of NYHA function class and thrombus size. Surgery should be reserved only for patients in whom thrombolysis is contraindicated or has failed [20, 21, 24–26]. In case of failure of thrombolysis, surgery can be performed 24 h after discontinuation of thrombolysis administration. Earlier surgery can be undertaken on the basis of vital indication with high risk of bleeding despite substitution therapy.

After successful management of valve thrombosis, patients who had been anticoagulated properly have to maintain anticoagulation therapy at INR between 3.0 and 4.5 and antiaggregation comedication (acetylsalicylic acid) is usually recommended [21]. Patients with known poor compliance to anticoagulation therapy should be given bioprosthesis at reoperation.

9.4 Paraprosthetic Leak

Paraprosthetic leak is a pathological communication through the patient's annulus outside of the sewing ring (Fig. 9.14). After closure of the valve, paraprosthetic blood regurgitation of various degrees of severity occurs through this communication. Paraprosthetic regurgitation is always pathological and has to be distinguished from transvalvular regurgitation, which is in minimal quantity present in all prostheses. Transvalvular "physiological" regurgitation volume of an implanted valve varies between 5 and 10% of systolic volume and is hemodynamically insignificant.

The paraprosthetic leak results from tearing of (cutting through) the sutures or imperfect healing of the sewing ring

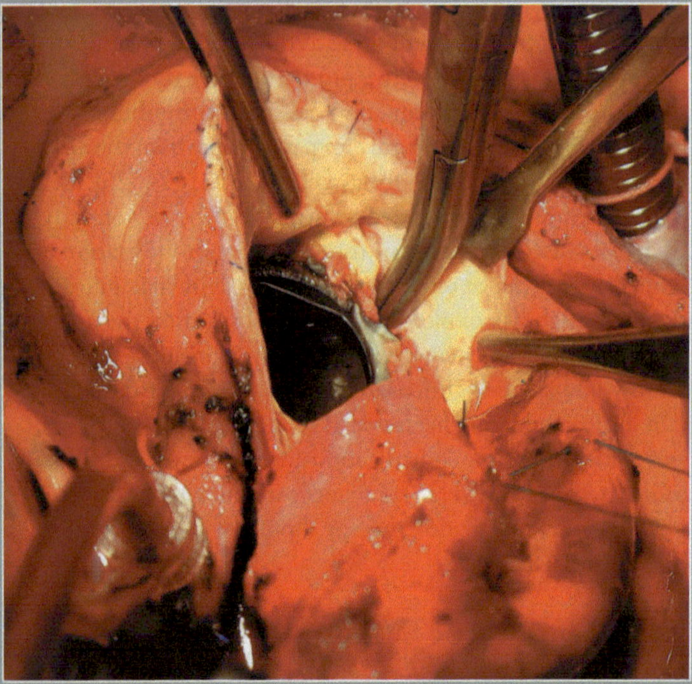

Fig. 9.14 Paraprosthetic leak in the area of original commissure between right and non-coronary aortic cusp

to the patient's annular tissue, or is due to infective loosening of the sutures. Insignificant leaks are present in a form of slit-like dehiscence, whereas severe leaks may occupy up to half, occasionally even more, of the annular circumference.

Occurrence of paraprosthetic leak is related to the following:

1. Poor-quality annulus (extensive calcifications, periannular abscess, etc.)
2. Actions of the surgeon (e.g., choosing suboptimal technique of valve fixation, insufficient debridement of the calcified annulus)
3. Infection (e.g., resulting from native valve endocarditis or secondary infection leading to early or late prosthetic endocarditis)
4. Material of the sewing ring (e.g., a higher incidence of paraprosthetic leak was reported with the first-generation Omniscience valves with Dacron sewing ring in the 1980s [27]. For that same reason a Silzone valve, which had the sewing ring impregnated with silver to prevent infection, was withdrawn from the market in 2000) [28].

The incidence of hemodynamically significant leaks that necessitate reoperation is reported to be between 0 and 5% (mostly 1–2% of the operated patients). With regard to its etiology, paraprosthetic leak is classified as non-infective and infective (resulting from infective endocarditis). In cases of leak several months or years after operation, infectious etiology has always to be suspected. This underscores the importance of a detailed postoperative echocardiography analysis of the valve prosthesis, which serves as a referential for future comparison. Clinical course of prosthetic endocarditis is associated with development of paraprosthetic leak, which gradually worsens with the progression of infection.

Diagnosis of paraprosthetic leak is based on auscultatory findings (regurgitation murmur), echocardiography, or angiocardiography. If the leak occupies a substantial portion of the annulus, a pathological tilting of the contrast ring can be seen at cinefluoroscopy.

Indication criteria for reoperation are similar to those for initial operation of incompetent valves and include onset of subjective complaints, enlargement of left ventricular dimensions, and verification of significant paraprosthetic regurgitation by means of echocardiography, angiocardiography, or by dilution quantification at catheterization.

Surgical treatment consists of explantation of the valve and its replacement by a new valve. Minor and accessible non-infective leaks can be treated by suturing the dehiscence with pledgeted mattress sutures. Paraprosthetic leaks in the area of the former non-coronary cusp can be closed by transaortic mattress sutures with pledgets placed externally (Fig. 9.15).

Risk of reoperation for paraprosthetic leak is reported to be between 5 and 10% for patients in stable condition (assuming non-infective leaks).

9.5 Prosthetic Valve Endocarditis

Infection of an implanted heart valve is the most serious complication after heart valve replacement either in early or late postoperative course (Figs. 9.16–9.18).

Incidence of prosthetic endocarditis is reported in the literature to be most often between 0.2 and 0.8% for each year of life with an implanted valve [29]. Diagnosis of

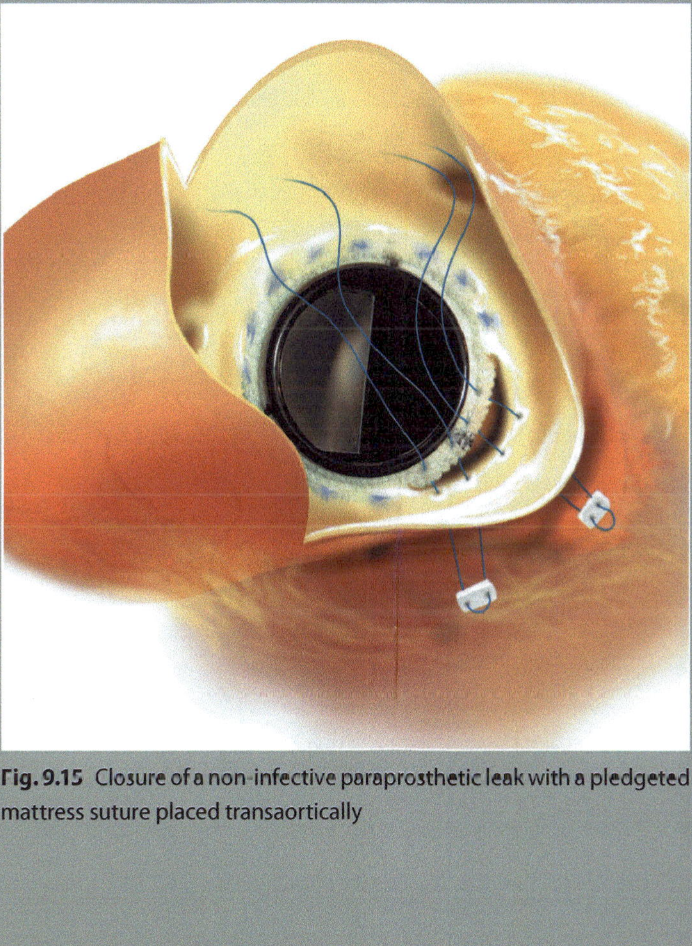

Fig. 9.15 Closure of a non-infective paraprosthetic leak with a pledgeted mattress suture placed transaortically

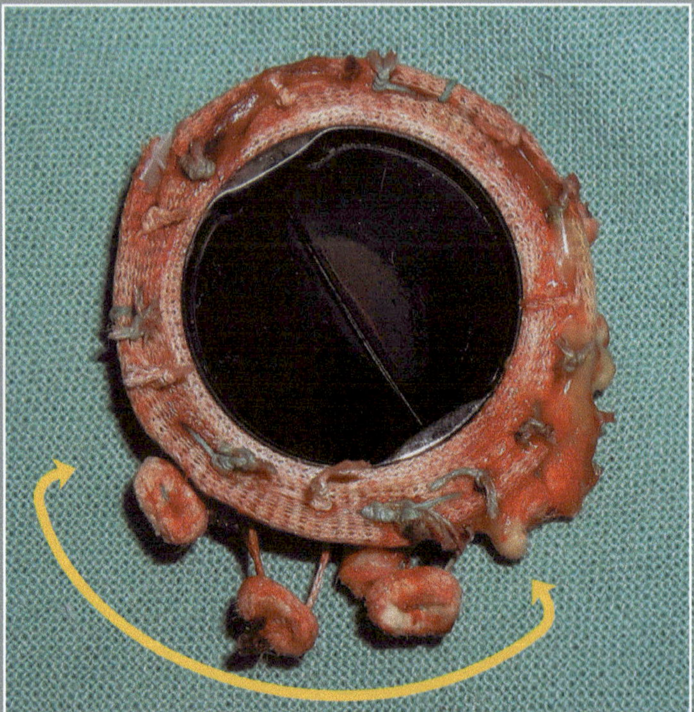

Fig. 9.16 Bileaflet valve explanted due to prosthetic endocarditis with extensive paraprosthetic leak. The extent of infective dehiscence (leak) is marked

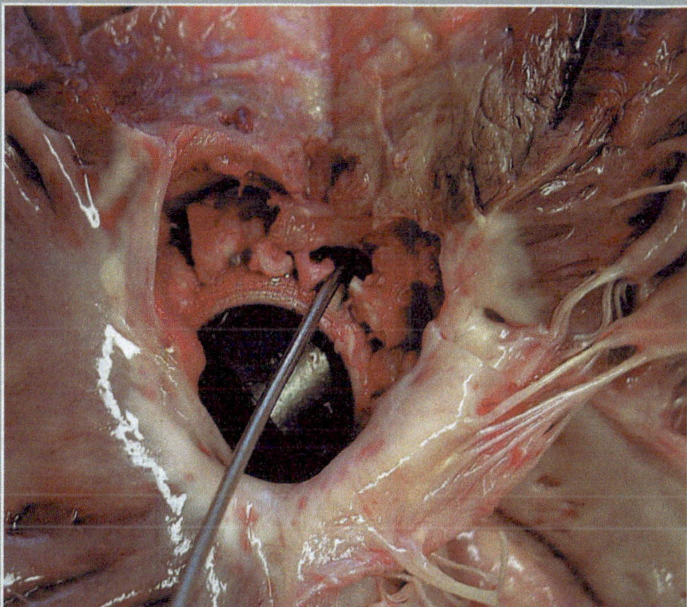

Fig. 9.17 Prosthetic endocarditis of aortic valve (postmortem finding). View from the left ventricle. Multiple periannular abscesses and paraprosthetic leaks

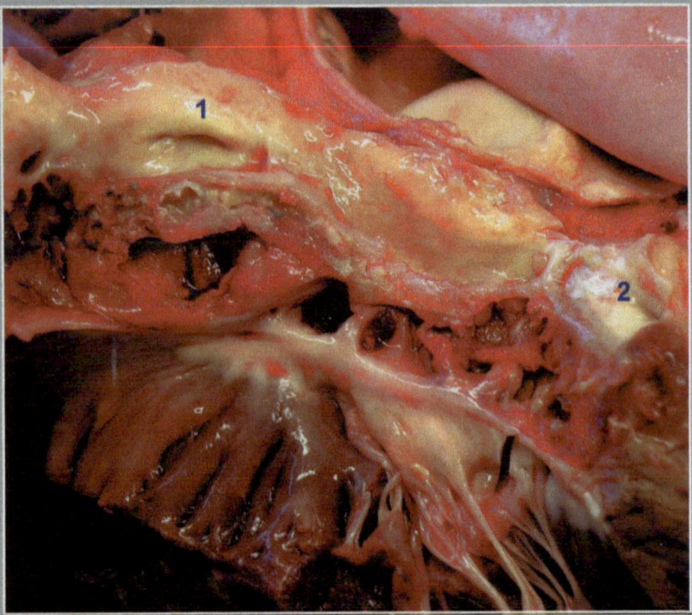

Fig. 9.18 Extensive, almost circular abscesses in the aortic annulus due to prosthetic endocarditis. *1* Right coronary ostium, *2* left coronary ostium

prosthetic endocarditis is based on septic condition of the patient, positive hemocultures, detection of vegetations, and abscess or paraprosthetic leak on echocardiography, auscultatory findings, and clinical development of heart failure. Other alarming signs include septic embolizations, conduction disorders, and also septal perforations. Large vegetations may interfere with tilting motion of the poppet (especially in mitral position). Considerable risk of embolization is present with vegetations larger than 10 mm.

Therapy is always initiated with conservative treatment with intravenous administration of high-dose bactericide antibiotics according to results of hemocultures. Should conservative therapy fail, radical surgical treatment has to be undertaken promptly, despite its higher operative risk, before development of complications which would further increase the risks of such surgery (e.g., heart failure, periannular abscess, perforation, conduction disorders, and embolization). Infection that is deep-seated in the fabric of the sewing ring and has already led to paraprosthetic leak or abscess formation can hardly be cured by conservative treatment.

Indications for surgery are severe congestive heart failure, persistent sepsis despite 1 week of antibiotic therapy, progression of perivalvular pathology (annular abscess, paravalvular leak, new conduction abnormalities, false aneurysm, pathological communication), large mobile vegetations, fungal and staphylococcal etiology, and valve obstruction with vegetation (Fig. 9.19) [14, 30–32].

Risk of reoperation for prosthetic endocarditis still remains very high. In large cohorts, the 30-day mortality rate is reported to be 13–69%. Mortality due to early prosthetic endocarditis is substantially higher than that of late endocar-

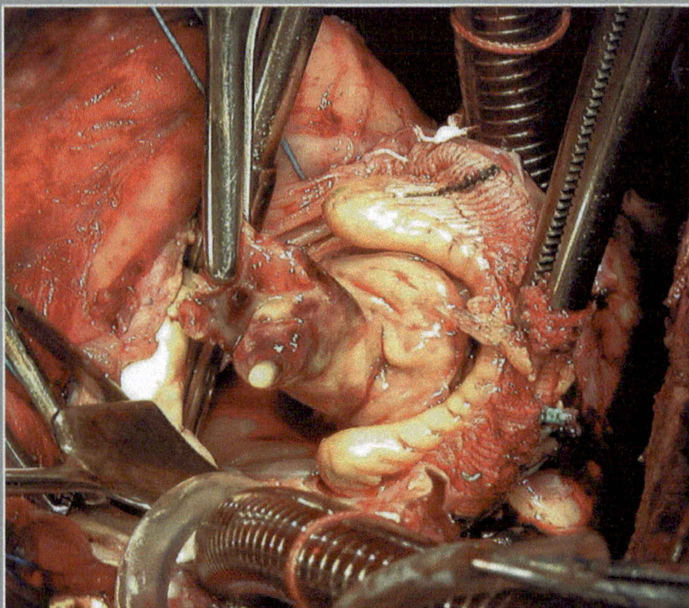

Fig. 9.19 Bioprosthesis 1 year after implantation into tricuspid orifice because of infective endocarditis in a drug addict. Prosthetic endocarditis in a patient who failed to stop his drug abuse resulted in obstruction of the orifice by vegetation

ditis. In recent years mortality rates have gradually decreased and presently vary around 20% [29, 30, 32, 33].

The seriousness of prosthetic endocarditis accentuates the necessity of preventive measures (a) preoperatively (e.g., eradication of focal infection), (b) perioperatively (e.g., strict asepsis, antibiotic prophylaxis, early extraction of catheters and cannulas), and (c) postoperatively (e.g., antibiotic treatment of every potential bacteremia).

References

1. Abdulali SA, Silverton NP, Schoen FJ et al. (1984) Late outcome of patients with Braunwald–Cutter mitral valve replacement. Ann Thorac Surg 38:579–585
2. Basta LL, Wolfson P, Kioschos JM et al. (1974) Clinical and angiographic features of Beall-valve-disc variance. J Cardiovasc Surg (Torino) 15:679–683
3. Huber S, Burckhardt D, Raeder EA et al. (1980) Complications in patients with cloth-covered Starr–Edwards prostheses. J Cardiovasc Surg (Torino) 21:19–24
4. Jonas RA, Garratt-Boyes BG, Kerr AR et al. (1982) Late follow-up of the Braunwald–Cutter valve. Ann Thorac Surg 33:554–561
5. Joob AW, Kron IL, Craddock GB et al. (1985) A decade of experience with the Model 103 and 104 Beall valve prostheses. J Thorac Cardiovasc Surg 89:444–447
6. Sezai A, Hata M, Niino T et al. (2007) Prophylactic reoperation after mitral valve replacement with the Starr–Edwards ball valve: a report of four cases. Ann Thorac Cardiovasc Surg 13:316–321
7. Winter TQ, Reis RL, Glancy DL et al. (1972) Current status of the Starr–Edwards cloth-covered prosthetic cardiac valves. Circulation 45:I14–I24
8. Birkmeyer JD, Marrin CA, O'Connor GT (1992) Should patients with Bjork–Shiley valves undergo prophylactic replacement? Lancet 340:520–523

9. Blackstone EH, Kirklin JW (1992) Recommendations for prophylactic removal of heart valve prostheses. J Heart Valve Dis 1:3–14
10. van der Graaf Y, de Waard F, van Herwerden LA et al. (1992) Risk of strut fracture of Bjork–Shiley valves. Lancet 339:257–261
11. Lin SS, Tiong IY, Asher CR et al. (2000) Prediction of thrombus-related mechanical prosthetic valve dysfunction using transesophageal echocardiography. Am J Cardiol 86:1097–1101
12. Rizzoli G, Guglielmi C, Toscano G et al. (1999) Reoperations for acute prosthetic thrombosis and pannus: an assessment of rates, relationship and risk. Eur J Cardiothorac Surg 16:74–80
13. Vitale N, Renzulli A, Agozzino L et al. (1997) Obstruction of mechanical mitral prostheses: analysis of pathologic findings. Ann Thorac Surg 63:1101–1106
14. Bonow RO, Carabello BA, Kanu C et al. (2006) ACC/AHA 2006 guidelines for the management of patients with valvular heart disease. A report of the American College of Cardiology/American Heart Association Task Force on Practice Guidelines (writing committee to revise the 1998 Guidelines for the Management of Patients With Valvular Heart Disease); developed in collaboration with the Society of Cardiovascular Anesthesiologists; endorsed by the Society for Cardiovascular Angiography and Interventions and the Society of Thoracic Surgeons. Circulation 114:e84–e231
15. Ozkokeli M, Sensoz Y, Ates M et al. (2005) Surgical treatment of left-sided prosthetic valve thrombosis: short- and long-term results. Int Heart J 46:105–111
16. Roudaut R, Roques X, Lafitte S et al. (2003) Surgery for prosthetic valve obstruction. A single-center study of 136 patients. Eur J Cardiothorac Surg 24:868–872
17. Roudaut R, Lafitte S, Roudaut MF et al. (2003) Fibrinolysis of mechanical prosthetic valve thrombosis: a single-center study of 127 cases. J Am Coll Cardiol 41:653–658
18. Das M, Twomey D, Al Khaddour A et al. (2007) Is thrombolysis or surgery the best option for acute prosthetic valve thrombosis? Interact Cardiovasc Thorac Surg 6:806–811

19. Durrleman N, Pellerin M, Bouchard D et al. (2004) Prosthetic valve thrombosis: twenty-year experience at the Montreal Heart Institute. J Thorac Cardiovasc Surg 127:1388–1392
20. Lengyel M, Fuster V, Keltai M et al. (1997) Guidelines for management of left-sided prosthetic valve thrombosis: a role for thrombolytic therapy. Consensus Conference on Prosthetic Valve Thrombosis. J Am Coll Cardiol 30:1521–1526
21. Lengyel M, Horstkotte D, Voller H et al. (2005) Recommendations for the management of prosthetic valve thrombosis. J Heart Valve Dis 14:567–575
22. Tong AT, Roudaut R, Ozkan M et al. (2004) Transesophageal echocardiography improves risk assessment of thrombolysis of prosthetic valve thrombosis: results of the international PRO-TEE registry. J Am Coll Cardiol 43:77–84
23. Vahanian A, Baumgartner H, Bax J et al. (2007) Guidelines on the management of valvular heart disease: The Task Force on the Management of Valvular Heart Disease of the European Society of Cardiology. Eur Heart J 28:230–268
24. Caceres-Loriga FM (2008) Prosthetic valve thrombosis: Is it time for a new consensus conference? Eur J Echocardiogr 9:413–414
25. Caceres-Loriga FM, Perez-Lopez H, Morlans-Hernandez K et al. (2006) Thrombolysis as first choice therapy in prosthetic heart valve thrombosis. A study of 68 patients. J Thromb Thrombolysis 21:185–190
26. Nagy A, Denes M, Lengyel M (2009) Predictors of the outcome of thrombolytic therapy in prosthetic mitral valve thrombosis: a study of 62 events. J Heart Valve Dis 18:268–275
27. Fananapazir L, Clarke DB, Dark JF et al. (1983) Results of valve replacement with the Omniscience prosthesis. J Thorac Cardiovasc Surg 86:621–625
28. Tozzi P, Al-Darweesh A, Vogt P et al. (2001) Silver-coated prosthetic heart valve: a double-bladed weapon. Eur J Cardiothorac Surg 19:729–731
29. Edwards MB, Ratnatunga CP, Dore CJ et al. (1998) Thirty-day mortality and long-term survival following surgery for pros-

thetic endocarditis: a study from the UK heart valve registry. Eur J Cardiothorac Surg 14:156–164
30. Mahesh B, Angelini G, Caputo M et al. (2005) Prosthetic valve endocarditis. Ann Thorac Surg 80:1151–1158
31. Horstkotte D, Follath F, Gutschik E et al. (2004) Guidelines on prevention, diagnosis and treatment of infective endocarditis executive summary; the task force on infective endocarditis of the European society of cardiology. Eur Heart J 25:267–276
32. Tornos P, Iung B, Permanyer-Miralda G et al. (2005) Infective endocarditis in Europe: lessons from the Euro heart survey. Heart 91:571–575
33. Romano G, Carozza A, Della Corte A et al. (2004) Native versus primary prosthetic valve endocarditis: comparison of clinical features and long-term outcome in 353 patients. J Heart Valve Dis 13:200–209

Results of Heart Valve Surgery

10 Results of Heart Valve Surgery

Before surgery, the patient has to be given accurate information about the nature of his or her disease, expected natural history of the disease without operation, and the estimated risk of surgical procedure. The average in-hospital mortality rate, drawn from large patient cohorts [1–9] (Table 10.1), is approximately 3% for isolated aortic valve replacement, 6% for isolated mitral valve replacement, and 1–2% for mitral valve repair. The published mortality rate for concomitant aortic and mitral valve replacement is 9%, and 6% for aortic valve replacement with concomitant mitral valve repair. The mortality rate for tricuspid valve surgery(usually for mitral–tricuspid valve disease) is approximately 10%. Aortic valve replacement with concomitant coronary bypass grafting has the expected mortality rate of approximately 6%, whereas the mortality rate for mitral valve replacement combined with coronary bypass grafting ranges between 10 and 12%. The mortality rate for mitral valve repair with concomitant coronary bypass grafting is about 6–8%.

All these mortality estimates increase in patients over 70 years as well as in cases of urgent surgery, reoperation, active endocarditis, pulmonary hypertension (systolic pressure >60 mmHg), low ejection fraction, long-term diabetes mellitus, and serious renal, pulmonary, neurological or atherosclerotic disease. Risk of operation in patients without the abovementioned risk factors is lower than the average estimates, whereas risk of surgery in elderly and polymorbid patients exceeds the given data.

Prediction of mortality for a given patient can be calculated more precisely by EuroSCORE (**Euro**pean **S**ystem for **C**ardiac **O**perative **R**isk **E**valuation) [10]. It has to be

J. Dominik and P. Zacek, *Heart Valve Surgery: An Illustrated Guide*,
DOI 10.1007/978-3-642-12206-4_10,

Table 10.1 Hospital mortality rates of heart valve surgery.

Procedure	Germany 2004–2008		Author J. D. 1978–2008		USA 2000–2008	
	n	%	n	%	n	%
AVR	57 056	**3.7**	735	**2.1**	125 545	**3.3**
MVR	10 251	**7.9**	319	**6.0**	38 881	**5.7**
MVP	12 877	**2.1**	124	**0.8**	37 592	**1.7**
AVR + MVR	3 647	**12.2**	105	**8.6**	9 849	**9.7**
AVR + MVP	3 974	**5.4**	30	**6.6**		
TVR, TVP	6 632	**9.0**	130	**9.2**	39 416	**10.1**
AVR + CABG	40 829	**6.3**	361	**5.3**	119 579	**5.5**
MVR + CABG	4 756	**12.9**	63	**9.5**	24 505	**11.3**
MVP + CABG	8 440	**8.5**	15	**6.7**	37 562	**7.1**

AVR aortic valve replacement, *MVR* mitral valve replacement, *MVP* mitral valve plasty, *TVR* tricuspid valve replacement, *TVP* tricuspid valve plasty, *CABG* coronary artery bypass grafting. (From [2, 4–8])

realized, however, that both additive and logistical EuroSCORE calculations take into account some important patient risk factors, but they ignore the extent of necessary surgical procedure [11, 12]. In valve surgery, EuroSCORE thus forecasts exactly the same probability of death for one valve procedure as for extensive complex procedures (e.g., aortic valve replacement with concomitant mitral valve repair, tricuspid valve repair, and coronary bypass grafting). EuroSCORE therefore works well predominantly for isolated coronary surgery and for single-valve surgery.

No less important than the early results of the heart valve surgery are the long-term outcomes. In the long term the patient is jeopardized by infrequent, but life-threatening, valve dysfunctions as well as thromboembolic and bleeding complications resulting usually from inadequately maintained anticoagulation therapy. After valve-sparing operations, failure of repair can occur during long-term follow-up. After heart valve surgery, before discharge, all patients have to undergo a detailed cardiological checkup, including echocardiography examination, which serves later as a referential for future checkups and eventual decision making in case of subsequent complications.

References

1. Unger F, Rainer WG, Horstkotte D et al. (2000) Standards and concepts in valve surgery. J Cardiovasc Surg (Torino) 41:585–593
2. STS Adult Cardiac Surgery Database (2009) Executive summary. http://www.sts.org/documents/pdf/ndb/2ndHarvestExecutiveSummary_2009.pdf. Accessed December 2009.
3. Brown JM, O'Brien SM, Wu C et al. (2009) Isolated aortic valve replacement in North America comprising 108,687 patients in 10 years: changes in risks, valve types, and outcomes in the Society of Thoracic Surgeons National Database. J Thorac Cardiovasc Surg 137:82–90
4. Gummert JF, Funkat A, Beckmann A et al. (2006) Cardiac surgery in Germany during 2005: a report on behalf of the German Society for Thoracic and Cardiovascular Surgery. Thorac Cardiovasc Surg 54:362–371
5. Gummert JF, Funkat A, Beckmann A et al. (2008) Cardiac surgery in Germany during 2007: a report on behalf of the German Society for Thoracic and Cardiovascular Surgery. Thorac Cardiovasc Surg 56:328–336

6. Gummert JF, Funkat A, Beckmann A et al. (2009) Cardiac surgery in Germany during 2008. A report on behalf of the German Society for Thoracic and Cardiovascular Surgery. Thorac Cardiovasc Surg 57:315–323
7. Gummert JF, Funkat A, Beckmann A et al. (2007) Cardiac surgery in Germany during 2006: a report on behalf of the German Society for Thoracic and Cardiovascular Surgery. Thorac Cardiovasc Surg 55:343–350
8. Gummert JF, Funkat A, Krian A (2005) Cardiac surgery in Germany during 2004: a report on behalf of the German Society for Thoracic and Cardiovascular Surgery. Thorac Cardiovasc Surg 53:391–399
9. Vahanian A, Baumgartner H, Bax J et al. (2007) Guidelines on the management of valvular heart disease: The Task Force on the Management of Valvular Heart Disease of the European Society of Cardiology. Eur Heart J 28:230–268
10. Nashef SA, Roques F, Michel P et al. (1999) European system for cardiac operative risk evaluation (EuroSCORE). Eur J Cardiothorac Surg 16:9–13
11. Jin R, Grunkemeier GL (2005) Additive vs logistic risk models for cardiac surgery mortality. Eur J Cardiothorac Surg 28:240–243
12. Jin R, Grunkemeier GL (2006) Does the logistic EuroSCORE offer an advantage over the additive model? Interact Cardiovasc Thorac Surg 5:15–17

Recommended Monographs and Guidelines on Heart Valve Surgery

Recommended Monographs and Guidelines on Heart Valve Surgery

Monographs on Heart Valve Surgery

1. Cohn LM (2007) Cardiac surgery in the adult, 3rd edn. McGraw--Hill Medical, London
2. Doty D (1997) Cardiac surgery. Operative technique. Mosby, New York
3. Gardner TJ, Spray T (2004) Operative cardiac surgery, 5th edn. Hodder Arnold, London
4. Henein MY (2009) Valvular heart disease in clinical practice. Springer, Berlin Heidelberg New York
5. Chikwe J, Beddow E, Glenville B (2006) Cardiothoracic surgery. Oxford University Press, London
6. Ng CHK, Nesser J, Poncengruber C et al. (2003) Modern mitral valve repair. Springer, Berlin Heidelberg New York
7. Khonsari S, Sintek CF (2008) Cardiac surgery: safeguards and pitfalls in operative technique, 4th edn. Lippincott, Philadelphia
8. Kirklin JW, Barrat-Boyes BG (2003) Cardiac surgery, 3rd edn. Churchill Livingstone, Philadelphia
9. Otto CM, Bonow RO (2009) Valvular heart disease. Saunders, Philadelphia
10. Savage EB, Bolling S (2006) Atlas of mitral valve repair. Lippincott Williams and Wilkins, Baltimore
11. Sellke F, Ruel M (2009) Atlas of cardiac surgical techniques. Saunders Elsevier, Philadelphia
12. Turina M et al. Multimedia manual of cardiothoracic surgery collections. http://www.mmcts.org. Accessed December 2009.
13. Yuh DD, Vricella LA, Baumgartner WA (2007) The Johns Hopkins manual of cardiothoracic surgery. McGraw-Hill Medical, New York
14. Wahlers T, Wittwer T, Adams DH (2008) Cardiac surgical operative atlas. Lehmans Media, Berlin

15. Zacek P, Dominik J, Kubis P (2005) Interactive cardiac surgery. DVD-ROM. Springer, Berlin Heidelberg New York

Guidelines on Heart Valve Disease

1. Bonow RO, Carabello BA, Chatterjee K et al. (2008) 2008 Focused update incorporated into the ACC/AHA 2006 guidelines for the management of patients with valvular heart disease. A report of the American College of Cardiology/American Heart Association Task Force on Practice Guidelines (Writing Committee to Revise the 1998 Guidelines for the Management of Patients With Valvular Heart Disease); endorsed by the Society of Cardiovascular Anesthesiologists, Society for Cardiovascular Angiography and Interventions, and Society of Thoracic Surgeons. Circulation 118:e523–e661
2. Bonow RO, Carabello BA, Kanu C et al. (2006) ACC/AHA 2006 guidelines for the management of patients with valvular heart disease. A report of the American College of Cardiology/American Heart Association Task Force on Practice Guidelines (writing committee to revise the 1998 Guidelines for the Management of Patients With Valvular Heart Disease); developed in collaboration with the Society of Cardiovascular Anesthesiologists; endorsed by the Society for Cardiovascular Angiography and Interventions and the Society of Thoracic Surgeons. Circulation 114:e84–e231
3. Dunning J, Versteegh M, Fabbri A et al. (2008) Guidelines on antiplatelet and anticoagulation management in cardiac surgery. Eur J Cardiothorac Surg 34:73–92
4. Horstkotte D, Follath F, Gutschik E et al. (2004) Guidelines on prevention, diagnosis and treatment of infective endocarditis executive summary. The Task Force on Infective Endocarditis of the European Society of Cardiology. Eur Heart J 25:267–276
5. Nishimura RA, Carabello BA, Faxon DP et al. (2008) ACC/AHA 2008 guideline update on valvular heart disease: focused update on infective endocarditis. A report of the American College of Cardiology/American Heart Association Task Force on

Practice Guidelines; endorsed by the Society of Cardiovascular Anesthesiologists, Society for Cardiovascular Angiography and Interventions, and Society of Thoracic Surgeons. Circulation 118:887–896
6. Unger F, Rainer WG, Horstkotte D et al. (2000) Standards and concepts in valve surgery. J Cardiovasc Surg (Torino) 41:585–593
7. Vahanian A, Alfieri OR, Al-Attar N et al. (2008) Transcatheter valve implantation for patients with aortic stenosis: a position statement from the European Association of Cardio-Thoracic Surgery (EACTS) and the European Society of Cardiology (ESC), in collaboration with the European Association of Percutaneous Cardiovascular Interventions (EAPCI). Eur J Cardiothorac Surg 34:1–8
8. Vahanian A, Baumgartner H, Bax J et al. (2007) Guidelines on the management of valvular heart disease. The Task Force on the Management of Valvular Heart Disease of the European Society of Cardiology. Eur Heart J 28:230–268

Index

Index

A

C

D

E

P

R

MIX
Papier aus verantwortungsvollen Quellen
Paper from responsible sources
FSC® C105338

If you have any concerns about our products,
you can contact us on
ProductSafety@springernature.com

In case Publisher is established outside the EU,
the EU authorized representative is:
Springer Nature Customer Service Center GmbH
Europaplatz 3, 69115 Heidelberg, Germany

Printed by Libri Plureos GmbH
in Hamburg, Germany